Improving Outcomes in Oral Cancer

Deepak Kademani
Editor

Improving Outcomes in Oral Cancer

A Clinical and Translational Update

Springer

Editor
Deepak Kademani
Department of Oral and Maxillofacial Surgery
North Memorial Medical Center
Minneapolis, MN
USA

ISBN 978-3-030-30093-7 ISBN 978-3-030-30094-4 (eBook)
https://doi.org/10.1007/978-3-030-30094-4

This Springer imprint is published by the registered company Springer Nature Switzerland AG
The registered company address is: Gewerbestrasse 11, 6330 Cham, Switzerland

To my patients who have given me the privilege to care for them and taught me so much about the human spirit

Contents

1 Oral Epithelial Dysplasia

Kenneth Wan and Deepak Kademani

1.1 Introduction

In general histopathology terms, dysplasia is a disordered growth that encompasses an abnormality in the maturation of cells within tissues and the development of cytological atypia within cells. When dysplasia occurs in the epithelium of the oral cavity, the WHO have termed it oral epithelial dysplasia (OED), defining it as a precancerous lesion of stratified squamous epithelium, characterized by cellular atypia and loss of normal maturation and stratification short of carcinoma in situ. It is a histologically proven oral premalignant lesion that is associated with a signifi cant higher risk of malignant transformation. An OED may be part of a clinically apparent lesion, such as leukoplakia, eythroplakia, erytholeukoplakia, lichen planus and submucosal fibrosis, actinic chelitis, and chronic hyperplastic candidiasis. These lesions are termed "oral potentially malignant disorders" (OPMD) by the 2005 WHO workshop and are referred to a variety of clinical lesions, conditions, or systemic disorders, which result in an increased risk of cancer development in the oral cavity compared to normal mucosa in a healthy patient. Recently, the term, "potentially premalignant oral epithelial lesions" (PPOEL), has been described in the literature to replace OPMD. For a lesion to be described as an oral epithelial dysplasia, there must be a biopsied and histopathologically reported foci of dysplasia.

1.2 Grading and Classification of OED

OED is a condition comprising of a spectrum of tissue changes, with several grading systems established to classify into arbitrary levels of severity, hence diagnosis is extremely subjective [1, 2]. The relevant diagnostic criteria have been revised several times and many systems of classification exist, each with their own biases [3]. These are generally based on the histopathological classification of premalignant lesions of other mucosal sites, which frequently develop SCC.

For example, squamous intraepithelial neoplasia (SIN) is an oral adaptation of a system used for classifying precursor lesions of the uterine cervix and have been used for grading OED in the older literature [3]. While the SIN system has its advantages, it has been rejected for use in the oral cavity and oropharynx due to the emphasis placed on tissue thickness due to hyperkeratinization, which is not considered to carry a higher risk of malignancy than normal tissue in the oral cavity [4, 5]. Furthermore, the SIN system suggests an

K. Wan
Department of Oral and Maxillifacial Surgery, North Memorial Health, Robbinsdale, MN, USA

D. Kademani (✉)
Oral and Maxillofacial Surgery and Hospital Dentistry, Head and Neck Oncologic and Reconstructive Surgery, North Memorial Medical Center, Minneapolis, MN, USA
e-mail: Deepak.Kademani@northmemorial.com

D. Kademani (ed.), *Improving Outcomes in Oral Cancer*,
https://doi.org/10.1007/978-3-030-30094-4_1

inevitable progression to malignancy, which is not the case of OEDs in the oral cavity [6].

In the Ljubljana grading system, lesions are categorized into simple hyperplasia, basal/parabasal hyperplasia, atypical hyperplasia, or carcinoma in situ. It is an alternative system based on another anatomical site but adapted for the oral cavity and oropharynx [7]. Originally utilized in the context of laryngeal precursor lesions, it is considered beyond the scope of the histopathological changes which occur in the oral cavity and oropharynx [3].

Another grading systems include the Smith and Pindborg, which utilizes 13 histological features that are standardized by a set of photographs. After comparing with the photographic standard, the feature is graded as none, slight, or marked and given a score. The scores are added to achieve the epithelial atypia index (EAI) score (maximum possible is 75), and depending upon the EAI, the dysplasia is graded as no dysplasia, mild, moderate, or severe.

Currently, the 2005 WHO Classification is most widely used for classification of tissue dysplasia. A range of cellular and architectural changes in the tissue is assessed and classified into a specific grade of dysplasia (Tables 1.1 and 1.2).

Issues with intraobserver reproducibility and interobserver agreement plagues all the aforementioned grading system, with the Ljubljana and Smith & Pindborg system faring worse than the WHO system. Merely determining the presence of OED appears to be a challenge, with one US study reporting a Kappa value of 0.51 (moderate strength of agreement) between three oral pathologists when asked to assess OED presence and absence [8]. Intraexaminer reliability varied greatly among the pathologists, with one scoring a Kappa value as low as 0.22 (slight strength of agreement) [8]. Another study reported Kappa agreement scores of 0.15 and 0.41 between six pathologists in determining the presence of OED among 120 slides [9]. Lumerman et al. reports an interexaminer reliability of only 54% [10].

Considering the low consistency between diagnoses, it is expected that this would be a major limitation among most studies, and this has resulted in remaining controversy surrounding the predictive value of OED.

Table 1.1 List of architectural and cytological changes associated with oral epithelia dysplasia, 2005 WHO Classification

Architecture	Cytology
Irregular epithelial stratification	Abnormal variation in nuclear size (anisonucleosis)
Loss of polarity of basal cells	Abnormal variation in nuclear shape (nuclear pleomorphism)
Drop-shaped rete ridges	Abnormal variation in cell size (anisocytosis)
Increased number of mitotic figures	Abnormal variation in cell shape (cellular pleomorphism)
Abnormal superficial mitoses	Increased nuclear-cytoplasmic ratio
Dyskeratosis	Increase nuclear size
Keratin pearls within rete pegs	Atypical mitotic figures
	Increase number and size of nucleoli
	Hyperchromasia

Table 1.2 Classification of oral epithelial dysplasia, 2005 WHO classification

Hyperplasia	Increased cell number; the architecture shows regular stratification without cellular atypia
Mild epithelial dysplasia	Architectural disturbance limited to the lower third of the epithelium accompanied by cytological atypia
Moderate epithelial dysplasia	Architectural disturbance extending into the middle third of the epithelium with consideration of the degree of cytologic atypia
Severe epithelial dysplasia	Greater than two-thirds of the epithelium showing architectural disturbance with associated cytologic atypia or architectural disturbance extended into the middle-third of the epithelium with sufficient cytologic atypia
Carcinoma in situ	Full-thickness architectural abnormalities in the viable cellular layer accompanied by pronounced cytologic atypia; atypical mitotic figures and abnormal superficial mitoses

1.3 Clinical Presentation of OED

OED within the oral cavity may present in a range of clinical lesions, rendering it not possible to diagnose without invasive biopsy. Clinically, OEDs may appear as homogenous lesion (clinically provisionally diagnosed as homogenous leukoplakia or keratosis), nonhomogenous (clinically provisionally diagnosed as nonhomogenous leukoplakia, eythroplakia, speckled leukoplakia), lichenoid (clinically provisionally diagnosed as oral lichen planus or oral lichenoid tissue reaction), or others (lesions which are diagnosed as nonspecific ulcerations/erosions/atrophies, angiogranuoloma, frictional keratosis, leukoedema). In several studies, nonhomogenous clinical appearance was highly associated with dysplasia, and over 80% of provisional nonhomogenous lesions were dysplastic or malignant on biopsy.

Lesions that display redness or surface irregularity are more likely to be dysplastic [11]. Erythroplakia is reported to carry the greatest rate of OED of any oral mucosal lesion, with greater than 90% exhibiting dysplastic characteristics on biopsy [12], and a vast majority of these undergo malignant transformation [2]. In a study of 166 leukoplakias, a nonhomogeneous clinical appearance was found to be associated with presence of OED on histopathological assessment, and they were more likely to develop oral SCC on follow-up [13].

In respect to the clinical features of OED, one study has found that all lesions that displays any degree of OED were associated with some form of leukoplakic appearance [14]. In the same study, severe dysplasia was diagnosed mostly in mixed red and white lesions; however, this was not statistically significant. Comparably, lesions which exhibited redness had a greater tendency to present with moderate dysplasia in contrast to clinically white lesions; however, the rate of severe dysplasia was equal between white and mixed red and white lesions, indicating that these findings may be due to sample variation [11]. Tissue redness as a feature of malignant progression can also be appreciated in relation to OLP, where it has been reported that erosive and ulcerative types are at risk of malignancy [15].

Lichenoid dysplasia is a term to describe lesions that on histopathology are primarily dysplastic in nature but exhibit some features of OLP [16]. Oral lichen planus is assumed to be potentially malignant and may of undertaking malignant transformation; however, controversy does exist. Up to 3% of OLP cases have been reported to undergo malignant transformation [17]. Krutchkoff et al. argue that OLP in itself is not potentially malignant, and that associations with transformation are due to inaccurate and overdiagnosis [16].

1.4 Risk Factors for OED

OED has a high association with the male gender [18–21]. Studies have demonstrated that males are more at risk because of greater levels of exposure to risk habits such as alcohol and tobacco consumption [4].

[I]It is well established in the literature that smoking is highly associated with the development of PPOELs and malignancies in the oral cavity [4]. In respect to the development of OED, the exposure and the level of exposure of tobacco to the oral epithelium is significantly associated with the development of dysplastic tissue changes. In one study, those who were identified as current smokers had an odds ratio of 4.1 for developing OED when compared to those who never smoked [22]. Of 173 OED cases in a retrospective study, the author found that half of the patients who reported tobacco usage presented with some degree of OED on biopsy [14]. Another study reported that severe and moderate dysplasia in particular arose at a higher rate among smokers, with approximately 77% of severe dysplasia occurring in tobacco users [23].

It is recognized in the literature that alcohol and tobacco act synergistically as a risk factor for oral SCC [24–26], but conflicting evidence exists to support alcohol's role in the development of OED. A paper by Morse et al. reported that they did not find any significant association between alcohol consumption and development of OED [27] while a previous study by the same groups of authors observed that consumption of seven or more alcoholic beverages a week increased the risk of detecting OED on biopsy of a PPOEL by two times [27]. In another study, 50% the PPOELs presenting with dysplasia occurred in individuals who reported regular consumption [28]. The carcinogenicity of alcohol is thought to be due to the metabolism of ethanol to mutogenic acetaladehyde in the oral cavity.

The most high-risk area for development of oral SCC and OED, as agreed on by many authors, is the floor of the mouth and the tongue, particularly the lateral border [1, 29, 30]. This is owing to the fact that a greater level of carcinogenic exposure is present as tobacco, and alcoholic products dissolve in the saliva and settle on the floor of the oral cavity [29]. In addition, due to the thinner and nonkeratinized epithelium of these sites, tissue penetration and a more potent level of carcinogenic exposure is possible. Also contributing may be the differing embryonic origins of these site and response to carcinogens [29]. In a study by Barnes et al. that examined the clinical features of OED, it was reported that severe dysplasia was more likely to form on the lateral tongue and floor of the mouth, compared to the rest of the oral cavity [4]. Pereira et al. also has a similar finding, with severe dysplasia occurring most often on the floor of mouth and tongue.

1.5 Relationship Between OED and PPOEL

Leukoplakia, erythroplakia, oral lichen planus, oral submucosa fibrosis, and actinic chelitis are recognized potential premalignant oral epithelial lesion.

Leukoplakia is defined as any "white plaque of questionable risk having excluded other known disease and disorders that carry no increased risk of cancer". The can be grouped in to homogenous or nonhomogenous (erythro-leukoplakia). A subtype of leukoplakia, proliferative verrucous leukoplakia has the highest rate of malignant transformation of any oral white patch lesion. The proportion of biopsied leukoplakia cases positive for OED has been reported as 15%, and the proportion of cases that will undergo malignant transformation is 1% [2, 4].

Erythroplakia is defined as a fiery red patch that cannot be characterized clinically or pathologically as any other definable disease. The proportion of biopsied erythroplakia cases positive for OED is reported as 91%, and the proportion of cases that will undergo malignant transformation is 100% [2, 4, 12].

Oral lichen planus (OLP) is considered by some authors to be a PPOEL; however, controversy does exist about this inclusion [13]. OLP is a chronic inflammatory disease thought to be immune-mediated and have some genetic predisposition; however, the exact etiology is not known. The proportion of biopsied OLP cases positive for OED that will undergo malignant transformation has been reported as 1–3.2% [2, 4].

Oral submucous fibrosis (OSF) is a chronic mucosa disease of the upper digestive tract [11, 20]. Fibrosis of the lamina propria and submucosal layers of the mucosal lining of the oral cavity, oropharynx, and, at times, the esophagus, resulting in loss of tissue mobility and limited oral opening, is its histopathological characteristic. The proportion of biopsied OSF cases positive for OED is 7–25%, and the proportion of cases that will undergo malignant transformation is 1–8% [2, 4, 31].

Actinic cheilitis is a keratotic condition of the lip vermillion which is considered to be potentially malignant. Patients may present with various clinical signs and symptoms, the most commonly reported being dryness of the lip, atrophy, erythema, ulceration, edema, and blurring of the vermillion border. Proportion of biopsied OSF cases positive for OED is 100% [4, 32].

1.6 Detection and Diagnosis

The gold standard test for diagnosis of OED is histopathological from specimens taken from a formal tissue biopsy [33–35]. There are no reported chairside adjunctive tests currently that have reported higher sensitivity and specificity numbers that trumps the combination of clinical examination and tissue biopsy [33]. There is a myriad of adjunctive tests available for the clinician's armamentarium, with the pros of being non/minimally invasive and causing little to no morbidity but with a tradeoff for giving appreciable levels of false positives and negatives. These adjunctive tests should only be used in situations where the clinician is unsure after clinical examination whether to go ahead with a tissue biopsy or to find areas within a large homogenous lesion to incisional biopsy that will yield a specimen with more advanced atypia or dysplasia. They should not be used when the lesion is clinically frankly dysplastic or cancerous where a formal biopsy would be indicated. We describe several more common adjunctive tests below.

Metachromatic dyes that have high affinity for nucleic acids, such as toluidine blue can be used as an aid to detect high-grade dysplasia and malignant lesion based on the premise that they produce higher levels of nucleic acids compared with normal tissue. The intention is to guide the clinician to areas for biopsy, but overall, toludine blue has poor sensitivity and specificity (57–81% and 56–67%, respectively) [33, 36]. The figures are better with increasing severity of dysplasia, such as severe dysplasia/carcinoma in situ but are poor in mild and moderate dysplasia.

Another minimally invasive detection technique is brush cytology/biopsy that required the clinician to use a dedicated brush to collect a transepithelial and exfoliated cell sample, which is then fixed on a histology slide and submitted for specialized computer-aided scanning analysis. As the transepithelial array of cells are architecturally disordered, it can only detect the presence of cellular atypia and not able to differentiate invasive carcinoma from carcinoma in situ. Apart from its high cost, it is in limited use in clinical practice owing to inconsistent sensitivity and specificity figures in the literature (range 73–100% and 32–94%, respectively) [37, 38].

There is evidence to suggest that light-reflecting properties of oral mucosal changes in a progressive and predictable manner from the spectrum of normal to frankly malignant oral epithelial tissue. Autofluorescence and chemiluminescence diagnostic/screening tools take advantage of this assumption for them to be marketed to clinicians for use, with a myriad of commercial brands available for sale. The tools' specificity and sensitivity functioning statistics are generally not promising with one systemic review's reporting rates of 0–100% and 0–75% for chemiluminescence and 30–100% and 15.3–100% for autofluorescence, respectively [33, 39]. It was purported that sensitivities of 100% published in some of the papers where owing to lesions that were clinically obvious by routine visual examination [40, 41]. From a specificity standpoint, both autofluorescence and chemiluminescence performed suboptimally in differentiating dysplasia/malignancy, inflammation, and reactive from each other. An alternative, modified chemilumninescence method that takes advantage of dysplastic and malignant cells expressing a different glycan residue, which can then be conjugated with a proprietary fluorescent lectin has shown promising results, with an in vivo study yielding sensitivity and specificity of 89% and 82%, respectively [42–44].

Dysplastic and malignant cells generally have depleted or negligible glycogen content compared to healthy mucosa. Lugol's iodine solution, which contains iodine and potassium iodide in an aqueous solvent will bind to normal mucosa and have low affinity for dysplastic/malignant tissue. The literature has shown that it is a useful adjunct in obtaining clear margins for dysplasia/intraepithelial neoplasm during tumor resections (32% clear margins in the control group versus 4% in the Lugol's solution group) [45].

1.7 Human Papillomavirus and Dysplasia

There are over 160 genotypes of human papilloma virus and some subtypes are risk factors for development of oropharyngeal and oral squamous cell carcinoma. Specifically, 16 and 18 have been described as high risk for the development of oropharyngeal carcinoma [46, 47]. HPV-derived oncogenes, E6 and E7, causes epithelial malignant transformation by repressing p53 and Rb tumor suppressor gene functions [46]. The prevalence of HPV is 0.9–12% in clinical normal mucosa, and in an immunocompetent host, the infection is usually cleared within 2 years [48]. Perseverance of the virus past the 2 year mark augments the likelihood of malignant genetic mutation and transformation. Controversy exist on the association and prevalence of HPV in PPOELs. A systematic review described an overall odds ratio of 3.87 between all PPOELs and aggregate HPV-DNA, and when dysplasia was the specific variable, the OR raised to 5.10 [46].

The prevalence of HPV subtypes 16 and 18 was reported to be 25% in oral and oropharyngeal dysplasia in one meta-analysis [49]. HPV-driven dysplasia have been described as being unique in histopathological studies as they are characterized by karyorrhexis and apoptosis [47]. Chemoprevention and HPV vaccination is anticipated to reduce the prevalence and incidence of oropharyngeal/oral squamous cell carcinoma.

1.8 Field Cancerization and OED

OED presents the initial steps of field cancerization, when early cellular and architectural changes affect the mucosal epithelium. Field cancerization describes the multistep and sequential process of carcinogenesis of epithelial tumors. This process was first described by Slaughter et al. after microscopic examination of almost 800 oral and pharyngeal cancers revealed that tissue abnormalities extended beyond the clinically obvious tumor [50]. This suggested that cancers arise from patches or fields of genetically abnormal cells which display features of malignancy but remain noninvasive. These fields develop from a single mutated stem cell which divides and differentiates to produce similarly abnormal daughter cells. Uncontrolled cell division allows for the growth and development of this field which replaces the overlying normal tissue [51]. Histopathologically, this field is diagnosed as OED and is considered potentially malignant.

1.9 Malignant Transformation

There is a myriad of widely varying figures in the literature relating to the malignant transformation rate of OED to OSCC; this may be owing to when effect of confounding factors such as exposure to risk factors not considered, classification of clinical lesions being varied between studies, and, as previously outlined, the classification of dysplasia is not an exact science. The malignant transformation rate of OED varies vastly in the literature, with a range of 6–36% [52]. Current variables in the literature that affect the MTR are the site of the lesion; tongue and FOM being at the higher end of the MTR spectrum along with the grade of the dysplasia [1]. There are conflicting reports with respect to grading severity being correlated with MTR [23, 53, 54]. A predominance of the contemporary literature supports the hypothesis that MTR is correlated with the presence of OED and it severity [1]. On the otherhand, there are some studies not supporting the relationship between MTR and grade of dysplasia, such as Dost et al.'s paper, involving biopsy-proven OED in 368 individuals, which came to a conclusion that the severity of dysplasia, graded according the 2005 WHO classification and the Kujan et al. binary system, was not correlated with the risk of malignant transformation [23].

In a retrospective study of biopsy specimens collected over 20 years, Cowen et al. [55] demonstrated that a relationship existed between the presence of OED and malignancy. However, the authors failed to undertake a statistical analysis of their findings. A similar retrospective study was conducted in the UK, and a significant relationship between OED grading and oral SCC development was found [56]. The annual transformation rate of severe dysplasia was 5.6%, compared with 0.3% of nondysplastic PMDs. This is further corroborated by Schepman et al. [13], who concluded that leukoplakia which presented with moderate to severe OED, had a significantly higher predisposition to developing a malignancy. Silverman et al. [17] reported a malignant transformation rate of 36% for lesions which present with OED. Small sample size however is a shortcoming of this study, which puts into doubt the validity of these results; only 22 lesions which presented with some degree of OED were included in the aforementioned study. Another study from Australia has reported that 4.7% of OEDs progressed to oral cancer in a mean time of 3.3 years, and it also suggested that mild grades of OED were just as likely to transform into OSCC as severe-grade OEDs. This is in stark contrast to Mehanna's meta-analysis that showed mild/moderate OEDs had a malignant transformation of 10% versus severe OED/CIS which has a rate of 24%.

These findings differ from those from Asian countries such as Taiwan and India, which tend to conclude that OED does not affect malignant potential. Prospective evaluation of 1458 Taiwanese patients presenting with a PPOEL revealed that in over 10 years of follow-up, no cases of severe OED developed a malignancy [57]. While results show that those patients presenting with OED transformed at a higher rate than those without, this was not statistically significant, indicating SCC development is unaffected by dysplastic features. The estimated annual malignant transformation rate of 3.02% is considered particularly low in light of other research; however, the authors suggest this to be due to broader inclusion criteria, incorporating a wider variety of PPOELs. Comparative studies tend to limit analysis to a particular type of lesion, such as leukoplakia [13, 17, 29, 58]. A smaller scale study also conducted in Taiwan found similar results [59].

Difficulty arises when comparing the results of these studies, as differing study design, inclusion criteria, and statistical analyses affect the findings. Several studies restrict inclusion criteria to certain types of PPOELs, most commonly leukoplakias [13, 17, 58], which limit the generalisability of malignant transformation rates, which themselves are calculated via differing means. Varying definitions of PPOELs also affect selection criteria, particularly those with a focus on leukoplakia, the diagnostic criteria of which has been revised several times. Older studies tend to follow the classification of the time, so conditions such as frictional keratosis, which have no risk of malignancy above normal healthy mucosa, were included as leukoplakias, affecting overall study outcomes [2].

1.10 Molecular Markers Associated with Development and Progression of OED/PPOEL

Research of complex molecular mechanisms underpinning oral behavior, development, and progression of oral cancers has been vast and progressing at a rapid pace in the past several decades.

Despite this, our current cognizance of the critical molecular process that heralds and drives dysplastic or potentially premalignant epithelial lesions' progression to oral squamous cell carcinoma is still lacking [60]. As such, the development of clinically applicable prognostic and diagnostic markers and targeted therapies that eventuate in improved prognosis and survival of head and neck cancer patients has not been fruitful to date.

A comprehensive description of all molecules studied is beyond the scope of this chapter. The majority of the molecules explored are associated with critical cellular and molecular oncogenic processes or the term "hallmarks of cancer" coined by Hanahan and Weinberg [61]. These processes involve sustained cell proliferation, evasion of growth suppression, resistance to apoptosis, replicative immortality, angiogenesis, invasion, and metastasis as well as emerging "hallmarks" such as evasion of immune system surveillance, reprogramming of cellular metabolism, and enabling molecular characteristics (genomic instability and tumor-promoting inflammation) [61].

Of note are markers relating to epigentetic events, which is an emerging area in research. These epigenetic events include histone sumoylation and acetylation, microRNA and long encoding RNA post-transcriptional regulation (upregulation, downregulation, or overprogression or underexpression) and DNA methylation [60].

DNA Hypermethylation. In approximately 40% of OED cases, p16 gene hypermethylation is detected and a corresponding proportion progresses to OSCC. In addition, during the progression of mild to severe OED, hypermethylation of the p15 and 16 gene has been documented. MGMT gene methylation is described to be greater than 50–80% of OL. Oral lichen planus without dysplastic features can be distinguished from those with dysplasia by detection of methylation of TSPYLS5, NKX2-3, RBP4, TRPC4, CMTM3, CLDN11, and MAP6 genes. Methylated HOXA9, EDNRB, and DCC (deleted in colorectal cancer) were correlated with malignant or premalignant oral lesions. Methylated zinc finger protein 582 (ZNF582, transcription factor on chromosome 19) has also been suggested as a biomarker for oral dysplasia and cancer [60].

Histone Modification. Tumor invasion and oncological transformation can be the result of histone modification that has triggered deregulation of chromatic-based process. An example of this is lysine modification on H3 histone at specific position Lys9, Lys4, Lys18, and Lys27 that become methylated and/or acetylated as is observed in some oral squamous cell carcinoma lesion. Papillon-Cavanagh et al. [62] have demonstrated diminished H3-K36 methylation characterizes a subset of head and neck SCC, but all studies have thus far addressed only SCCs, and data on PPOELs or dysplasia are deficient.

Micro-RNA. Cellular noncoding mirco-RNA, in concert with other factors, regulates the cellular protein expression and functions. Reports of association between miRNA profiles and oral premalignant/dysplasia are few. MiR-31 was reported as being augmented in some potentially premalignant oral epithelial lesions, such as hyperkeratotic and hyperplastic lesions, which are deemed less likely to progress to SCC compared to OED. Cervigne et al. have reported that overexpression of miRNA-345, miRNA-21, and miRNA-181b was essential to malignant transformation. Increase in lesion severity during progression was associated with elevated expression of miRNA-345, miR-181b, and miR-21 [63].

1.11 Management

1.11.1 Prevention

In the management of premalignancy, primary prevention should be the first armamentarium utilized, and any modifiable risk factors for OED should be eliminated in order to prevent and arrest the progression of premalignancy to malignancy. Patients should be counseled on tobacco use cessation and limit alcohol intake. Risk stratifying is extremely important in order to identify high-risk individuals and then to provide appropriate screening and counseling. From a systemic review, the predicted attributable lifetime risk for developing oral squamous cell carcinoma if an individual smoked solely, consumed alcohol solely, or in used tobacco and alcohol in combination was 25%, 18%, and 40%, respectively [64]. The correlation between development of OED that may progress to oral squamous cell carcinoma with tobacco use and alcohol consumption risk is dose-dependent and cumulative over an individual's lifetime. A meta-analysis study involving 5338 patients who received surgical excision/resection of oral squamous cell carcinoma, 30% were found positive for all HPV subtypes, 18% for HPV18, and 25% for HPV16 [65]. Although the link between HPV as a causative factor in oral squamous cell carcinoma is not as strong as for oropharyngeal carcinoma, the HPV vaccine may play a role in secondary prevention. Other prevention strategies include early detection of PPOELs and prevention of malignant transformation [33].

1.11.2 Surgical Management

Surgery management of OED involving excision using scalpel, excision, or ablation using laser or cryosurgery is reported. There are no RCTs comparing the efficacies of these in respect to recurrence, progression to malignancy. Surgery in the form of excision and/or laser ablation is at present, the most accepted mode of treatment [54, 66–68].

Cryosurgery have limited use in treatment of OED and have been reported to yield higher rates of recurrence and malignant transformation [69]. Surgical excision with a scalpel blade is a consistent modality and common in surgical practice as it is cost effective, simple to use, and provides a surgical specimen with margins that is undamaged by heat of a laser, which allow for accurate histopathological examination [52]. Excision of large OED lesion with a blade may produce undesirable cicatricial healing, this can be overcome by placing a split thickness skin graft in the surgical bed [69].

CO_2 lasers are used frequently in the surgical management of OED. The mechanism of CO_2 laser involved applied focal, collimated energy that augments the temperature of the target tissue to greater than 100 °C, culminating in the phase change of water to steam. Adjustable power of laser permits its use as a surgical knife or ablative agent (5–25 W). Laser can be used defocused to ablate the tissue and permit hemostasis, and the site is left deepithelialized to heal by secondary intention. CO_2 laser creates a unique wound, in that it is only a few tenth of mm deep with limited removal of healthy tissue. Meltzer suggests recurrence of leukoplakia with laser is only 10% compared with scalpel at 34% [70]. Other advantages include cellular destruction by ablation minimizes release of inflammatory mediators compared with a scalpel, hence patient is reported to have less pain and swelling; blood vessels with diameter of the lumen less than half of a millimeter are sealed off, producing a less bloody field; and limited wound contracture. The main criticism is that the vaporized tissue is not available for histological exam, but this can be overcome somewhat by taking multiple incision biopsy specimens prior to lasering. Another disadvantage of laser ablation is that epithelial migration is delayed, and the surgical wound may take longer to heal [70].

The general consensus is that the presence of OED predisposes a lesion to undergo malignant transformation; logic would follow that the severity would have an impact, as the more severe the dysplasia is, the more genetically aberrant and therefore histopathologically similar to an SCC. Regardless of this supposed multistep progression model, current practice sees some clinicians forgoing active treatment of milder lesions, which are monitored rather than excised [1, 6]. This is somewhat supported by the literature, which reports the risk of a mildly dysplastic lesion progressing to cancer being less than 5% [6]. More severe tissue changes are reported to progress to SCC in as low as 7% of cases [6]. Distinguishing between these levels of severity in itself presents a challenge, with subjectivity unavoidable in the process of classifying a continuous scale of tissue change. In contrast, there is literature to support the notion that irrespective of the grade of OED, all biopsy-proven OED should be treated by excision or laser ablation, instead of the "wait and watch" approach some clinicians take for mild dysplasia. The management of mild and moderate OED remains controversial, and there is no concrete well-designed RCTs that give support either way. Owing to the higher risk of malignant transformation of severe OEDs and CIS, the accepted convention treatment is surgical excision with or without reconstruction. Diagram 1 depicts our departments protocol in the management of mild, moderate, and severe/CIS OEDs [71] (Fig. 1.1).

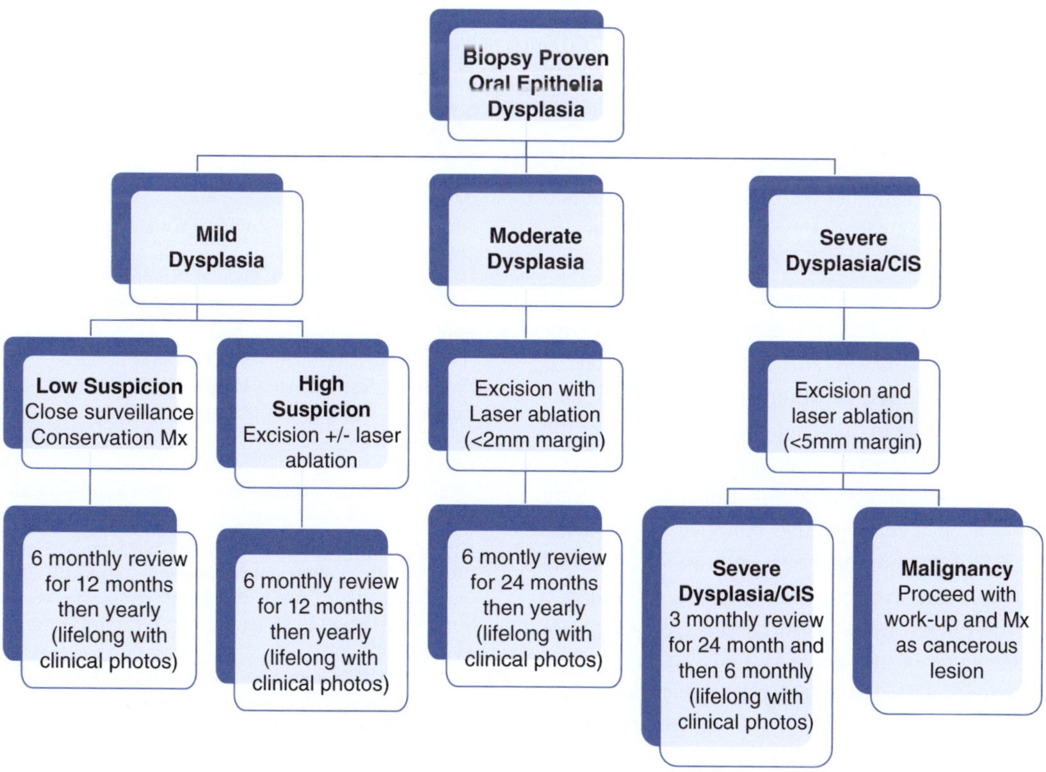

Fig. 1.1 Authors' algorithm for management of oral epithelial dysplasia

1.11.3 Medical Treatments

Medical treatments have no supporting evidence at this time. Topical bleomycin, systemic retinoic acid, and lycopene may help to resolve OED in the short term, but there is no evidence exists to support that they prevent malignant transformation [35]. There is also poor evidence in support of photodynamic therapy or using COX inhibitors or attenuated virus as mouthwash therapy to treat OED [35].

1.12 Follow-Up and Recurrence After Excision or Ablation of OED

For those individuals diagnosed with OED, at present, widely accepted standardized or guidelines on the frequency of surveillance, and clinical follow-up do not exist [35]. Despite this, clinical surveillance ought to be sufficiently frequent; especially in moderate and severely dysplastic lesions [54, 67]. This should be contingent from the notion of field cancerization, variable interval to malignant transformation, and rate of recurrence. Surveillance of a patient should be individualized according to the lesion (site of lesion, degree of dysplasia) and the patient's risk factors (alcohol/tobacco uses, age, gender) [1, 53]; some authors recommend that continued surveillance is mandatory long term, as long as 20 years to life-long after excision [35, 71].

Despite surgical modalities of treatment, an appreciable risk of recurrence and malignant transformation still persists. Excision of OEDs is reported to diminish the rate of recurrence by close to 50% but does not eradicate the risk [72]. Holmstup et al. reported a recurrence rate of 13% and malignant transformation rate of 12% in a retrospective study of 94 patients, who had nonhomogenous or homogenous oral leukoplakias excised; their clinical surveillance period ranged from 1.5 to 18 years. Seventy-one percentage of the excised leukoplakias exhibited oral epithelial dysplasia, and 7 years was the mean time to malignant transformation [72]. Nankivell reported a lower recurrence rate of 5% after surgical excision of OEDs. In cohort study by Thomson et al. that looked at PPOEL excised with CO_2 lasers, of the 590 patients, there was a persistence rate of 9% and malignant transformation rate of 16%. The mean surveillance duration was 7.3 years, and mean time for malignant transformation was 7 years [68].

Acknowledgement *Disclaimer*: All figures and tables submitted are original. We report no conflict of interest and no financial support was received.

References

1. Speight PM, Speight PM. Update on oral epithelial dysplasia and progression to cancer. Head Neck Pathol. 2007;1:61–6.
2. Van Der Waal I. Potentially malignant disorders of the oral and oropharyngeal mucosa; terminology, classification and present concepts of management. Oral Oncol. 2009;45:317–23.
3. Warnakulasuriya S, Reibel J, Bouquot J, Dabelsteen E. Oral epithelial dysplasia classification systems: predictive value, utility, weaknesses and scope for improvement. J Oral Pathol Med. 2008;37:127–33.
4. Barnes L, Eveson JW, Reichart P, Sidransky D, editors. World Health Organisation classification of tumours pathology and genetics of head and neck tumours. Lyon: IARC Press; 2005.
5. Warnakulasuriya S, Johnson NW, van der Waal I. Nomenclature and classification of potentially malignant disorders of the oral mucosa. J Oral Pathol Med. 2007;36:575–80.
6. Bouquot JE, Speight PM, Farthing PM. Epithelial dysplasia of the oral mucosa—diagnostic problems and prognostic features. Curr Diagn Pathol. 2006;12:11–21.
7. Hellquist H, Cardesa A, Gale N, Kambic V, Michaels L. Criteria for grading in the Ljubljana classification of epithelial hyperplastic laryngeal lesions. A study by members of the Working Group on Epithelial Hyperplastic Laryngeal Lesions of the European Society of Pathology. Histopathology. 1999;34:226–33.
8. Brothwell DJ, Lewis DW, Bradley G, et al. Observer agreement in the grading of oral epithelial dysplasia. Commun Dent Oral. 2003;31:300–5.
9. Abbey LM, Kaugars GE, Gunsolley JC, et al. Intraexaminer and interexaminer reliability in the diagnosis of oral epithelial dysplasia. Oral Surg Oral Med Oral Pathol Oral Radiol Endod. 1995;80:188–91.
10. Lumerman H, Freedman P, Kerpel S. Oral epithelial dysplasia and the development of invasive squamous cell carcinoma. Oral Surg Oral Med Oral Pathol Oral Radiol. 1995;79:321–9.

11. Jaber MA, Porter SR, Speight P, Eveson JW, Scully C. Oral epithelial dysplasia: clinical characteristics of western European residents. Oral Oncol. 2003;39:589–96.
12. Hashibe M, Mathew B, Kuruvilla B, et al. Chewing tobacco, alcohol, and the risk of erythroplakia. Cancer Epidem Biomar. 2000;9:639–45.
13. Schepman KP, van der Meij EH, Smeele LE, van der Waal I. Malignant transformation of oral leukoplakia: a follow-up study of a hospital-based population of 166 patients with oral leukoplakia from The Netherlands. Oral Oncol. 1998;34:270–5.
14. Pereira J, Carvalho Mde V, Henriques AC, et al. Epidemiology and correlation of the clinicopathological features in oral epithelial dysplasia: analysis of 173 cases. Ann Diagn Pathol. 2011;15:98–102.
15. Barnard NA, Scully C, Eveson JW, Cunningham S, Porter SR. Oral cancer development in patients with oral lichen planus. J Oral Pathol Med. 1993;22:421–4.
16. Krutchkoff DJ, Eisenberg E. Lichenoid dysplasia: a distinct histopathologic entity. Oral Surg Oral Med Oral Pathol Oral Radiol Endod. 1985;60:308–15.
17. Silverman S Jr, Bahl S. Oral lichen planus update: clinical characteristics, treatment responses, and malignant transformation. Am J Dent. 1997;10:259–63.
18. Epstein JB, Wan LS, Gorsky M, Zhang L. Oral lichen planus: progress in understanding its malignant potential and the implications for clinical management. Oral Surg Oral Med Oral Pathol Oral Radiol Endod. 2003;96:32–7.
19. Silverman S Jr, Gorsky M, Lozada-Nur F, Giannotti K. A prospective study of findings and management in 214 patients with oral lichen planus. Oral Surg Oral Med Oral Pathol Oral Radiol Endod. 1991;72:665–70.
20. Silverman S Jr, Gorsky M, Lozada-Nur F. A prospective follow-up study of 570 patients with oral lichen planus: persistence, remission, and malignant association. Oral Surg Oral Med Oral Pathol Oral Radiol Endod. 1985;60:30–4.
21. Silverman S, Bhargava K, Smith LW, Malaowalla AM. Malignant transformation and natural history of oral leukoplakia in 57,518 industrial workers of Gujarat, India. Cancer. 1976;38:1790–5.
22. Morse DE, Katz RV, Pendrys DG, et al. Smoking and drinking in relation to oral epithelial dysplasia. Cancer Epidem Biomar. 1996;5:769–77.
23. Dost F, Cao KA, Ford P, Farah C, et al. Malignant transformation rate of oral epithelial dysplasia: a real-world evaluationof histopathological grading. Oral Surg Oral Med Oral Pathol Oral Radiol Endod. 2014;117:323–52.
24. Ogden GR, Wight AJ. Aetiology of oral cancer: alcohol. Brit J Oral Max Surg. 1998;36:247–51.
25. Zygogianni AG, Kyrgias G, Karakitsos P, et al. Oral squamous cell cancer: early detection and the role of alcohol and smoking. Head Neck Oncol. 2011;3:2.
26. Znaor A, Brennan P, Gajalakshmi V, et al. Independent and combined effects of tobacco smoking, chewing and alcohol drinking on the risk of oral, pharyngeal and esophageal cancers in Indian men. Int J Cancer. 2003;105:681–6.
27. Morse DE, Psoter WJ, Cleveland D, et al. Smoking and drinking in relation to oral cancer and oral epithelial dysplasia. Cancer Cause Contr. 2007;18:919–29.
28. Dost F, Cao KA, Ford P, Farah C, et al. A retrospective analysis of clinical features of oral malignant and potentially malignant disorders with and without oral epithelial dysplasia. Oral Surg Oral Med Oral Pathol Oral Radiol Endod. 2013;116:725–33.
29. Zhang L, Cheung KJ Jr, Lam WL, et al. Increased genetic damage in oral leukoplakia from high risk sites: potential impact on staging and clinical management. Cancer. 2001;91:2148–55.
30. Napier SS, Speight PM. Natural history of potentially malignant oral lesions and conditions: an overview of the literature. J Oral Pathol Med. 2008;37:1–10.
31. Cox SC, Walker DM. Oral submucous fibrosis. A review. Aust Dent J. 1996;41:294–9.
32. Savage NW, McKay C, Faulkner C. Actinic cheilitis in dental practice. Aust Dent J. 2010;55(Suppl 1):78–84.
33. Rhodus NL, Kerr AR, Patel K. Oral cancer: leukoplakia, premalignancy, and squamous cell carcinoma. Dent Clin N Am. 2014;58(2):315–40.
34. Panwar A, Lindau R, Wieland A. Management for premalignant lesions of the oral cavity. Expert Rev Anticancer Ther. 2014;14(3):349–57.
35. Brennan M, et al. Management of oral epithelial dysplasia: a review. Oral Surg Oral Med Oral Pathol Oral Radiol Endod. 2007;103(Suppl):S19.e1–12.
36. Portugal LC, Wilson KM, Biddinger PW, et al. The role of toluidine blue in assessing margin status after resection of squamous cell carci-nomas of the upper aerodigestive tract. Arch Otolaryngol Head Neck Surg. 1996;122:517–9.
37. Gupta S, et al. Clinical correlative study on early detection of oral cancer and precancerous lesions by modified oral brush biopsy and cytology followed by histopathology. J Cancer Res Ther. 2014;10(2):232–8.
38. Babshet M, et al. Efficacy of oral brush cytology in the evaluation of the oral premalignant and malignant lesions. J Cytol. 2011;28(4):165–72.
39. Rashid A, Warnakulasuriya S. The use of light-based (optical) detection systems as adjuncts in the detection of oral cancer and oral potentially malignant disorders: a systematic review. J Oral Pathol Med. 2015;44(5):307–28.
40. Liviu Feller JL. Oral squamous cell carcinoma epidemiology, clinical presentation and treatment. Cancer Ther. 2012;3:263–8.
41. Gillenwater A, Papadimitrakopoulou V, Richards-Kortum R. Oral premalignancy: new methods of detection and treatment. Curr Oncol Rep. 2006;8(2):146–54.
42. McCullough MJ, Farah CS. The role of alcohol in oral carcinogenesis with particular reference to alcohol-containing mouthwashes. Aust Dent J. 2008;53:302–5.
43. Baeten J, et al. Chairside molecular imaging of aberrant glycosylation in subjects with suspicious oral lesions using fluorescently labeled wheat germ agglutinin. Head Neck. 2018;40(2):292–301.

44. Baeten J, et al. Molecular imaging of oral premalignant and malignant lesions using fluorescently labeled lectins. Transl Oncol. 2014;7(2):213–20.
45. McMahon J, et al. Use of Lugol's iodine in the resection of oral and oropharyngeal squamous cell carcinoma. Br J Oral Maxillofac Surg. 2010;48(2):84–7.
46. Syrjanen S, et al. Human papillomaviruses in oral carcinoma and oral potentially malignant disorders: a systematic review. Oral Dis. 2011;17(Suppl 1):58–72.
47. Woo SB, Cashman EC, Lerman MA. Human papillomavirus-associated oral intraepithelial neoplasia. Mod Pathol. 2013;26(10):1288–97.
48. Lerman MA, et al. HPV-16 in a distinct subset of oral epithelial dysplasia. Mod Pathol. 2017;30(12):1646–54.
49. Jayaprakash V, et al. Human papillomavirus types 16 and 18 in epithelial dysplasia of oral cavity and oropharynx: a meta-analysis, 1985–2010. Oral Oncol. 2011;47(11):1048–54.
50. Slaughter DP, Southwick HW, Smejkal W. Field cancerization in oral stratified squamous epithelium; clinical implications of multicentric origin. Cancer. 1953;6:963–8.
51. Braakhuis BJ, Tabor MP, Kummer JA, Leemans CR, Brakenhoff RH. A genetic explanation of Slaughter's concept of field cancerization: evidence and clinical implications. Cancer Res. 2003;63:1727–30.
52. Mehanna HM, et al. Treatment and follow-up of oral dysplasia – a systematic review and meta-analysis. Head Neck. 2009;31:600–9.
53. Amagasa T, Yamashiro M, Uzawa N. Oral premalignant lesions: from a clinical perspective. Int J Clin Oncol. 2011;16(1):5–14.
54. Goodson ML, et al. Oral precursor lesions and malignant transformation—who, where, what, and when? Br J Oral Maxillofac Surg. 2015;53(9):831–5.
55. Cowan CG, Gregg TA, Napier SS, McKenna SM, Kee F. Potentially malignant oral lesions in northern Ireland: a 20-year population-based perspective of malignant transformation. Oral Dis. 2001;7:18–24.
56. Warnakulasuriya S, Kovacevic T, Madden P, et al. Factors predicting malignant transformation in oral potentially malignant disorders among patients accrued over a 10-year period in South East England. J Oral Pathol Med. 2011;40(9):677–83.
57. Hsue SS, Wang WC, Chen CH, et al. Malignant transformation in 1458 patients with potentially malignant oral mucosal disorders: a follow-up study based in a Taiwanese hospital. J Oral Pathol Med. 2007;36:25–9.
58. Banoczy J. Follow-up studies in oral leukoplakia. J Maxillofac Surg. 1977;5:69–75.
59. Ho PS, Chen PL, Warnakulasuriya S, et al. Malignant transformation of oral potentially malignant disorders in males: a retrospective cohort study. BMC Cancer. 2009;9:260.
60. Nikitakis N, Pentenero M, Georgaki M, Poh C, et al. Molecular markers associated with development of potentially premalignant oral epithelial lesions: current knowledge and future implications. Oral Surg Oral Med Oral Pathol Oral Radiol Endod. 2008;125:650–69.
61. Hanahan D, Weinberg RA. Hallmarks of cancer: the next generation. Cell. 2011;144:646–74.
62. Papillon-Cavanagh S, Lu C, Gayden T, et al. Impaired H3 K36 methylation defines a subset of head and neck squamous cell carcinomas. Nat Genet. 2017;49:180–5.
63. Cervigne NK, Reis PP, Machado J, et al. Identification of a microRNA signature associated with progression of leukoplakia to oral carcinoma. Hum Mol Genet. 2009;18:4818–29.
64. Radoi L, Luce D. A review of risk factors for oral cavity cancer: the importance of a standardized case definition. Community Dent Oral Epidemiol. 2013;41(2):97–109, e78–91.
65. Kansy K, Thiele O, Freier K. The role of human papillomavirus in oral squamous cell carcinoma: myth and reality. Oral Maxillofac Surg. 2014;18(2):165–72.
66. Mogedas-Vegara A, et al. Oral leukoplakia treatment with the carbon dioxide laser: a systematic review of the literature. J Craniomaxillofac Surg. 2016;44(4):331–6.
67. Field EA, et al. The management of oral epithelial dysplasia: the Liverpool algorithm. Oral Oncol. 2015;51(10):883–7.
68. Thomson PJ, et al. Interventional laser surgery for oral potentially malignant disorders: a longitudinal patient cohort study. Int J Oral Maxillofac Surg. 2017;46(3):337–42.
69. Kademani D. Surgical management of oral and mucosal dysplasia: the case for surgical excision. J Oral Maxillofac Surg. 2007;65:287–92.
70. Meltzer C. Surgical management of oral and mucosal dysplasia: the case for laser excision. J Oral Maxillofac Surg. 2007;65:293–5.
71. Awadallah M, Idle M, Patel K, Kademani D. Management update of potentially premalignant oral epithelial lesions. Oral Surg Oral Med Oral Pathol Oral Radiol. 2018;125(6):628–36.
72. Holmstrup P, et al. Long-term treatment outcome of oral premalignant lesions. Oral Oncol. 2006;42(5):461–74.

2 Chemoprevention in Oral Cancer

Jeffrey Y. Tsai and Jasjit K. Dillon

2.1 Introduction

Chemoprevention is the concept of preventing, delaying, or reversing the progression of premalignant lesions to invasive cancer. This can be achieved through the use of natural, synthetic, or biologic agents [1]. Studies have been reported in the literature regarding the utility of agents such as systemic and topical retinoids, bleomycin, cyclooxygenase inhibitors, and phytochemical-enriched products in decreasing the clinical presence of oral premalignant lesions, as well as in preventing second primary tumors that may arise through field cancerization of the oral cavity [2, 3]. Population-based studies have revealed possible reduction in the relative risk of developing head and neck cancers with the ingestion of certain nutrients (e.g., carotenoids [4]) or medications (e.g., NSAIDs [5]). Thus, the idea that chemoprevention can be utilized to prevent or even reverse premalignant disease of the oral cavity in high-risk individuals has attracted a great deal of scientific inquiry.

As described by Bauman in 2016 [6], finding effective chemoprevention strategies against head and neck squamous cell carcinoma has been made more difficult by several factors, including the lack of preclinical oral carcinogenesis models allowing for the identification of biomarkers that can be targeted by chemoprevention. Based on the multistep carcinogenesis model of progression from hyperplasia to invasive cancer (hyperplasia, to dysplasia, to carcinoma in situ, to cancer), the identification of the molecular drivers of these pathways could reveal molecular targets that can halt this stepwise progression.

To date, there have been many compounds that have been studied for their potential in preventing progression of premalignant lesions to cancer in the oral cavity and/or prevention of second primary head and neck tumors. Further, with the advent of the identification of molecular biomarkers of oral cancer risk, molecularly targeted agents (e.g., epidermal growth factor [EGFR] inhibitors) have additionally been evaluated [7]. This chapter aims to provide the reader with an overview of the present literature of several chemoprevention agents that have been studied in clinical trials and provide commentary on potential future directions of research in this field. While chemoprevention of oral cancer has not yet entered the domain of routine clinical practice, it is an evolving field that may yet yield future therapeutics.

2.2 Antimutagens

Mutagens lead to the development of cancer through permanent changes in a cell's DNA, resulting in alterations to a gene product, defects

J. Y. Tsai · J. K. Dillon (✉)
Department of Oral and Maxillofacial Surgery, University of Washington, Seattle, WA, USA
e-mail: tsaijeff@uw.edu; dillonj5@uw.edu

D. Kademani (ed.), *Improving Outcomes in Oral Cancer*, https://doi.org/10.1007/978-3-030-30094-4_2

in cellular functions, and potentially the loss of cell growth control. In the case of oral squamous cell carcinoma, known mutagens include lifestyle agents (tobacco, alcohol, betel nut) and infectious agents (bacterial, candidiasis, human papilloma virus, herpes simplex virus). Compounds with antimutagenic properties exert their effect by either preventing the mutagen's effect on DNA (desmutagens) or by suppressing the process of mutation after genes are damaged by mutagens (bio-antimutagens). The major mechanisms of mutagenesis include chemical or enzymatic inactivation, prevention of formation of active species, scavenging of mutagens, and antioxidant or scavenging of free radicals [8].

2.2.1 *N*-Acetyl-L-Cysteine

A variant of the amino acid L-cysteine, *N*-acetyl-L-cysteine (NAC) is widely used for the treatment of acetaminophen toxicity via repletion of glutathione reserves. This increase in glutathione levels leads to support of the body's antioxidant system. As such, NAC has been found to have anti-inflammatory effects beneficial for the treatment of chronic obstructive pulmonary disease (COPD), influenza, and idiopathic pulmonary fibrosis [9].

NAC has been also investigated for its potential anticancer effects and has been demonstrated to suppress epidermal growth factor (EGF)-induced EGF receptor (EGFR) phosphorylation. Overexpression of EGFR has been demonstrated in greater than 80% of head and neck squamous cell carcinoma and is linked with high recurrence and low survival rates [10, 11]. An in vitro study performed by Lee et al. in 2012 [11] demonstrated that NAC induces cell cycle arrest and apoptosis in a human tongue squamous carcinoma cell line that expresses higher EGFR levels than other such cell lines. A murine model study performed by the same group demonstrated reduction in mean tumor volume relative to control animals. Taken together, NAC could be a potential anticancer adjuvant in EGFR overexpressing oral cancers.

Evidence demonstrating the effectiveness of NAC in chemoprevention of oral cancer in the form of randomized controlled trials (RCTs) has been less confirmatory. A large RCT performed in 2002 by the European Organization for Research and Treatment of Cancer (EORTC) investigated the effectiveness of Vitamin A and NAC as chemoprevention agents that may improve the prognosis of patients that were already treated for head and neck cancer or for lung cancer by preventing second primary tumors. Focusing on the arm that received NAC (600 mg daily for 2 years), no statistically significant difference in survival or event-free survival were found between these subjects as compared to subjects who did not receive NAC during the study time period of 2 years [12]. To date, no further RCTs evaluating the use of NAC in oral cancer chemoprevention have been published.

2.2.2 Topical Bleomycin

Bleomycin is an antibiotic that has been found to exhibit antitumoral effects through several mechanisms, including the scission of DNA via activated oxygen and inhibition of DNA ligase. The drug is often incorporated into the chemotherapy regimen for the treatment of Hodgkin's lymphoma and non-Hodgkin's lymphoma and can be administered intravenously, subcutaneously, intramuscularly, intralesionally, or topically [13]. Potential adverse effects include interstitial pneumonitis and mucocutaneous toxicity. The advantage of a locally administered formulation of bleomycin (and conceivably of any chemoprevention agent) is the ability to deliver a high local dose with low total systemic dose which may minimize toxicity [2].

The effectiveness of topical bleomycin in the treatment of oral premalignant lesions has been documented in investigational clinical studies. A systematic review of the literature on topical agents for oral cancer chemoprevention by Chau et al. in 2017 found five studies that utilized topical bleomycin in the treatment of oral premalignant lesions [2]. With a mean treatment duration of 2 weeks, the mean complete response rate (defined as no clinical and/or histopathologic evidence of leukoplakia) was 40.2%, 25%, and 8%

for patients receiving 1% topical bleomycin in DMSO, 0.5% topical bleomycin in DMSO, and placebo, respectively, thereby demonstrating a dose-dependent complete response rate. In one of the included studies by Epstein et al. in 1994, participants were randomized to 1% topical bleomycin in DMSO versus DMSO alone (placebo) [14]. These authors found that 100% of those receiving the 1% topical bleomycin in DMSO agent had an adverse effect, which included erythema, erosion, and discomfort at the site of application. Future clinical studies that evaluate the highest effective dose while producing the fewest adverse effects are needed.

2.2.3 Polyphenols

As a category, polyphenols are a broad group of phytochemicals found in plants, particularly fruits, seeds, and leaves. Polyphenols have been shown to exhibit a protective effect against reactive oxygen species and have been utilized in in vitro and clinical studies to examine their potential antimutagenic effect [15]. Within the broad category of plant-derived dietary polyphenols, tea and tea extracts (e.g., from green tea) have been utilized in epidemiological and clinical studies examining their potential to suppress the development of oral cancer.

2.2.3.1 Green Tea Extract

Preclinical models have demonstrated that the polyphenol epigallocatechin 3-gallate (EGCG), found in high amounts in green tea extract, arrests cells in the G_0/G_1 phase, regulates apoptosis, and blocks angiogenesis through the phosphorylation of vascular endothelial growth factor receptor (VEGFR) and inhibition of VEGF secretion in tumor cells [15, 16]. A phase II randomized, placebo-controlled trial of green tea extract in patients with high-risk oral premalignant lesions was published in 2009 by Tsao et al. [17], which demonstrated a potential partial or complete regression of oral premalignant lesions in subjects administered oral green tea extract over a period of 12 weeks. While the results of the study did not reach statistical significance (perhaps due to small sample sizes), they demonstrated a possible dose–response to green tea extract, whereby subjects administered higher doses of green tea extract had higher rates of clinical response. Of the biomarkers examined in this study, stromal VEGF expression was downregulated in subjects receiving higher doses of green tea extract, suggesting a possible mechanistic action of green tea extract causing inhibition of angiogenesis [17]. While the study did demonstrate possible effect of green tea extract on clinical response of oral premalignant lesions, this clinical response was not associated with a decreased risk of progression to oral cancer. Further studies demonstrating the effectiveness and therapeutic dosing of green tea extract in preventing oral cancer are needed.

2.2.3.2 Curcumin

A yellow coloring agent found in turmeric, curcumin has been studied as a potential agent in the chemoprevention of colon, breast, prostate, and oral cancers. In vitro studies have demonstrated its ability to downregulate nuclear factor-kappa B (NF-κB) and cyclooxygenase-2 (COX-2) in oral premalignant and cancer cells [18, 19]. Chronic exposure to carcinogens causes inflammation and exposure to reactive oxygen species that contribute to aberrant activation of NF-κB and development of squamous cell carcinoma, thus making curcumin a potential agent of study. A recent prospective cohort study by Rai in 2010 [18] demonstrated possible antioxidant effect of curcumin by increasing serum and salivary concentrations of vitamin C and E in patients with oral leukoplakia, lichen planus, and submucous fibrosis. The poor bioavailability of curcumin due to biotransformation in the gut and enterohepatic cycling of metabolites has made the clinical study of curcumin as a chemoprevention agent more difficult, and high-quality randomized trials are necessary to determine curcumin's potential use as a systemic agent of chemoprevention in oral cancer.

2.3 Antiproliferatives

Antiproliferative agents exert their chemoprotective effect by preventing the proliferation of cells. A select review of antiproliferative agents that have been utilized in clinical studies is described and includes retinoids, carotenoids, anti-inflammatories, and ligands of peroxisome proliferator-activated receptor gamma (PPAR-γ).

2.3.1 Retinoids

Included in this group are vitamin A (retinol) and vitamin A analogues (e.g., isotretinoin), which exert their effects through the modulation of gene expression, apoptosis, and cell proliferation [20, 21]. Retinol enters a cell and is eventually converted to retinoic acid via oxidation, which then binds to nuclear receptors that regulate the expression of genes. Retinoids have been used in the induction treatment of malignancies such as lymphoma.

The effects of vitamin analogs on the remission of oral leukoplakia was clinically demonstrated first by Koch et al. in 1978 [22], with a confirmatory randomized controlled trial by Hong et al. in 1986 [23] verifying the effectiveness of oral isotretinoin in the treatment of oral premalignant lesions. This randomized controlled trial also demonstrated relapse of oral premalignant lesions with discontinuation of isotretinoin therapy. A follow-up study on high-dose isotretinoin by Hong et al. in 1990 [3] demonstrated a significant reduction in the development of second primary head and neck squamous cell carcinoma tumors in subjects receiving high-dose isotretinoin (50–100 mg/m^2 of body-surface area per day). As with the previous clinical trial, toxicity with high doses of oral isotretinoin was a barrier to therapy compliance, with severe skin dryness, cheilitis, hypertriglyceridemia, and conjunctivitis leading to reduction or discontinuation of isotretinoin. The results from a randomized clinical trial published by Khuri et al. in 2006 [24] could not demonstrate the efficacy of low-dose (30 mg/day) isotretinoin in reducing the rates of second primary tumors, suggesting that combination therapies or retinoid receptor agonists may be avenues for further research.

As highlighted by the challenges associated with the systemic administration of isotretinoin, long-term patient adherence to therapy may be hampered by toxic effects associated with therapy. In addition, low-dose isotretinoin appears ineffective in reducing recurrence rates of head and neck squamous cell carcinoma [24]. Thus, the local delivery of isotretinoin in the oral cavity has attracted consideration for its potential as a chemoprevention agent against oral cancer. While studies demonstrating the effectiveness of topical retinoids in preventing oral cancer are scarce, a recent study by Kadakia et al. in 2016 [25] summarized a single institution's 15-year experience with isotretinoin rinse as a chemoprophylaxis against recurrence for patients previously treated for oral cavity squamous cell carcinoma, in situ disease, or dysplasia. All subjects were treated with reconstituted 0.2% isotretinoin rinses twice daily, for 1 min duration each, following completion of ablative therapy. Patients who used the medication for a minimum of 12 months were included in the analysis. The difference between recurrence among subjects using isotretinoin rinses compared to the control group was statistically significant, whereby subjects treated with isotretinoin rinse had lower rates of recurrence of disease. Individual group analysis revealed that the recurrence rate was statistically decreased in subjects with multiple oral cavity early-stage cancerous foci or multifocal dysplasia, whereas patients with squamous cell carcinoma in situ or patients with dysplasia following treatment of oral cavity squamous cell carcinoma did not have this response to treatment. This finding suggests a potential benefit of topical isotretinoin use in patients with multiple lesions (consistent with field cancerization), with less or no benefit to those with a single isolated lesion [25].

While these results are promising, caution should be taken prior to the widespread administration of retinoids for the chemoprophylaxis of cancer. A randomized Phase III trial of isotretinoin investigating its effects in preventing second primary tumors in non-small-cell lung cancer patients demonstrated a higher risk of mortality among those with squamous first primaries and in current smokers [26]. Further, a systematic review of antioxidants for primary and secondary prevention by Bjelakovic et al. in 2007 [27] demonstrated that Vitamin A supplementation could increase mortality. Further investigations regarding the safety and efficacy of retinoids are needed, particularly in light of evidence suggesting the potential for harm.

2.3.2 Carotenoids

Carotenoids are a broad group of organic pigments found in various plants. Various carotenoids have Vitamin A activity and can be converted to retinol, thus providing an antiproliferative effect. Others exhibit antioxidant effects, decreasing DNA damage from reactive oxygen species [4]. These properties have prompted investigations into carotenoids and their potential chemopreventive effects in various cancers, including head and neck cancers. A systematic review of the effect of dietary carotenoid intake and the risk of head and neck cancer by Leonici et al. in 2015 [4] demonstrated a reduction in the rate various head and neck cancers. Specifically, dietary beta-carotene intake resulted in a relative risk reduction of 46% for oral cavity cancer. Dietary lycopene intake demonstrated a 26% reduction in the rate of oral and pharyngeal cancer [28].

Conversely, potential harm has been demonstrated from the administration of beta-carotene in populations at high risk for lung cancer. Two randomized clinical trials in particular demonstrated an increased rate of lung cancer in subjects administered beta-carotene: the Beta-Carotene and Retinol Efficiency Trial (CARET) and the Alpha-Tocopherol, Beta-Carotene cancer prevention study (ATBC study), both published in 1996 [26]. These findings are possibly attributed to the high doses of supplements provided. Further study is required to understand why dietary carotenoid intake (including beta-carotene) may have a protective effect against oral cancer, whereas supplementation with beta-carotene appears to cause harm.

2.3.3 Nonsteroidal Anti-inflammatory Drugs (NSAIDs)

The rationale for using NSAIDs for chemoprevention of oral cancer developed from the realization that many malignancies, including head and neck squamous cell carcinoma, exhibit increased prostaglandin synthesis [29]. These prostaglandins facilitate the pathogenesis of malignancies by affecting cell proliferation, angiogenesis, immune surveillance, and apoptosis. The increased synthesis of prostaglandins may be a consequence of increased expression of cyclooxygenase-2 (COX-2) in tumor cells. Experimental data have previously demonstrated that COX-2 is involved in several mechanisms important to carcinogenesis, including apoptosis, inflammation and immunosuppression, angiogenesis, and metastasis. Increased amounts of COX-2 are also seen in oral leukoplakia and head and neck squamous cell carcinoma [29]. Thus, COX-2 inhibition (as with NSAIDs) is a potential strategy in preventing head and neck cancer.

A metanalysis of prospective cohort and case-control studies published by Shi et al. in 2017 [30] examined the association of NSAID use with the relative risk of developing head and neck cancers, including oral cancer. Their analysis revealed a statistically significant reduction in the relative risk of head and neck cancers in the included populations taking NSAIDs, and further subgroup analysis revealed that this relationship was seen with aspirin, COX-2 inhibitor, ibuprofen, and other NSAID use. Further, the results of their metanalysis also suggest a dose–response relationship between NSAID use and relative risk reduction of head and neck cancer, whereby increasing NSAID use was associated with a greater reduction in relative risk.

Randomized clinical trials assessing the effect of topical or systemic COX-2 inhibition on oral premalignant lesions have thus far have been unable to demonstrate a clinical or histologic response to treatment versus placebo [31, 32]. Further, these medications have also been demonstrated to cause potential harm. High use of regular strength aspirin was associated with an elevated risk of small-cell lung cancer, a finding not seen with low-dose aspirin or nonaspirin NSAIDs [26]. Use of selective COX-2 inhibitors may be associated with an increased risk of cardiovascular events [33]. Thus, the potential benefit of COX-2 inhibition in preventing head and neck cancer must be balanced with the potential for adverse effects.

2.3.4 Ligands of Peroxisome Proliferator-Activated Receptor gamma (PPAR-γ)

Upon activation via ligand binding, PPAR-γ heterodimerizes with retinoic acid receptors and controls the expression of genes involved in metabolic pathways, including for lipid biosynthesis and glucose metabolism [34]. Synthetic ligands of PPAR-γ (such as the thiazolidinedione class of medications) have been developed for the treatment of type II diabetes mellitus as they increase insulin sensitivity. Activation of PPAR-γ may have an antiproliferative and proapoptotic action. In vitro studies have demonstrated a proportional decrease in COX-2 expression with increased PPAR-γ expression, suggesting an anti-inflammatory mechanism as well [34]. Such preclinical data suggest that ligands of PPAR-γ may serve a role in the chemoprevention of various cancers, including squamous cell carcinoma of the head and neck.

A retrospective cohort analysis by Govindarajan and Siegel in 2017 [35] examined the incidence of head and neck cancers across diabetic male veterans taking thiazolidinediones (TZDs) across ten Veterans Affairs medical centers. When adjusted for several confounding variables, individuals with TZD exposure showed a large and statistically significant reduction in the incidence of developing head and neck cancer compared to individuals managing their diabetes through diet alone. This relationship remained statistically significant if the patient was taking TZD in addition to other oral antidiabetic agents. Importantly, this study population included only diabetic male veterans, thus potentially limiting the generalizability of these findings. A randomized clinical trial assessing the effects of the TZD pioglitazone on the clinical and histologic response of oral leukoplakia in nondiabetic subjects is currently underway [34].

2.4 Future Directions

The selection of oral cancer chemoprevention agents for clinical investigation has been historically based on epidemiological and laboratory data [6]. Once selected, these agents are then studied on populations believed to be at high risk of developing oral cancer. Clinical trials have therefore focused on patients with oral premalignant lesions as these patients have an elevated risk of developing invasive cancer and have lesions that are accessible for clinical and histological examination.

Evidence of clinical and histological reversal of oral premalignant lesions has often been the desired outcome of chemoprevention trials. However, oral premalignant lesions as a broad category encompass pathologies with varying natural histories that can include spontaneous regression. Further, clinical or histological response of oral premalignant lesions does not necessarily correlate with the prevention of invasive cancer [6]. Thus, the identification of molecular markers that can be measured and can correlate with disease risk and progression may aid in selecting high-risk populations and therapeutics suitable for clinical trial.

Such an approach to a randomized clinical trial was utilized by William et al. in 2016 [7] for the Erlotinib Prevention of Oral Cancer (EPOC) study. Erlotinib is an inhibitor of epidermal growth factor receptor (EGFR) tyrosine kinase, therefore inhibiting the action of EGFR upon binding. As discussed previously, overexpression of EGFR has been demonstrated in many head and neck squamous cell carcinomas, and EGFR amplification is associated with oral premalignant lesion transformation to invasive cancer. The investigators chose to select subjects at high risk of oral premalignant lesion transformation to invasive cancer based on specific loss of heterozygosity (LOH) patterns associated with increased risk of such transformation [7, 36]. Rather than selecting clinical and/or histologic regression of the lesions as the primary endpoint, the authors chose to focus on cancer-free survival. While the trial did not yield an improvement in cancer-free survival in subjects treated with erlotinib, this study is notable for being the first chemoprevention trial to prospectively validate LOH as a molecular marker for oral premalignant lesion progression to malignant disease [6, 7].

While much focus has been placed on the genomic sequencing and molecular profiling of head and neck invasive squamous cell carcinoma, less of this attention has been placed on the identification of molecular profiles of oral premalignant lesions. Identifying such profiles serially from premalignancy to invasive carcinoma would aid in the development of predictive molecular markers and targeted therapies [37]. Possible molecular pathways that may warrant further study include Notch-1 (second-most commonly mutated gene in head and neck SCC), Stat-3 (found to be a constitutively activated oncogenic transcription factor in head and neck SCC), chemokine receptor 7 (CCR7, upregulated expression associated with tumor cell survival), nuclear factor-kappa B (NF-κB), and cyclooxygenase-2 (COX-2) [37].

2.5 Conclusions

Despite the identification of several agents that may prevent the development of oral squamous cell carcinoma via in vitro, animal, and epidemiological studies, evidence of the clinical effectiveness of these agents remains limited, and more high-quality, long-term randomized clinical trials are necessary [38]. Several factors make the clinical study of chemoprevention agents difficult, including toxicity of therapy, limited bioavailability of agents, and still-unknown molecular basis of the disease and its progression to invasive cancer.

The recurrence of oral premalignant lesions with discontinuation of the chemoprevention agent (as seen with green tea extract and retinoids) suggests a transitory prevention benefit of such agents. Thus, long-term chemoprevention might be necessary in order to prevent progression to invasive cancer. In order for patients to tolerate such long-term therapy, the ideal agent should have low systemic toxicity with minimal side effects. Many of the chemoprevention agents discussed in this article present with evidence of potential harm with prolonged use at high doses (see Table 2.1). Reducing the systemic dose of the agent (as with isotretinoin) seems ineffective in preventing disease.

Topical therapy may be a strategy to avoid systemic toxicity, but this is not without its own

Table 2.1 List of chemoprevention agents discussed in this review, purported mechanism of action, clinical evidence for efficacy, and potential harm

Agent	Possible mechanism of action	Clinical evidence	Potential harm
N-acetylcysteine	• Support of body's antioxidant system via restoration of glutathione reserves [9] • Anti-inflammatory effect [9] • Suppression of EGFR [11]	• RCT in 2002 unable to demonstrate effectiveness in preventing second primary tumors in subjects previously treated for primary head and neck cancer [12]	• At high doses, can cause headache, urticaria, fever, anaphylactoid reaction [9] • Potentiates the effect of nitroglycerin [9]
Topical bleomycin	• Scission of DNA and inhibition of DNA ligase	• Systematic review demonstrated complete (40% of subjects) or partial (25% of subjects) response to treatment [2]	• With systemic administration, can cause interstitial pneumonitis and mucocutaneous toxicity • With topical administration, can cause localized erythema, erosion, and discomfort [13]
Green tea extract containing EGCG	• Regulation of apoptosis • Inhibition of VEGFR action [15, 16]	• Phase II trial in 2009 demonstrated possible partial or complete regression of oral premalignant lesions [17] • Downregulation of stromal VEGFR expression [17]	• Insomnia and gastrointestinal symptoms [17].

Table 2.1 (continued)

Agent	Possible mechanism of action	Clinical evidence	Potential harm
Curcumin	• Downregulation of NF-κB and COX-2	• Prospective cohort study in 2010 demonstrated possible antioxidant effect by increasing serum and salivary concentrations of Vitamin E and C [18]	• None reported in a 2003 review of curcumin use in human trials [39]
Retinoids	• Modulation of gene expression, apoptosis, and cell proliferation [20, 21]	• Randomized clinical trials in 1986 and 1990 demonstrate efficacy of high-dose isotretinoin in treating oral premalignant lesions and preventing second primary head and neck tumors [3, 23] • Low-dose isotretinoin has not been demonstrated to reduce rate of developing second primary tumors [24] • Possible efficacy as a topical rinse in preventing recurrence of disease [25]	• High systemic doses associated with severe skin dryness, cheilitis, hypertriglyceridemia, and conjunctivitis [3, 23] • Supplementation with Vitamin A may increase risk of mortality [26, 27]
Carotenoids	• Some carotenoids undergo conversion to retinol, providing antiproliferative effect • Antioxidant effect [4].	• Systematic review in 2015 demonstrated reduction in rate of head and neck cancer with dietary intake of carotenoids (including beta-carotene and lycopene) [4]	• Possible increase in lung cancer rate in high-risk populations taking beta-carotene [26].
NSAIDs	• COX-2 inhibition leading to anti-inflammatory effect and inhibition of prostaglandin synthesis [29]	• Metanalysis in 2017 shows possible reduction in relative risk of head and neck cancer in populations taking NSAIDs in a dose–response relationship [30] • Randomized clinical trials of topical and systemic NSAIDs unable to demonstrate a response in treating oral premalignant lesions [31, 32]	• High use of regular strength aspirin is associated with elevated risk of small-cell lung cancer [26] • Selective COX-2 inhibitors may be associated with increased risk of cardiovascular events [33]
Ligands of PPAR-γ	• Antiproliferative and proapoptotic effects • Anti-inflammatory effect via suppression of COX-2 [34]	• Retrospective cohort study in 2017 demonstrated that subjects with TZD exposure showed a reduction in the incidence of developing head and neck cancer [35]	• Abnormalities in liver function tests • Possible cardiovascular effects with glitazones • Possible increased incidence of bladder cancer [35]
Erlotinib	• Inhibitor of EGFR [7]	• Randomized clinical trial in 2016 demonstrated no improvement in cancer-free survival [7]	• Dermatologic effects, including mucositis [7]

EGFR epidermal growth factor receptor, *NSAIDs* nonsteroidal anti-inflammatory drugs, *PPAR-γ* peroxisome proliferator-activated receptor gamma, *EGCG* epigallocatechin 3-gallate, *VEGFR* vascular endothelial growth factor receptor, *NF-κB* nuclear factor-kappa B, *COX-2* cyclooxygenase-2, *TZD* thiazolidinediones challenges. Topical agents may still enter systemic circulation and cause side effects [2]. They can produce localized side effects that can limit compliance, as seen with topical bleomycin and retinoids. Selective topical application may not target additional at-risk mucosa from field cancerization [21].

Despite the difficulties in demonstrating clinical effectiveness of these agents in the chemoprevention of oral cancer, further elucidation of the molecular pathways responsible for the stepwise progression from hyperplasia to carcinoma may reveal new therapeutic targets and the specific populations that may be responsive to such treatments. With this deeper understanding of the disease, the field of chemoprevention in oral cancer may enter into an era of precision therapy.

References

1. Fotedar V, Fotedar S, Seam RK, Gupta MK. Oral cancer and chemoprevention. Int J Pharm Sci Invent. 2013;2(2):16–20.
2. Chau L, Jabra JT, Lai W, et al. Topical agents for oral cancer chemoprevention: a systematic review of the literature. Oral Oncol. 2017;67:153–9.
3. Hong WK, Lippman SM, Itri LM, et al. Prevention of second primary tumors with isotretinoin in squamous-cell carcinoma of the head and neck. N Engl J Med. 1990;323(12):795–801.
4. Leoncini E, Nedovic D, Panic N, et al. Carotenoid intake from natural sources and head and neck cancer: a systematic review and meta-analysis of epidemiological studies. Cancer Epidemiol Biomark Prev. 2015;24(7):1003–11.
5. Wilson JC, Murray LJ, Hughes CM, et al. Non-steroidal anti-inflammatory drug and aspirin use and the risk of head and neck cancer. Br J Cancer. 2013;108:1178–81.
6. Bauman JE, Grandis J. Oral cancer chemoprevention – the end of EPOC, the beginning of an epoch of molecular selection. JAMA Oncol. 2016;2(2):178–9.
7. William W, Papadimitrakopoulou V, Lee JJ, et al. Erlotinib and the risk of oral cancer: the erlotinib prevention of oral cancer (EPOC) randomized clinical trial. JAMA Oncol. 2016;2(2):209–16.
8. Bhattacharya S. Natural antimutagens: a review. Res J Med Plant. 2011;5(2):116–26.
9. Millea PJ. N-Acetylcysteine: multiple clinical applications. Am Fam Physician. 2009;80(3):265–9.
10. Lee MF, Chan CY, Hung HC, et al. N-acetylcysteine (NAC) inhibits cell growth by mediating the EGFR/Akt/HMG box-containing protein 1 (HBP1) signaling pathway in invasive oral cancer. Oral Oncol. 2013;49:129–35.
11. Temam S, Kawaguchi H, El-Naggar AK, et al. Epidermal growth factor receptor copy number alterations correlate with poor clinical outcome in patients with head and neck squamous cancer. J Clin Oncol. 2007;25(16):2164–70.
12. van Zandwijk N, Dalesio O, Pastorino U, et al. EUROSCAN, a randomized trial of vitamin A and N-acetylcysteine in patients with head and neck cancer or lung cancer. J Natl Cancer Inst. 2000;92(12):977–86.
13. Surber C, Elsner P, Farage MA. Topical applications and the mucosa. Curr Probl Dermatol. 2011;40:71–82.
14. Epstein JB, Wong FL, Millner A, Le ND. Topical bleomycin treatment of oral leukoplakia: a randomized double-blind clinical trial. Head Neck. 1994;16(6):539–44.
15. Ding Y, Yao H, Yao Y, et al. Protection of dietary polyphenols against oral cancer. Nutrients. 2013;5:2173–91.
16. Gomes de Moura CF, Noguti J, Pacheco de Jesus GP, et al. Polyphenols as chemopreventive agent in oral carcinogenesis: putative mechanisms of action using in-vitro and in-vivo test systems. Eur J Cancer Prev. 2013;22;467–72.
17. Tsao AS, Liu D, Martin J, et al. Phase II randomized, placebo-controlled trial of green tea extract in patients with high-risk oral premalignant lesions. Cancer Prev Res (Phila). 2009;2(11):931–41.
18. Rai B, Kaur J, Jacobs R, Singh J. Possible action mechanism for curcumin in pre-cancerous lesions based on serum and salivary markers of oxidative stress. J Oral Sci. 2010;52(2):251–6.
19. Patel JB, Shah FD, Joshi GM, Patel PS. Clinical significance of inflammatory mediators in the pathogenesis of oral cancer. J Can Res Ther. 2016;12:447–57.
20. Sheth SH, Johnson DE, Kensler TW, Bauman JE. Chemoprevention targets for tobacco-related head and neck cancer: past lessons and future directions. Oral Oncol. 2015;51:557–64.
21. Foy JP, Bertolus C, William W, Saintigny P. Oral premalignancy: The roles of early detection and chemoprevention otolaryngol. Clin North Am. 2013;46(4):579–97.
22. Koch HF. Biochemical treatment of precancerous oral lesions: the effectiveness of various analogues of retinoic acid. J Maxillofac Surg. 1978;6:59–63.
23. Hong WK, Endicott J, Itri LM, et al. 13-cis-retinoic acid in the treatment of oral leukoplakia. N Engl J Med. 1986;315(24):1501–5.
24. Khuri FR, Lee JJ, Lippman SM, et al. Randomized phase III trial of low-dose isotretinoin for prevention of second primary tumors in stage I and II

head and neck cancer patients. J Natl Cancer Inst. 2006;98(7):441–50.
25. Kadakia S, Badhey A, Milam M, et al. Topical oral cavity chemoprophylaxis using isotretinoin rinse: a 15-year experience. Laryngoscope. 2017;127:1595–9.
26. Potter JD. The failure of cancer chemoprevention. Carcinogenesis. 2014;35(5):974–82.
27. Bjelakovic G, Nikolova D, Gluud LL, Simonetti RG, Gluud C. Mortality in randomized trials of antioxidant supplements for primary and secondary prevention systematic review and meta-analysis. JAMA. 2007;297(8):842–57.
28. Lu R, Dan H, Wu R, et al. Lycopene: features and potential significance in the oral cancer and precancerous lesions. J Oral Pathol Med. 2011;40:361–8.
29. Lin DT, Subbaramaiah K, Shah JP, et al. Cyclooxygenase-2: a novel molecular target for the prevention and treatment of head and neck cancer. Head Neck. 2002;24:792–9.
30. Shi J, Leng W, Zhao L, et al. Nonsteroidal anti-inflammatory drugs using and risk of head and neck cancer: a dose–response meta analysis of prospective cohort studies. Oncotarget. 2017;8(58):99066–74.
31. Mushine JL, Atkinson JC, Greer RO, et al. Randomized, double-blind, placebo-controlled phase IIB trial of the cyclooxygenase inhibitor ketorolac as an oral rinse in oropharyngeal leukoplakia. Clin Cancer Res. 2004;10:1565–73.
32. Papadimitrakopoulou VA, William W, Dannenberg AJ, et al. Pilot randomized phase II study of celecoxib in oral premalignant lesions. Clin Cancer Res. 2008;14(7):2095–101.
33. Bertagnolli MM. Chemoprevention of colorectal cancer with cyclooxygenase-2 inhibitors: two steps forward, one step back. Lancet Oncol. 2007;8:439–43.
34. Burotto M, Szabo E. PPARγ in head and neck cancer prevention. Oral Oncol. 2014;50(10):924–9.
35. Govindarajan R, Siegel ER. The effect of exposure to thiazolidinediones on the development of head-and-neck cancer in patients with diabetes mellitus. Transl Res Oral Oncol. 2017;2:1–5.
36. Rosin MP, Cheng X, Poh C, et al. Use of allelic loss to predict malignant risk for low-grade oral epithelial dysplasia. Clin Cancer Res. 2000;6:357–62.
37. Bhatia A, Burtness B. Novel molecular targets for chemoprevention in malignancies of the head and neck. Cancers. 2017;9:113.
38. Lodi G, Franchini R, Warnakulasuriya S, et al. Interventions for treating oral leukoplakia to prevent oral cancer. Cochrane Database Syst Rev. 2016;7:Art. No.: CD001829.
39. Chainani-Wu N. Safety and anti-inflammatory activity of curcumin: a component of tumeric (Curcuma longa). J Alternat Compl Med. 2003;9(1):161–8.

3 Diagnostic Adjuncts for Screening and Surveillance in Head and Neck Cancer

James Murphy and Mohammed Qaisi

3.1 Introduction

Head and neck cancer is the seventh most common cancer worldwide and the incidence is increasing in the developed world largely due to the human papilloma virus (HPV) epidemic and its effect on oropharyngeal carcinoma [1]. The majority of head and neck cancers are diagnosed at a late stage which has implications for prognosis. The eighth edition of the American Joint Commission on Cancer staging for head and neck cancer factored HPV status into the staging algorithm, which would lead to downstaging of some p16-positive tumors, but despite this, a significant proportion of head and neck cancers tend to present at later stages [2]. Screening programs have been shown to be valuable in certain cancers like cervical carcinoma and colon cancer. With regards to head and neck cancer and specifically oral cancer, screening by visual exam has only been shown to be of epidemiological benefit when undertaken in high-risk populations such as in the Indian subcontinent [3]. In lower risk populations, malignant lesions detected during a non-symptom-driven exam have been shown to be diagnosed on average at a statistically significant earlier clinical and pathological stage [4]. In contradiction to this, though, the United States Preventative Services Task Force (USPSTF) currently states evidence is insufficient to assess the balance of benefits and harms of screening for oral cancer in asymptomatic adults [5]. The American Academy of Family Physicians has stated it concurs with the USPSTF recommendation [6]. The USPSTF position statement, however, does not apply to dental professionals or otolaryngologists. The American Cancer Society, American Head & Neck Society, and the American Dental Association all stress the importance of regular oral cavity examination looking for suspicious lesions without advocating for any diagnostic screening adjuncts [7, 8].

The difficulty that arises with visual examination is potentially malignant lesions can look non worrisome on clinical exam, and benign lesions can look suspicious, especially to the nontrained eye or those who infrequently see head and neck cancer. The gold standard to diagnose head and neck cancer is biopsy and histopathological evaluation. Tissue biopsy is not without its inherent issues, among which include sampling error by the clinician obtaining the biopsy and interpretive error by the pathologist [9]. Pathological interpretive error is particularly high when dysplastic lesions are being evaluated [10]. Furthermore, patients tend to resent tissue biopsy and may be a factor in late presentation of head and neck can-

J. Murphy (✉) · M. Qaisi
Division of Oral and Maxillofacial Surgery, Department of Surgery, John H. Stroger, Jr. Hospital of Cook County, Chicago, IL, USA
e-mail: james.murphy@cookcountyhhs.org; mqaisi@cookcountyhhs.org

D. Kademani (ed.), *Improving Outcomes in Oral Cancer*,
https://doi.org/10.1007/978-3-030-30094-4_3

cer for fear of having to undergo tissue biopsy. As a means of mitigating this, various diagnostic and screening adjuncts have been created to diagnose and facilitate surveillance of the head and neck cancer patient.

A diagnostic and screening adjunct needs to conform to a number of elements if it is to be considered useful and viable. The most important ones are:

- Simple to use.
- Inexpensive.
- Minimally invasive.
- Detects early disease that is likely to progress.
- High sensitivity with low false-negative results.

Unfortunately, the current gold standard of the scalpel biopsy does not meet a number of these criteria. From the physician's perspective, its accuracy is overshadowed by patients' misgivings about its invasiveness. It is hoped that the diagnostic and screening adjuncts described below may conform more to the elements of an ideal test, and that combined with a thorough clinical exam, they may be helpful in early detection and the decision making of obtaining a scalpel biopsy. These techniques will be discussed in the following sections.

3.2 Vital Staining

3.2.1 Toludine Blue

Toludine blue, also known as tolonium chloride, is a vital dye of the thiazine group which has an affinity to bind to the nucleic acids of DNA. This premise forms the logic of using it as a diagnostic and screening aid in head and neck cancer, in that it preferentially stains neoplastic cells with their comparatively high turnover rate. Unfortunately, therein lies the main disadvantage of toludine blue as it cannot reliably distinguish between inflammatory, regenerative epithelium, and exposed connective tissue, which also have high cell turnover rates. Studies show toluidine blue to have good sensitivity rates but questionable specificity rates in the detection of oral cancer and oral premalignant lesions [11, 12]. Even if it has a potential benefit as a diagnostic aid in malignant lesion detection, research data suggest it is of very questionable benefit in detecting dysplasia [13].

The application method of toluidine blue to evaluate for suspicious lesions within the oral cavity differs slightly between practitioners. The authors follow the following regimes depending on if an isolated area is being evaluated or the entire oral cavity is being assessed. With regards to when an isolated area or lesion of the oral cavity is being evaluated, the authors wipe the area gently with a moist 0.9% normal saline-soaked gauze to remove any surface debris. Acetic acid 1% is used to gently wipe the area with a cotton tip applicator for 20 s, and then 1% toluidine blue is subsequently applied with a cotton-tipped applicator for 20 s. The area is then assessed with areas of greater intensity of blue staining being regarded as more suspicious and potentially deserving of tissue biopsy. Toludine blue can also be used to evaluate the entire oral cavity. The authors' regime for this is the patient rinses with 15 ml of 0.9% normal saline for 30 s to remove debris. Following this, the patient rinses with 1% acetic acid 15 ml for 30 s and then after expectorating the patient rinses with 15 ml of 1% toluidine blue for 30 s. Finally the patient once again rinses 1% acetic acid for 30 s to remove mechanically retained stain. The oral cavity is then assessed with areas of more intense blue staining deserving of greater evaluation and consideration for tissue biopsy.

From a practical perspective, toluidine blue may be of benefit as a diagnostic adjunct when used to direct biopsy of a clinically evident suspicious lesion isolating areas of more intense staining and theoretically minimizing selection error or for monitoring for recurrent disease in altered oral mucosa tissue. Epstein et al. recommended the use of toluidine blue as a diagnostic screening adjunct in high-risk populations when used by expert providers [14]. This caveat limits its usefulness as a diagnostic screening adjunct among the majority of community-based practitioners as it is of questionable value in detecting oral premalignant disease in this population [15]. The reported ranges of sensitivity and specificity of toluidine blue in the literature is not ideal at 57–81% and 56–67%, respectively [16]. It has also been noted that toluidine blue becomes more sensitive and specific as lesion severity of dysplasia increases or in frankly malignant lesions. This is a limitation that needs to be appreciated when used as a diagnostic adjunct. Toludine blue use as an adjunct does not eliminate the need for scalpel biopsy.

3.2.2 Lugol's Iodine

Another screening adjunct is Lugol's iodine. Lugol's iodine aids in detecting suspicious lesions in nonkeratinized mucosa based on the fact that glycogen within the cell binds to the iodine component of this vital stain. Preneoplastic cells tend to be more metabolically active with a high cell turnover, thus leaving these cells with depleted glycogen stores when compared to normal tissues. Because of the depleted glycogen, these cells do not stain with the lugol's iodine and remain relatively white compared to normal tissue which stains mahogany brown.

Lugol's iodine has been shown to be useful as an intraoperative guide in determining where to resect head and neck malignant and dysplastic lesions [17] (Fig. 3.1a, b). In that study by McMahon et al., the rate of carcinoma, carcinoma in situ (CIS), or dysplasia present at margins was 32% following resection with a 1 cm margin based solely on visual clues. When lugol's iodine was used to guide the resection margins, the rate of dysplasia or CIS at the margin dropped to 4%. In addition to aiding with margins, lugol's iodine may be helpful as a screening adjunct in the identification and diagnosis of oral malignant and premalignant lesions [18]. In a comparative study, the sensitivity/specificity of toluidine blue was 0.93/0.63 compared to 0.88/0.84 with lugol's iodine [19]. This higher specificity of lugol's iodine is a noteworthy finding.

Like toludine blue, there is practitioner variation in the application of lugol's iodone. The authors' protocol involves rinsing the oral cavity with 0.9% normal saline for 30 s. Cotton-tipped applicators are then used to apply 1% lugol's iodine to individual nonkeratinized anatomic subunits of the oral cavity. Multiple passes of lugol's iodine-soaked cotton-tipped applicators are generally used on an individual anatomic subunit. Following application of the lugol's iodine, suction is used to remove any excess pooled lugol's iodine. The anatomic subunit is then evaluated. A mahogany brown color is considered nonsuspicious but an off-white area should be viewed with suspicion and consideration given to tissue biopsy.

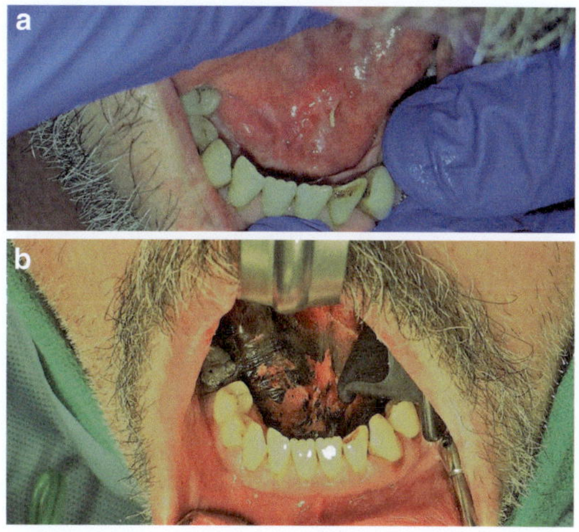

Fig. 3.1 (**a**) Lesion floor of mouth before lugols application. (**b**) Lesion floor of mouth after lugols application

Lugol's iodine is relatively inexpensive and easy to use and may be considered as a diagnostic adjunct in conjunction with a thorough exam for screening and surveillance of head and neck cancer. Like toluidine blue, lugol's iodine does not replace a thorough clinical exam or the need for a scalpel biopsy for clinically suspicious lesions.

3.3 Visual Light-Based Adjuncts

3.3.1 Chemiluminescence

ViziLite® is the most well-known within this category, although it now comes as ViziLite Plus® which requires its use in combination with toluidine blue. Microlux DL® is another example, although it is not well researched in the peer-reviewed literature.

The method to use chemiluminescene in the evaluation of the oral cavity for suspicious lesions is as follows: The oral cavity is rinsed with 1% acetic acid for 1 min to remove surface glycoprotein and cause cellular dehydration which facilitates exposure of the cellular elements to the luminescence. Upon completion of the prerinse, the chemiluminescent blue-white light in the spectral wavelength of 490–510 nm is applied to evaluate the tissues. The blue-white light is generated either via an interaction between acetylsalicylic acid and hydrogen peroxide (ViziLite Plus®) or by a battery-powered light-emitting diode (Microlux DL®) (Fig. 3.2a, b). Upon examination of the oral mucosa in a darkened room using manufacturer specific eyewear, normal epithelium appears light blue, whereas abnormal epithelium appears white. Toludine blue is then applied to the lesion that appears abnormal with the ViziLite Plus® system.

Unfortunately, the sensitivity and specificity of chemiluminescence is relatively poor with a lack of good evidence to support the use of this adjunct in screening and surveillance of head and neck cancer at present [20, 21]. Mehrotra et al. noted 102 innocuous clinically evident lesions on conventional oral exam. These lesions were then examined with ViziLite following which the lesions were biopsied. Histopathological examination revealed three dysplasias and one malignancy, none of which were identified with the ViziLite [22]. Chemiluminescence appears to be better at detecting and evaluating suspicious white lesions as opposed to red lesions [23]. For many, chemiluminescence is currently not a beneficial diagnostic adjunct [24].

3.3.2 Tissue Fluorescence Imaging

The ideology behind this diagnostic adjunct is that abnormal tissues of the oral cavity have an altered structure (e.g., hyperkeratosis, hyperchromatin, increased cellular/nuclear pleomorphism), altered metabolism, and potentially changes in the subepithelial stroma which subsequently alter the interaction of the tissue with light compared to normal oral mucosal tissues. Various systems are on the market including VELscope®, Sapphire Plus®, Identafi®, Bio/Screen®, DOE SE Kit®, OralID®, and ViziLite PRO®, with VELscope® being the most studied [25] (Fig. 3.3a, b).

The process to use tissue fluorescence imaging to detect suspicious lesions of the oral cavity involves the application of an intense blue light in the wavelength of 390–460 nm and viewing the effect on tissue through the device viewer or special eyewear to create a narrow band filter. Normal oral mucosa appears pale green using this technique, but abnormal tissues appear dark due to a loss of fluorescence. The phenomenon of diascopic fluorescence has been described with this modality [26]. Tissues with loss of fluorescence but which completely blanch on the application of pressure and return to normal fluorescence pattern should be considered negative

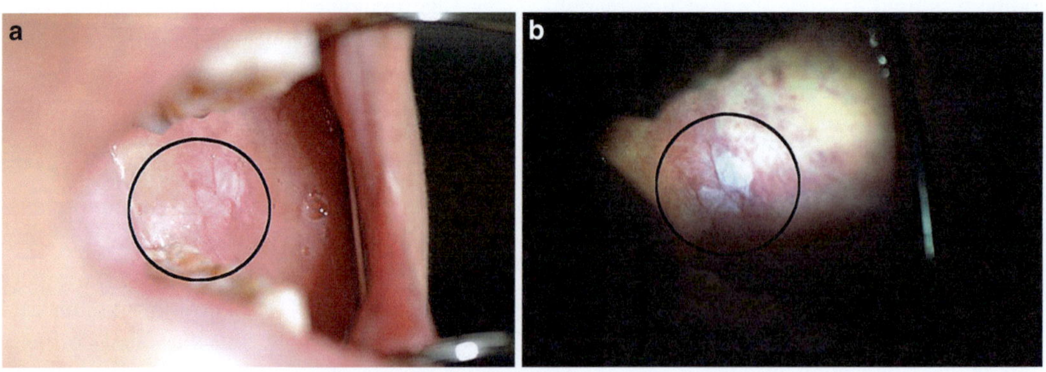

Fig. 3.2 (**a**) Clinical suspicious lesion before Microlux Dx use. (**b**) Microlux Dx highlighting suspicious lesion. (Courtesy of Addent Inc.)

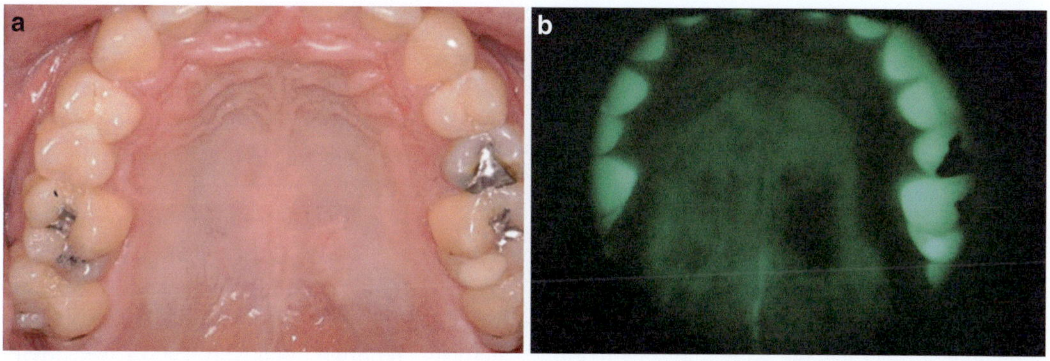

Fig. 3.3 (**a**) Clinical photo of palate with possible suspicious lesion. (**b**) VELscope highlighting suspicious lesion of palate. (Courtesy of LED Dental)

for loss of fluorescence. Therefore, a degree of experience and interpretive acumen is necessary in utilizing this diagnostic and screening adjunct.

Tissue fluorescence imaging has been shown in a retrospective case–control observational study to significantly reduce the rate of local recurrence when used as an intraoperative surgical aid to determine resection margins for high-grade dysplastic lesions and early-stage oral squamous cell carcinoma [27]. Encouraging data are present in the literature with regard to using this technique in screening and surveillance of oral cancer; however, it is limited by false-positive results [11, 28, 29]. More worrisome than the false positives with this diagnostic adjunct is the fact that keratin is autofluorescent which has implications that potentially malignant and frankly malignant lesions may be missed in hyperkeratotic tissues such as proliferative verrucous leukoplakia [30]. The importance of subjective interpretation and the recognition that it is a diagnostic adjunct to be used in combination with a thorough clinical oral exam cannot be overstated.

3.4 Exfoliative-Based Techniques

3.4.1 Brush Biopsy

The screening of cervical cancer with the Pap Smear test, a brush biopsy-based cytology screening technique, is routinely heralded as the champion screening test for malignancy. The principle behind this screening method has been adapted for the oral cavity to obtain transepithelial tissue samples using a specialized brush which is subsequently analyzed for cytomorphological abnormalities. Early following the introduction of this diagnostic adjunct, there were multiple peer-reviewed articles extolling its virtue. Among its fanfare introduction, it even featured on the cover of the Journal of the American Dental Association in October 1999. In the accompanying article, Sciubba reported a 100% sensitivity and specificity with this diagnostic adjunct following a multicenter trial [31]. The titles of letters to the Editor of the Journal of the American Dental Association in 2002 responding to negative criticism of the technique included "Brush Biopsy 'Saves Lives,'' "Brush Biopsy 'Bridges the Gap,'' and "Overwhelmingly Positive" [32–34]. Unfortunately, the initial hype masked a significant flaw that permeated early studies looking at this adjunct, in that a scalpel biopsy was only performed on those with an abnormal or positive result. Therefore, confidence in the negative predictive value of this adjunct is compromised. Currently it is believed the sensitivities and specificities vary between 71–100% and 27–100%, respectively, for this diagnostic adjunct [35].

The OralCDx Brush Test® system obtains a full transepithelial specimen sample using a sampling brush. The harvested specimen can be scanned and analyzed microscopically by means of a computer-based imaging system, OraScan®, to get one of the following results—"negative or benign", "positive", or "atypical". The test has also been adapted for the evaluation of laryngo-pharyngeal lesions based on the same principles (EndoCDx LP—Laryngeal®). Abnormal or positive results should undergo scalpel biopsy and histopathological evaluation.

When properly performed, this diagnostic and screening adjunct has the potential to be helpful and accurate. Research experience and results suggest that the technique is good at diagnosing clinically suspicious lesions correctly which will ultimately need a scalpel biopsy, but the fact the majority of studies do not take scalpel biopsy of samples taken from questionable sites or sites of low clinical suspicion, for which this technique should be primarily used for, means an element of doubt over the true usefulness of this product remains. The encouraging results for brush biopsy in a recent meta-analysis from the Cochrane Collaboration cannot fully allay this concern [36]. The technique may have usefulness but further rigorous study with comparison to the gold standard of scalpel biopsy and histopathological examination from more innocuous lesions needs to be performed and reported before fully embracing this technique as a diagnostic and screening adjunct.

3.4.2 DNA-Image Cytometry

Like OralCDx Brush Test®, DNA-image cytometry is a computer-assisted analysis of exfoliative cells. DNA-image cytometry has been proposed as a diagnostic adjunct capable of very early detection of malignant transformation of squamous epithelial cells. The method behind this involves the assessment of exfoliative cells for chromosomal DNA-aneuploidy, an abnormal nuclear DNA finding. It is theorized that the finding of DNA-aneuploidy is a sensitive and effective method of detecting very early malignant transformation within head and neck epithelium before cytology and histopathology can detect any such changes [37]. A brush biopsy specimen is obtained, but unlike the previously discussed cytological evaluation of the sample with the aid of Papanicolaou staining, Feulgen staining is used for DNA-image cytometry. The assessment of the stained specimen with 566 nm monochromatic light allows an analysis of DNA-aneuploidy of the specimen. The findings of the test may document DNA-diploidy, DNA-polyploidy, or DNA-aneuploidy, with DNA-aneuploidy needing further evaluation and workup. A recent meta-analysis reported relatively good sensitivity (89%) and specificity (99%) along with an impressive diagnostic odds ratio of 446, but the fact only five DNA-image cytometry studies met the inclusion criteria of the meta-analysis cannot be ignored [38]. Therefore, even though the ideology behind this technique makes logical sense, it is understudied at present to be recommended as a reliable diagnostic and screening adjunct for head and neck cancer.

3.5 Molecular Biology

Advancements in molecular biology and data from the Human Genome Project and Cancer Genome Atlas open the possibility of diagnosis and screening for head and neck cancer with the application of this knowledge. Saliva is seen as a readily available source from which to obtain samples which can be tested for potential biomarkers for oral malignant and premalignant conditions. Potential biomarkers include but are not limited to proteinaceous material, DNA, messenger RNA, microRNA, long noncoding RNA, nonorganic compounds, and metabolites. To date, over 100 potential biomarkers have been reported in the literature that may be useful in detecting oral/oropharyngeal malignant and premalignant conditions [39]. Unfortunately a lack of standardization with regards to collection, storage, and processing of samples as well as the natural variability of potential salivary biomarkers between subjects with oral/oropharyngeal malignant and premalignant conditions compared to those without, together with a lack of validity of this method mean that at present salivary biomarkers remain a focus of research interest without any evidence to support clinical application [40]. Screening of head and neck cancer has been performed on exfoliated cells and biopsy samples using molecular biology techniques analyzing them for loss of heterozygosity at various chromosome locations using microsatellite markers [41]. Unfortunately despite some promising candidate biomarkers being identified, this method at present is not clinically useful as a diagnostic or screening adjunct in head and neck cancer.

3.6 In Vivo Microscopy

This modality, which is a potential diagnostic and screening adjunct for head and neck cancer, is currently undergoing scientific investigation. It incorporates some of the features of existing adjuncts with high-resolution microscopic imaging. Issues with the various modalities within this potential group of adjuncts include minimal data in the peer-reviewed literature and expense. Examples include multimodal imaging, optical coherence tomography, reflectance confocal microscopy, and multiphoton microscopy [42]. Multimodal imaging, reflectance confocal microscopy, and multiphoton microscopy make use out of fluorescence in order to highlight and evaluate areas/cells of interest. Optical coherence tomography is a technique in clinical use in ophthalmology [43]. The technique may have value in looking at epithelial architecture changes such as epithelial thickness, basement membrane continuity, and rete ridge arrangement that may be used to detect abnormalities suggestive of dysplasia and/or carcinoma. No in vivo microscopy technique is currently in clinical use as a diagnostic and screening adjunct for head and neck cancer, but they are the source of intense research interest.

3.7 Putting It All Together

In October 2017, the Journal of the American Dental Association once again featured a cover story on evaluating potentially malignant disorders of the oral cavity. The accompanying article presented one good practice statement and six clinical recommendations formulated by an expert panel convened by the American Dental Association Council on Scientific Affairs and the Center for Evidence-Based Dentistry [44]. The panel's good practice statement advocated that clinicians should obtain an updated medical, social, and dental history and perform an intraoral and extraoral conventional visual clinical exam in all adult patients. The synopsis of the clinical recommendations is that no available diagnostic adjuncts demonstrated sufficient diagnostic test accuracy to support their use in evaluating oral cavity lesions. The panel did state that in the exceptional circumstance of a patient refusing a scalpel biopsy or in cases where geographical limitations hinder access to care, cytological testing may be used to initiate the diagnostic process until a biopsy can be performed. A flow chart presented by the American Dental Association Council on Scientific Affairs and the Center for Evidence-Based Dentistry, which can be used as a guideline, of how best to incorporate the panel's good practice statement and clinical recommendations in the evaluation of the patient with a potentially malignant condition of the oral cavity (Fig. 3.4).

Similarly the American Head & Neck Society position statement on early detection of premalignant oral cancer states that the gold standard for detecting potentially premalignant lesions is a thorough examination combined with biopsy where needed [45]. Their conclusion with regards to the different screening adjuncts discussed in this chapter is that they have not yet become widely adopted as part of the existing standard of care, and they may warrant additional consideration in the future.

The authors' thoughts are consistent in that there is no substitute for a good oral head and neck exam; however, if screening adjuncts help or motivate dental providers to examine patients, then they may be utilized. Caution has to be taken when interpreting the results of these diagnostic adjuncts due to the limitations discussed and with the understanding that an exam and biopsy super-

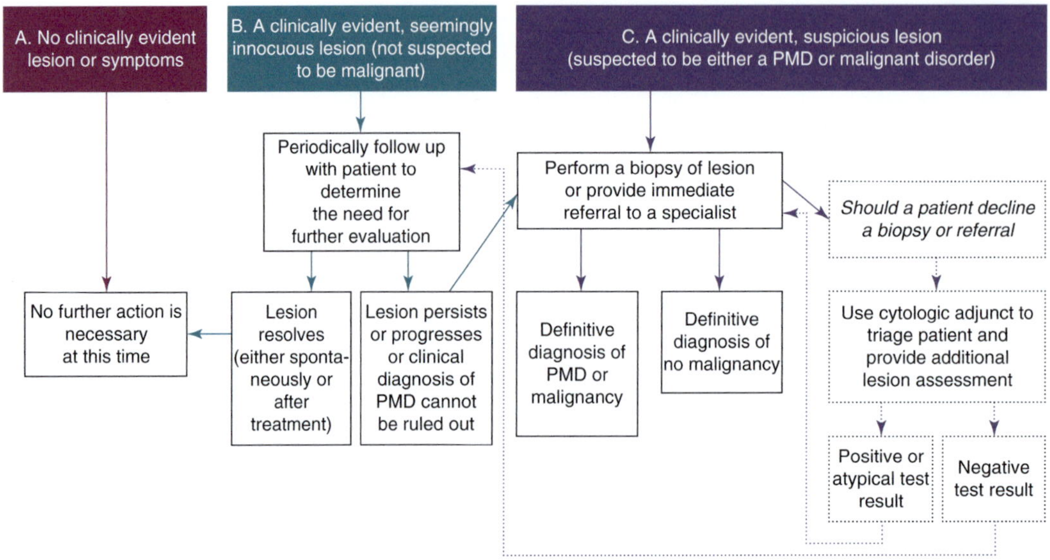

Fig. 3.4 American Dental Association Council on Scientific Affairs and the Center for Evidence-Based Dentistry flow chart

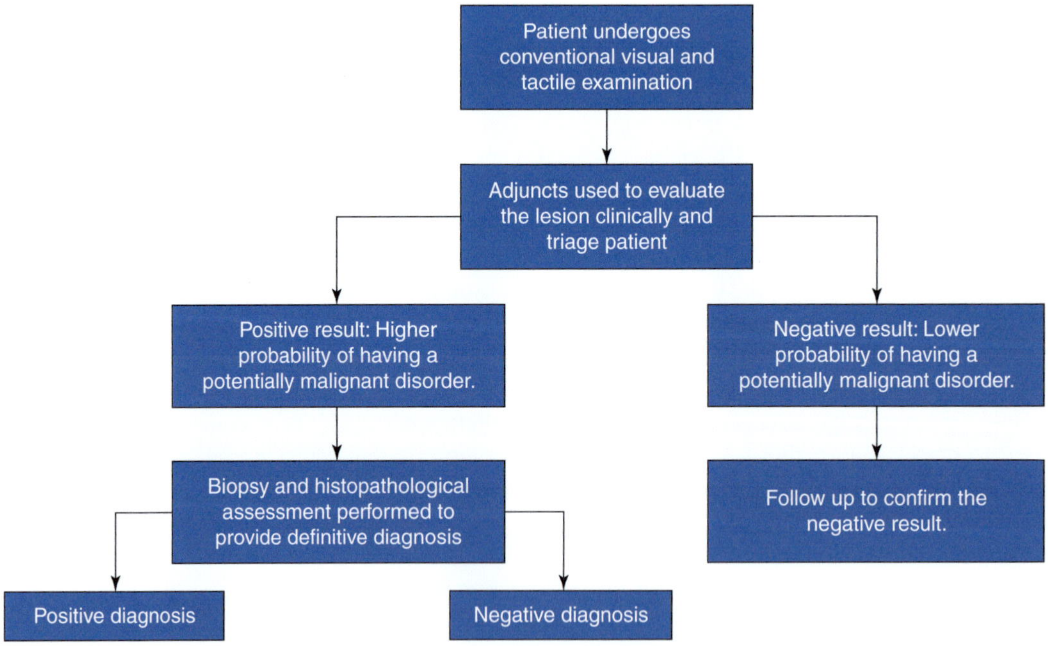

Fig. 3.5 Algorithm for the Incorporation of Diagnostic Adjuncts into Clinical Practice

sede diagnostic adjuncts. A suggestive algorithm for the incorporation of diagnostic adjuncts is shown in Fig. 3.5. It is important to understand the risk of false negatives with any diagnostic adjunct being used, and if any doubt exists regarding a suspicious oral lesion, an incisional biopsy with histopathological examination is the current standard of care.

3.8 Conclusion

To the head and neck surgeon, the potential utility of a reliable, valid, and accurate diagnostic and screening adjunct for the head and neck cancer patient is clear. Current adjuncts suffer from suboptimal sensitivity, poor negative predictive values, expense, and lack of quality supportive research in the peer-reviewed literature corroborating manufacturer or marketing claims to allow them to receive a strong recommendation. Some have merits, but unanswered questions remain that need elucidating before they can be advocated for. At present a thorough head and neck history and examination by a competent, experienced physician/dentist with selective scalpel biopsy of suspicious lesions is the best method we have for diagnosing and screening of head and neck cancer.

Acknowledgement The authors have no conflict of interest to declare.

References

1. WHO. World cancer report 2014. Geneva: World Health Organization; 2014.
2. AJCC. AJCC cancer staging manual. 8th ed. New York, NY: Springer; 2016.
3. Sankaranarayanan R, Ramadas K, Thomas G, Muwonge R, Thara S, Mathew B, Rajan B, Trivandrum Oral Cancer Screening Study Group. Effects of screening on oral cancer mortality in Kerala, India: a cluster randomized controlled trial. Lancet. 2005;365:1927–33.
4. Holmes JD, Dierks EJ, Homer LD, Potter BE. Is detection of oral and oropharyngeal squamous cell cancer by a dental care provider associated with a lower stage at diagnosis. J Oral Maxillofac Surg. 2003;61:285–91.
5. https://www.uspreventiveservicestaskforce.org/Page/Document/RecommendationStatementFinal/oral-cancer-screening1.
6. https://www.aafp.org/patient-care/clinical-recommendations/all/oral-cancer.html.
7. American Cancer Society. American Cancer Society guidelines for the early detection of cancer. Atlanta, GA: American Cancer Society; 2013. Accessed at http://www.cancer.org/healthy/findcancerearly/cancerscreeningguidelines/american-cancer-society-guidelines-for-the-early-detection-of-cancer.
8. Rethman MP, Carpenter W, Cohen EE, Epstein J, Evans CA, Flaitz CM, et al. Evidence-based clinical recommendations regarding screening for oral squamous cell carcinomas. J Am Dent Assoc. 2010;141(5):509–20.
9. Lee JJ, Hung HC, Cheng SJ, Chiang CP, Liu BY, Yu CH, Jeng JH, Chang HH, Kok SH. Factors associated with underdiagnosis from incisional biopsy of oral leukoplakic lesions. Oral Surg Oral Med Oral Pathol Oral Radiol Endod. 2007;104:217–25.
10. Abbey LM, Kaugars GE, Gunsolley JC, Burns JC, Page DG, Svirsky JA, Eisenberg E, Krutchkoff DJ, Cushing M. Intraexaminer and interexaminer reliability in the diagnosis of oral epithelial dysplasia. Oral Surg Oral Med Oral Pathol Oral Radiol Endod. 1995;80:188–91.
11. Rosenberg D, Cretin S. Use of meta-analysis to evaluate tolonium chloride in oral cancer screening. Oral Surg Oral Med Oral Pathol. 1989;67:621–7.
12. Warnakulasuriya KA, Johnson NW. Sensitivity and specificity of Orascan® toluidine blue mouthrinse in the detection of oral cancer and precancer. J Oral Pathol Med. 1996;25:97–103.
13. Onofre MA, Sposto MR, Navarro CM. Reliability of toluidine blue application in the detection of oral epithelial dysplasia and in situ and invasive squamous cell carcinomas. Oral Surg Oral Med Oral Pathol Oral Radiol Endod. 2001;91:535–40.
14. Epstein JB, Güneri P. The adjunctive role of toluidine blue in detection of oral premalignant and malignant lesions. Curr Opin Otolaryngol Head Neck Surg. 2009;17:79–87.
15. Awan K, Yang Y, Morgan P, Warnakulasuriya S. Utility of toluidine blue as a diagnostic adjunct in the detection of potentially malignant disorders of the oral cavity—a clinical and histological assessment. Oral Dis. 2012;18:728–33.
16. Awadallah M, Idle M, Patel K, Kademani D. Management update of potentially premalignant oral epithelial lesions. Oral Surg Oral Med Oral Pathol Oral Radiol. 2018;125:628–36.
17. McMahon J, Devine JC, McCaul JA, McLellan DR, Farrow A. Use of Lugol's iodine in the resection of oral and oropharyngeal squamous cell carcinoma. Br J Oral Maxillofac Surg. 2010;48:84–7.
18. Petruzzi M, Lucchese A, Baldoni E, Grassi FR, Serpico R. Use of Lugol's iodine in oral cancer diagnosis: an overview. Oral Oncol. 2010;46:811–3.
19. Epstein JB, Scully C, Spinelli J. Toluidine blue and Lugol's iodine application in the assessment of oral malignant disease and lesions at risk of malignancy. J Oral Pathol Med. 1992;21:160–3.
20. Rashid A, Warnakulasuriya S. The use of light-based (optical) detection systems as adjuncts in the detection of oral cancer and oral potentially malignant disorders: a systematic review. J Oral Pathol Med. 2015;44:307–28.
21. Lingen MW, Kalmar JR, Karrison T, Speight PM. Critical evaluation of diagnostic aids for the detection of oral cancer. Oral Oncol. 2008;44:10–22.
22. Mehrotra R, Singh M, Thomas S, Nair P, Pandya S, Nigam NS, Shukla P. A cross-sectional study evalu-

ating chemiluminescence and autofluorescence in the detection of clinically innocuous precancerous and cancerous oral lesions. J Am Dent Assoc. 2010;141:151–6.

23. Epstein JB, Gorsky M, Lonky S, Silverman S Jr, Epstein JD, Bride M. The efficacy of oral lumenoscopy (ViziLite) in visualizing oral mucosal lesions. Spec Care Dentist. 2006;26:171–4.
24. Oh ES, Laskin DM. Efficacy of the ViziLite system in the identification of oral lesions. J Oral Maxillofac Surg. 2007;65:424–6.
25. Huber MA. Adjunctive diagnostic techniques for oral and oropharyngeal cancer discovery. Dent Clin N Am. 2018;62:59–75.
26. Bhatia N, Matias MAT, Farah CS. Assessment of a decision making protocol to improve the efficacy of VELscope™ in general dental practice: a prospective evaluation. Oral Oncol. 2014;50:1012–9.
27. Poh CF, Anderson DW, Durham JS, Chen J, Berean KW, MacAulay CE, Rosin MP. Fluorescence visualization-guided surgery for early-stage oral cancer. JAMA Otolaryngol Head Neck Surg. 2016;142:209–16.
28. Leston JS, Dios PD. Diagnostic clinical aids in oral cancer. Oral Oncol. 2010;46:418–22.
29. Awan KH, Morgan PR, Warnakulasuriya S. Evaluation of an autofluorescence based imaging system (VELscope™) in the detection of oral potentially malignant disorders and benign keratoses. Oral Oncol. 2011;47:274–7.
30. Pavlova I, Williams M, El-Naggar A, Richards-Kortum R, Gillenwater A. Understanding the biological basis of autofluorescence imaging for oral cancer detection: high-resolution fluorescence microscopy in viable tissue. Clin Cancer Res. 2008;14:2396–404.
31. Sciubba JJ. Improving detection of precancerous and cancerous oral lesions. Computer-assisted analysis of the oral brush biopsy US Collaborative OralCDx Study Group. J Am Dent Assoc. 1999;130:1445–57.
32. Eisen D. Brush biopsy 'saves lives'. J Am Dent Assoc. 2002;133:688.
33. Sciubba JJ. Brush biopsy 'bridges the gap'. J Am Dent Assoc. 2002;133:692.
34. Farran H. Overwhelmingly positive. J Am Dent Assoc. 2002;133:692.
35. Patton LL, Epstein JB, Kerr AR. Adjunctive techniques for oral cancer examination and lesion diagnosis. A systematic review of the literature. JADA. 2008;139:896–905.
36. Macey R, Walsh T, Brocklehurst P, Kerr AR, Liu JL, Lingen MW, Ogden GR, Warnakulasuriya S, Scully C. Diagnostic tests for oral cancer and potentially malignant disorders in patients presenting with clinically evident lesions. Cochrane Database Syst Rev. 2015;5:CD010276.
37. Kämmerer PW, Koch FP, Santoro M, Babaryka G, Biesterfeld S, Brieger J, Kunkel M. Prospective, blinded comparison of cytology and DNA-image cytometry of brush biopsies for early detection of oral malignancy. Oral Oncol. 2013;49:420–6.
38. Ye X, Zhang J, Tan Y, Chen G, Zhou G. Meta-analysis of two computer-assisted screening methods for diagnosing oral precancer and cancer. Oral Oncol. 2015;51:966–75.
39. Cheng YS, Rees T, Wright J. A review of research on salivary biomarkers for oral cancer detection. Clin Transl Med. 2014;3:3.
40. Kaur J, Jacobs R, Huang Y, Salvo N, Politis C. Salivary biomarkers for oral cancer and pre-cancer screening: a review. Clin Oral Investig. 2018;22:633–40.
41. Graveland AP, Bremmer JF, de Maaker M, Brink A, Cobussen P, Zwart M, Braakhuis BJ, Bloemena E, van der Waal I, Leemans CR, Brakenhoff RH. Molecular screening of oral precancer. Oral Oncol. 2013;49:1129–35.
42. Yang EC, Tan MT, Schwarz RA, Richards-Kortum RR, Gillenwater AM, Vigneswaran N. Noninvasive diagnostic adjuncts for the evaluation of potentially premalignant oral epithelial lesions: current limitations and future directions. Oral Surg Oral Med Oral Pathol Oral Radiol. 2018;125:670–81.
43. Adhi M, Duker JS. Optical coherence tomography – current and future applications. Curr Opin Ophthalmol. 2013;24:213–21.
44. Lingen MW, Abt E, Agrawal N, Chaturvedi AK, Cohen E, D'Souza G, Gurenlian J, Kalmar JR, Kerr AR, Lambert PM, Patton LL, Sollecito TP, Truelove E, Tampi MP, Urquhart O, Banfield L, Carrasco-Labra A. Evidence-based clinical practice guideline for the evaluation of potentially malignant disorders in the oral cavity: a report of the American Dental Association. J Am Dent Assoc. 2017;148:712–27.
45. https://www.ahns.info/wp-content/uploads/2017/05/Early-Detection-of-Pre-Malignant-Oral-Cancer-FINAL.pdf.

4 Current Updates in Staging and Prognosis in Oral Cancer

Paul Covello and D. David Kim

4.1 Introduction

Cancer staging helps define tumor burden, predict prognosis, direct treatment, evaluate outcomes, and guide research initiatives. Ultimately, the system is used to improve provider-to-patient and provider-to-provider communication. Oral squamous cell carcinoma (OSCC) has been reliably staged using the TNM system, which has been developed and maintained by the American Joint Committee on Cancer (AJCC) and the Union for International Cancer Control (UICC). In this update, data supporting the recent changes to the eighth edition of the AJCC staging system for OSCC, as well as other important prognostic considerations, will be presented.

P. Covello
Department of Oral and Maxillofacial Surgery, Geisinger Health, Wilkes-Barre, PA, USA

Division of Head and Neck Surgical Oncology and Microvascular Reconstruction, Department of Oral and Maxillofacial Surgery, Louisiana State University Health Sciences Center, Shreveport, LA, USA
e-mail: pcovello@geisinger.edu

D. D. Kim (✉)
Division of Head and Neck Surgical Oncology and Microvascular Reconstruction, Department of Oral and Maxillofacial Surgery, Louisiana State University Health Sciences Center, Shreveport, LA, USA
e-mail: DKim1@lsuhsc.edu

4.2 Changes to the American Joint Committee on Cancer (AJCC) Staging System

The TNM cancer classification system was developed in the 1940s by Pierre Denoix. Under his leadership, the Union for International Cancer Control (UICC) established the Committee on Clinical Stage Classification, which continued to develop the system. Since its foundation in 1959, the American Joint Committee on Cancer (AJCC) has also focused on defining and standardizing cancer classification. The first cancer staging manual from the AJCC was released in 1977. In 1987, the UICC and AJCC unified their TNM classification systems. Revisions are made every 6–8 years to accommodate advances in cancer research. In 2017, the eighth edition of the Cancer Staging Manual by the AJCC was released.

In the latest edition, depth of invasion (DOI) and extranodal extension (ENE) are used to further define staging categories. Essentially, the T stage increases by one for every 5 mm of tumor DOI until ≥10 mm, and the pathologic N stage increases by one with ENE. Of note, infiltration of tumor cells into the extrinsic tongue muscles is no longer used as a criterion for T4 staging, as DOI supersedes it. A comparison of the AJCC 7 and AJCC 8 TNM staging systems for OSCC is detailed in Table 4.1 [1]. Case examples are provided in Fig. 4.1.

D. Kademani (ed.), *Improving Outcomes in Oral Cancer*,
https://doi.org/10.1007/978-3-030-30094-4_4

Table 4.1 The TNM staging system for oral squamous cell carcinoma, as described by the seventh and eighth editions of the AJCC cancer staging manual

T category	AJCC 7 criteria	AJCC 8 criteria
TX	Primary cannot be assessed.	
T0	Primary tumor cannot be assessed	N/A
Tis	Carcinoma in situ	
T1	Size ≤2 cm	Size ≤2 cm *with DOI ≤ 5 mm*
T2	Size >2–4 cm	*Size < 2 cm with DOI 5–10 mm or* Size >2–4 cm *with DOI ≤ 10 mm*
T3	Size >4 cm	Size >4 cm *or DOI > 10 mm*
T4a	Lip: Tumor invades through cortical bone, inferior alveolar nerve, floor of mouth, or skin of face	
	Oral Cavity: Tumor invades *through* cortical bone of maxilla or mandible, *into deep muscle of tongue (genioglossus, hyoglossus, palatoglossus,* or *styloglossus),* maxillary sinus, or skin of the face	Oral Cavity: Tumor invades *through* cortical bone of maxilla or mandible, maxillary sinus, or skin of the face.
T4b	Invasion of masticator space, pterygoid plates, skull base, and/or encases the internal carotid artery.	

N category	AJCC 7 criteria	AJCC 8 clinical criteria	AJCC 8 pathological criteria
NX	Regional lymph nodes cannot be assessed		
N0	No regional lymph node metastasis		
N1	Single, ipsilateral ≤3 cm	Single, ipsilateral ≤3 cm *with ENE(−)*	
N2a	Single, ipsilateral >3 to ≤6 cm	Single, ipsilateral >3 - ≤6 cm *with ENE(−)*	– *Single, ipsilateral ≤ 3 cm with ENE(+)* – Single, ipsilateral >3 - ≤6 cm *with ENE(−)*
N2b	Multiple, ipsilateral ≤6 cm	Multiple, ipsilateral ≤6 cm *with ENE(−)*	
N2c	Multiple, bilateral, or contralateral ≤6 cm	Multiple, bilateral, or contralateral ≤6 cm *with ENE(−)*	
N3	Any >6 cm	N/A	
N3a	N/A	Any >6 cm with ENE(−)	
N3b	N/A	Any with clinically overt ENE(+)	– Single, ipsilateral >3 cm with ENE(+) – Multiple, ipsilateral, bilateral, or contralateral any size with ENE(+)

M category	Criteria
M0	No distant metastasis
M1	Distant metastasis

Stage	T	N	M
I	T1	N0	M0
II	T2	N0	M0
III	T3 T1–3	N0 N1	M0 M0
IVA	T4a T1–4a	N0–1 N2	M0
IVB	Any T T4b	N3 Any N	M0
IVC	Any	Any	M1

4.3 Depth of Invasion

Depth of invasion (DOI) is defined as the deepest point of tumor invasion, as measured from the *basement membrane* of adjacent normal mucosa. Tumor thickness, on the other hand, is measured from the *mucosal surface* of the tumor. Thus, in exophytic lesions, thickness may be greater than DOI, and in ulcerative lesions, DOI may be greater than thickness. An example is depicted in Fig. 4.2. Clinically, DOI is estimated to the examiner's best judgment as superficial (≤5 mm), moderate (>5 to ≤10 mm), or deep (>10 mm). If uncertainty arises, the lesser depth is assigned, according to the rec-

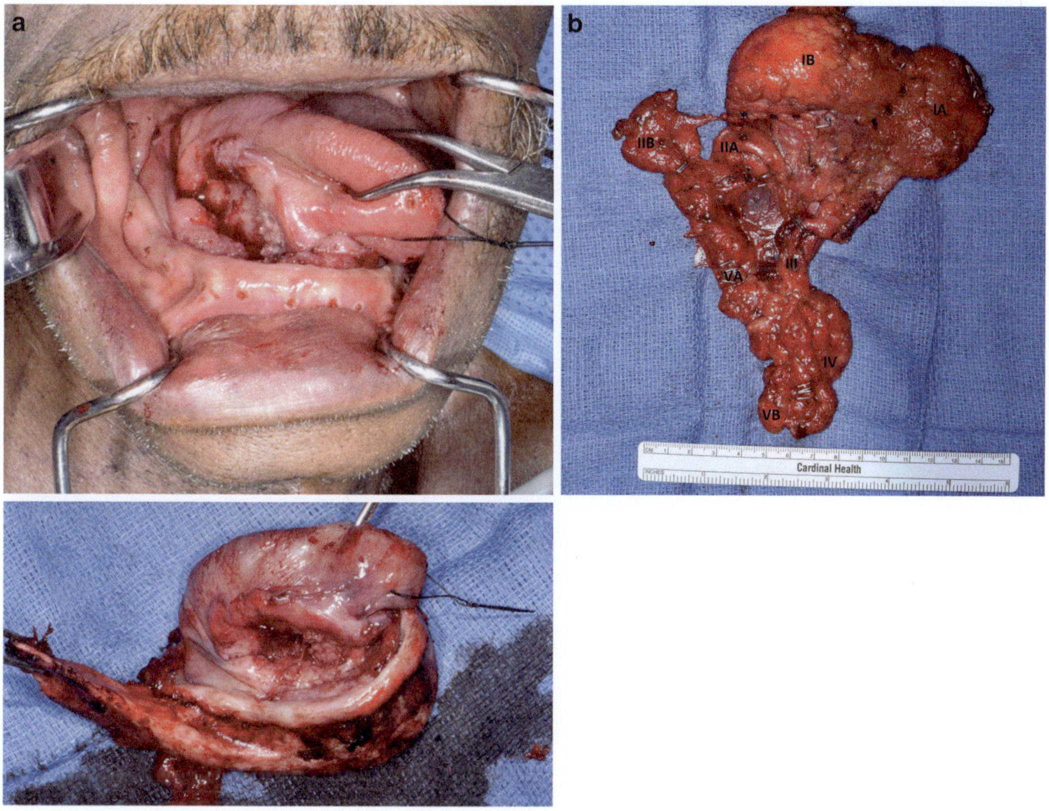

Fig. 4.1 (**a**) Case example. A 65-year-old male who presented with biopsy-proven squamous cell carcinoma of the right ventral tongue, extending into the floor of mouth without evidence of nodal disease. Final pathological evaluation demonstrated a 5.3 × 3.0 × 1.4 cm^3 moderately differentiated squamous cell carcinoma with a DOI of 15 and tumor extension into the glossus muscle, but no involvement of mandibular bone. Final pathological staging was noted to be pT4a according to the AJCC 7, but pT3 according to the AJCC 8. Difference in the T-staging system was due to the tumor extension into the extrinsic muscles of the tongue. Final staging did not alter the decision to perform adjuvant radiation therapy. (**b**) Case example. A 68-year-old female who presented with biopsy-proven squamous cell carcinoma of the right buccal mucosa with level 1B lymphadenopathy. Right neck dissection, levels I–V, depicted with 4 × 4 × 3 cm^3 lymph node indicated with dotted ink line in right level IB. 11/36 nodes found to be positive for carcinoma with evidence of ENE. Final pathological staging was noted to be pN2b according to the AJCC 7, but pN3b according to the AJCC 8. Difference in the N-staging system was due to ENE. The presence of ENE encouraged the use of adjuvant chemotherapy in addition to postoperative radiation

ommendations of the AJCC/UICC TNM staging manual [1]. Pathologically, DOI is assessed by establishing a "plumb line" from the horizon of the basement membrane of the adjacent squamous mucosa to the deepest point of tumor invasion, measured in millimeters [1].

When implemented retrospectively, incorporating DOI results in a pathologic upstaging of the T category in as many as 30% of patients, while demonstrating a significant correlation with 5-year disease-specific survival that was not noted using the former staging system [2, 3]. Due to the limited sample size attained from preoperative biopsies, exact quantitative measurements of DOI do not correlate well with those of the final postoperative specimens. However, when categorized as superficial (<4 mm) and deep (≥4 mm), sufficient agreement between pre- and postoperative samples allow for prognostication and treatment planning [4, 5]. For OSCC, a DOI of 4 mm or greater was found to be a strong pathologic predictor of local recurrence and mortality [6]. Critical primary tumor DOI in OSCC with a 20% or greater risk of occult nodal metastasis in clinical N0 disease was found to be 2 mm in the tongue, 3 mm in the floor of the mouth, and 4 mm

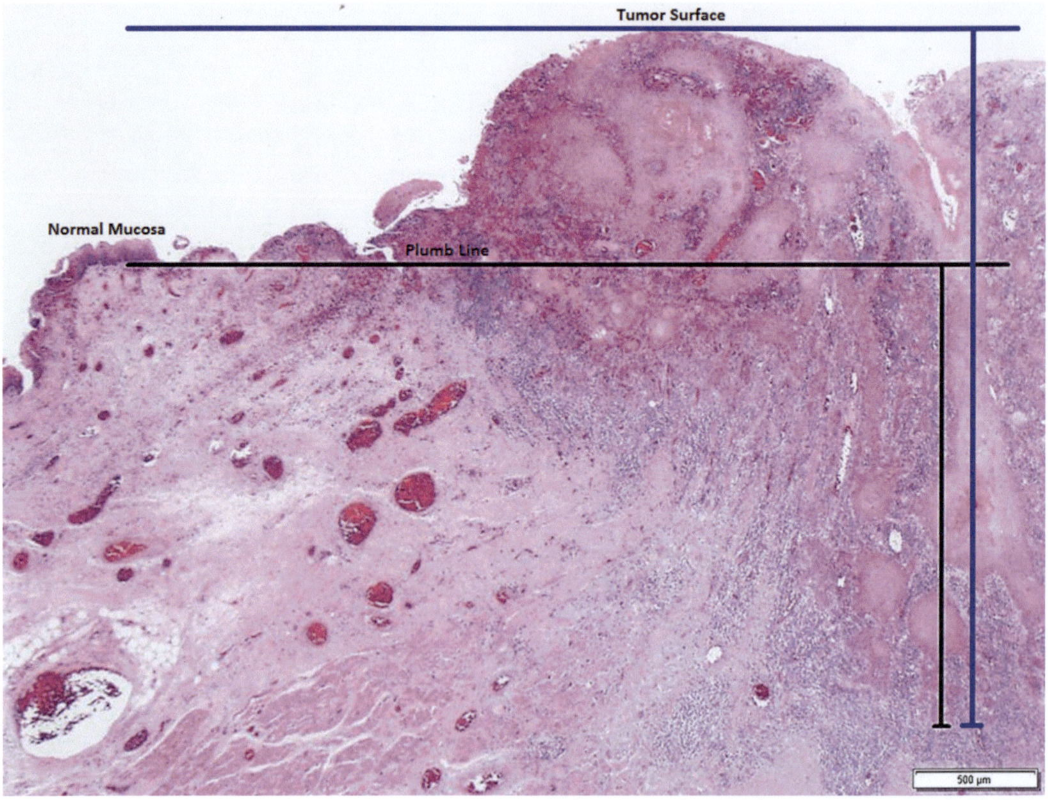

Fig. 4.2 Photomicrograph demonstrating the difference between DOI and tumor thickness in an exophytic lesion. The vertical black line depicts DOI, and the vertical blue line depicts tumor thickness. Photomicrograph by Ashley Flowers, MD, from Louisiana State University—Shreveport department of Pathology

in the retromolar trigone, alveolus, and hard palate [7]. Patients with a DOI > 4 mm have a nearly sixfold higher risk of lymph node metastasis [8]. Similarly, medullary bone invasion, but not cortical invasion alone, has been associated with poor local control, as well as decreased disease-specific and overall survival [9, 10]. Thus, erosion *through* cortical bone classifies a tumor as T4a, while superficial erosion of the alveolus does not.

4.4 Extranodal Extension

Extranodal extension (ENE) is defined as tumor infiltration that extends from the confines of the lymph node through the lymph node capsule into the surrounding connective tissue. Only unquestionable evidence of ENE, such as matted nodes, skin invasion, gross infiltration into surrounding deep tissues, and adjacent nerve dysfunction, in conjunction with strong radiographic evidence, should be used for clinical staging (Fig. 4.3) [1]. The two most common imaging modalities for the evaluation of cervical lymph node metastases are computed tomography (CT) and magnetic resonance imaging. Using the definition of "ill-defined nodal borders" for ENE, CT has a sensitivity of 61% and specificity of 95%, while MRI has a sensitivity of 40% and a specificity of 97% with an acceptable intrarater reliability [11]. With the presence of three or more ENE imaging criteria, including indistinct nodal margins, infiltration into adjacent tissues, irregular nodal enhancement, matted nodes, and central necrosis, improved specificity and PPV are possible (Fig. 4.4) [12].

Pathologically, only ENE >2 mm beyond the lymph node capsule microscopically is used to define nodal status [1]. Lewis et al. described a

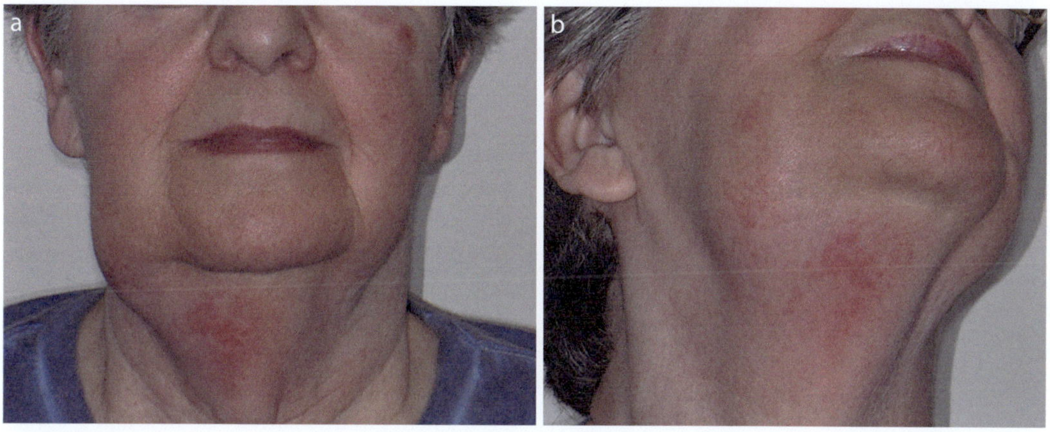

Fig. 4.3 Right level 1b lymphadenopathy, unquestionably matted to surrounding tissues with ENE confirmed on pathologic evaluation

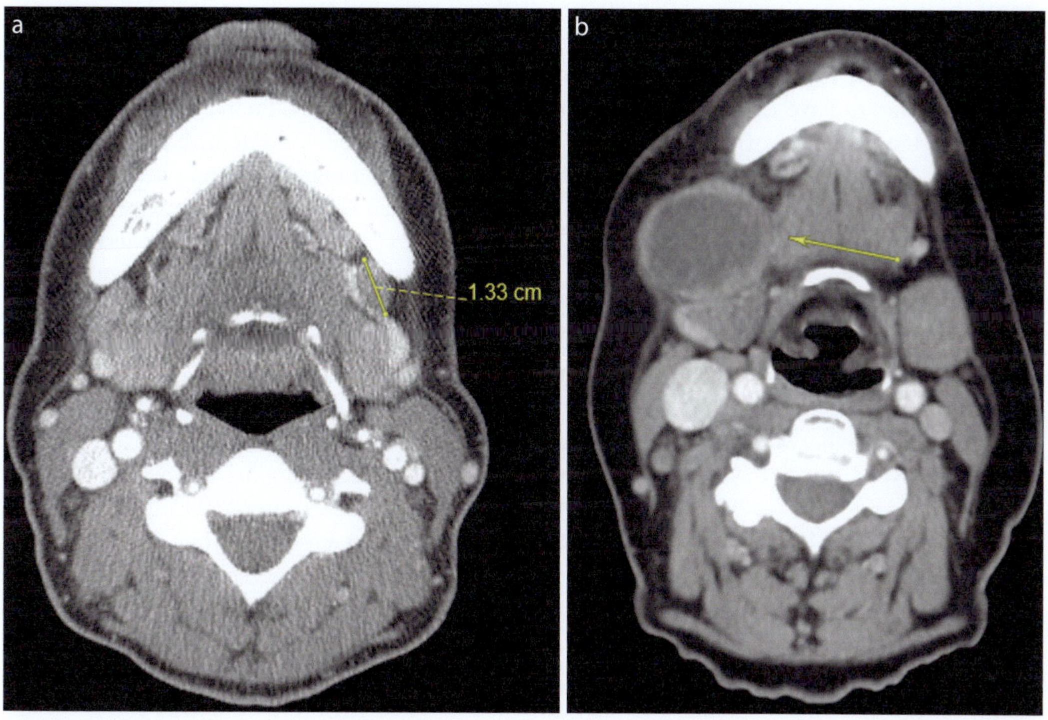

Fig. 4.4 (**a**) Left level 1b lymph node, 1.3 cm in greatest diameter with no evidence of ENE. Clinically, mobile lymphadenopathy reported. Radiographically, only central necrosis noted. (**b**) Right level 1b lymph node, 3.8 cm in greatest diameter with pathologically evident ENE. Clinically, fixed lymphadenopathy reported. Radiographically, infiltration into adjacent tissues (arrow), irregular nodal enhancement, and central necrosis noted

histological grading system for ENE, divided into four major groups [13]. A summary can be found in Table 4.2. However, internationally standardized histological grading criteria have not yet been defined or validated and are not included in the current AJCC cancer staging system.

ENE in patients with OSCC is associated with a significant decrease in 5-year disease-free survival, disease-specific survival, and

Table 4.2 Histological grading system for extranodal extension (ENE)

Extranodal extension	Description
Grade 0	Tumor confined to the lymph node (surrounded by lymphoid tissue)
Grade 1	Tumor reaching lymph node capsule (no intervening lymphoid tissue) with thickening of the overlying capsule
Grade 2	Tumor in perinodal tissue, limited to ≤1 mm beyond the capsule
Grade 3	Tumor in perinodal tissue, extending >1 mm beyond the capsule
Grade 4	Soft tissue metastasis. No residual nodal tissue or architecture

overall survival, as well as an increase in locoregional recurrence when compared to node-negative (N0) and ENE-negative patients of a similar cohort [14, 15]. Patients with ENE have also been found to have as high as a threefold increase in the incidence of distant metastases [16]. When implemented retrospectively, incorporating ENE has been shown to result in a pathologic upstaging of the N category in as many as 30% of patients, while demonstrating a significant correlation with 5-year disease-specific and overall survival that was not noted using the former staging system [17]. Of note, ENE is not associated with a negative impact in HPV-positive oropharyngeal squamous cell carcinoma [18].

4.5 Resection Margins

Most ablative surgeons perform wide local excision of the primary OSCC lesion and subsequently sample the remaining tumor bed margins via frozen section. Concordance between final and frozen specimen samples is 99% with a false-negative rate of 3.5% [19]. However, the concordance between tumor bed margins and the main specimen are low, likely due to sampling error. Thus, the margin obtained from the en-bloc specimen remains the only prognostically relevant margin in terms of local control [20].

Using a cutoff of 7 mm, the incidence of inadequate margins with intraoperative gross examination of the margin, measured from the tumor bed to the mucosal edge without stretching, has been reported to be similar to intraoperative frozen section with no difference in terms of disease-free survival and overall survival [21]. In fact, patients with involved intraoperative frozen margins in which an additional resection was performed demonstrated a 27% local recurrence rate, which was not statistically different from microscopically positive margins that were not cleared [19]. Conversely, intraoperative assessment of bony resection margins by cytological assessment has a sensitivity of 94% and specificity of 97%, resulting in a 60% relative risk reduction of residual carcinoma tissue in the final resection specimen that correlated with higher disease-free and overall survival [22].

A "close" margin is most commonly defined as being within 5 mm of the invasive tumor bed [23]. Regardless of additional adverse tumor features, the local control rate with surgery alone in patients with a margin <5 mm was found to be 91% with an 84% disease-specific survival at 5 years [24]. Stratification by categorization of margin status by 1 mm subunits was not found to be statistically significant. Patients with 0, 1, 2, and 3 additional adverse features (i.e., T3/T4 tumors, PNI, LVI, or multimodal involvement) had 5-year local control rates of 100%, 96%, 83%, and 71%, respectively [24].

Submillimeter margins, however, have been associated with 28% rate of local recurrence [25]. Nevertheless, a close margin (<5 mm) alone, without other negative prognostic indicators, does not warrant postoperative adjuvant therapy.

4.6 Sentinel Node Biopsy

Intraoperative lymphatic mapping with biopsy of the sentinel node in the regional basin is a minimally invasive manner of detecting metastatic disease [26]. The sentinel node is identified visually, following intralesion injection of methylene blue dye, or via gamma probe, following intralesion injection of Technetium-99m-labeled human serum (Fig. 4.5). The goal of sampling the SLN is to detect occult nodal metastasis with the inten-

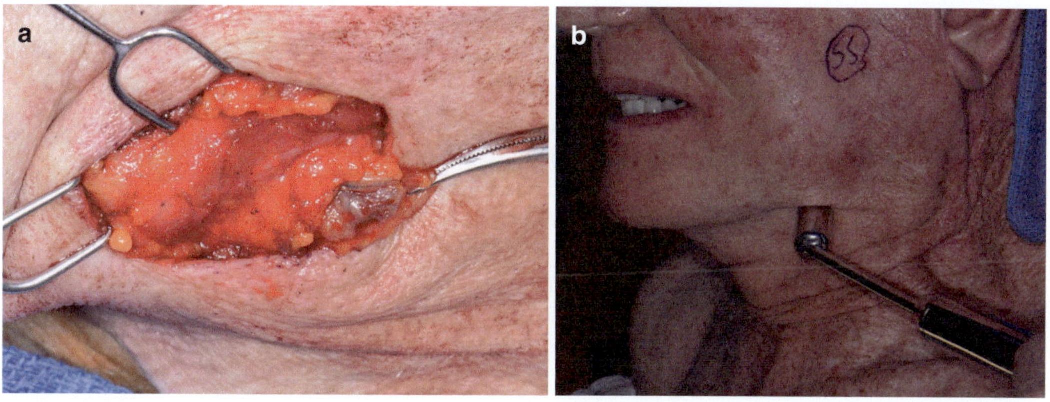

Fig. 4.5 Sentinel lymph node biopsy in left level 1b utilizing a combination of methylene blue (**a**) and gamma probe localization with Technetium-99m-labeled human serum (**b**)

tion of sparing the patient from the morbidity of an elective neck dissection or the potential locoregional recurrence during the postoperative observation period. SLNB for early AJCC Stage I and II OSCCs have demonstrated a detection rate of 98% with an overall sensitivity of 92%, specificity of 100%, and NPV of 96% [27–30]. Moreover, concordance of the SN status during intraoperative frozen sections with permanent histopathologic specimens is 97% [31].

4.7 Other Tumor-Specific Prognostic Factors

4.7.1 Perineural and Lymphovascular Invasion

Perineural invasion is defined as the presence of tumor cells within any of the three layers of nerve sheath or surrounding 33% of the nerve circumference [32]. PNI has been associated with a decrease in disease-specific and overall survival and increases in regional lymph node and distant metastasis, as well as locoregional recurrence [8, 33, 34]. In the absence of other adverse pathologic features, however, postoperative adjuvant radiation therapy was not found to significantly reduce the incidence of recurrence in PNI-positive patients [35–37].

Lymphovascular invasion is the presence of neoplastic cells in the wall and/or lumen of surrounding blood vessels and lymphatic channels. In clinically N0 patients, LVI is associated with locoregional recurrence and decreased overall survival [38–40]. Studies have yet to further elucidate the role of adjuvant therapy when LVI alone is detected.

4.7.2 Human Papilloma Virus

Squamous cell carcinoma that is related to transcriptionally active Human Papilloma Virus (HPV) has been shown to have distinct characteristics from HPV-negative carcinomas, particularly in the oropharynx. With the advent of various testing methods, it has been elucidated that 90% of OPSCC are caused by HPV, specifically subtype 16 [41]. Other high-risk subtypes include 18, 31, 33, 35, 39, 45, 51, 52, 56, 58, 59, 68, 69, 73, and 82. Furthermore, patients with oropharyngeal tumors in which HPV DNA is detected are generally younger with a lower number of cumulative pack-years of tobacco smoking, carrying a small primary tumor burden and better disease-specific and overall survival patterns [42]. Among HPV-positive OPSCC patients who receive radiochemotherapy, treatment outcomes are significantly better than those compared to the HPV-negative counterparts [43]. The impact that HPV testing has had on OPSCC has prompted a separate staging system, as defined by the eighth edition of the AJCC cancer staging manual, which is beyond the scope of this chapter.

HPV detection in sampled tissue can be accomplished using a variety of techniques, including polymerase chain reaction (PCR) assays, in situ hybridization (ISH), or immunohistochemistry (IHC) for the p16 protein [41, 44, 45]. At this time, no consensus on which testing method should be used has been reached. PCR for HPV DNA is highly sensitive, but expensive and cannot distinguish transcriptionally active from inactive HPV. Cross-contamination during PCR may also result in a relatively low specificity. PCR for the transcription-active oncogenes E6/E7 mRNA is highly sensitive and highly specific but requires fresh frozen tissue, remains technically challenging to perform, and is not readily available in all laboratories. ISH for DNA is highly specific but demonstrates a low sensitivity for detection, while ISH for and E6/E7 mRNA is still in development. IHC for p16 has demonstrated good concordance with ISH studies, particularly in oropharyngeal carcinomas, while being easier to interpret, highly sensitive, and more cost-effective [46]. To be interpreted as positive, p16 immunostaining must be nuclear (not cytoplasmic) with a intensity +2/+3 or greater with a distribution 75% or greater [1].

In early studies, HPV has been shown to be 2–3 times more likely to be detected in precancerous oral mucosa and nearly five times more likely to be detected in OSCC than in normal mucosa [47]. Recently, as many as 30% of OSCCs are HPV-positive, as elucidated by PCR and ISH techniques, with high-risk subtypes 16 and 18 found in 25% and 18% of samples, respectively [48]. Despite the presence of HPV DNA, active mRNA expression seems to be limited in OSCC [45]. Furthermore, p16 overexpression in IHC is not a reliable marker for the presence of transcriptionally active HPV in OSCC [49–51]. Unlike OPSCC, HPV-positive and HPV-negative OSCCs have not been shown to differ significantly in terms of pathogenesis, survival, or sensitivity to radiation therapy [43, 52]. To date, HPV has been consistently reported to have a minor role in oral oncogenesis.

Table 4.3 Histological patterns of invasion

Pattern of invasion	Definition
Type 1	Broad, pushing invasion with well-delineated infiltrating borders
Type 2	Broad, pushing "fingers,"cords, bands, and/or strands of infiltration with a stellate appearance
Type 3	Invasive islands of tumor cells (>15 per group)
Type 4	Invasive islands of tumor cells (<15 per group) and/or single cells

4.7.3 Pattern of Invasion

Byrne et al. previously described a histological malignancy grading system, in which a 4-point pattern of invasion was defined [53]. A brief summary can be found in Table 4.3. As the POI worsens, the risk for lymph node metastasis increases. Type 3 POI predicts lymph node metastasis with a sensitivity and specificity of 87% and 86%, respectively [8]. Brandwein-Gensler et al. subsequently introduced Type 5, a widely dispersed pattern of tumor infiltrate with ≥1 mm of normal tissue between tumor satellites and collapsed the grading system into two groups, cohesive (Types 1–3) and infiltrative (Types 4 and 5) [54]. Infiltrative POI is a strong pathologic predictor of locoregional recurrence and mortality from OSCC with a hazard ratio of 1.5 and 2.34, respectively [6].

4.7.4 Lymph Node Ratio

The ratio of tumor-laden nodes to the total number of nodes resected and examined has shown prognostic significance in OSCC. Generally, a selective neck dissection should include ≥10 lymph nodes, while a comprehensive neck dissection should include ≥15 lymph nodes. A lymph node ratio, >6% in tongue OSCC and >7% in buccal mucosa OSCC, correlates to a 4.8- and 10.3-fold increase in the risk of locoregional recurrence, respectively [55, 56]. Estimated 5-year overall survival rates were 65.3%, 49.9%, 41.1%, 29.7%, 18.5%, and 9.7% for groups with

0, 1, 2, 3, 4–6, 7–9, and 10 or more metastatic lymph nodes [16]. In these studies, the number of metastatic nodes demonstrated more importance than size or contralaterality.

4.8 Conclusion

The eighth edition of the Cancer Staging System by the AJCC appropriately emphasizes DOI and ENE as prognostic factors for OSCC, as both have been shown to correlate to locoregional control and 5-year survival. Factors that are not included in the staging system, but must be considered, include resection margins, PNI, LVI, WPOI, and LNR. Intraoperative margin evaluation and sentinel lymph node biopsy techniques are being further developed to aid in improving outcomes while minimizing surgical morbidity. Despite its impact on oropharyngeal cancer, HPV seems to play a minor role in the oncogenesis of OSCC.

Acknowledgements Photomicrograph in Fig. 4.2 by Ashley Flowers, MD—Assistant Professor, Department of Pathology, Louisiana State University Health Sciences Center, Shreveport, LA.

Conflicts of interest: There are no conflicts of interest to report.

References

1. Ridge JA, Lydiatt WM, Patel SG, Glastonbury CM, Brandwein-Gensler MS, Ghossein RA, et al. Lip and oral cavity. In: Amin MB, editor. AJCC cancer staging manual. 8th ed. NewYork, NY: Springer; 2017. p. 79–94.
2. Tirelli G, Gatto A, Boscolo Nata F, Bussani R, Piccinato A, Marcuzzo AV, et al. Prognosis of oral cancer: a comparison of the staging systems given in the 7th and 8th editions of the American Joint Committee on cancer staging manual. Br J Oral Maxillofac Surg. 2018;56(1):8–13.
3. Ebrahimi A, Gil Z, Amit M, Yen TC, Liao CT, Chaturvedi P, et al. Primary tumor staging for oral cancer and a proposed modification incorporating depth of invasion: an international multicenter retrospective study. JAMA Otolaryngol Head Neck Surg. 2014;140(12):1138–48.
4. Almangush A, Leivo I, Siponen M, Sundquist E, Mroueh R, Makitie AA, et al. Evaluation of the budding and depth of invasion (BD) model in oral tongue cancer biopsies. Virchows Archiv. 2018;472(2):231–6.
5. Tan WJ, Chia CS, Tan HK, Soo KC, Iyer NG. Prognostic significance of invasion depth in oral tongue squamous cell carcinoma. ORL. 2012;74(5):264–70.
6. Almangush A, Bello IO, Coletta RD, Makitie AA, Makinen LK, Kauppila JH, et al. For early-stage oral tongue cancer, depth of invasion and worst pattern of invasion are the strongest pathological predictors for locoregional recurrence and mortality. Virchows Archiv. 2015;467(1):39–46.
7. Brockhoff HC 2nd, Kim RY, Braun TM, Skouteris C, Helman JI, Ward BB. Correlating the depth of invasion at specific anatomic locations with the risk for regional metastatic disease to lymph nodes in the neck for oral squamous cell carcinoma. Head Neck. 2017;39(5):974–9.
8. Arora A, Husain N, Bansal A, Neyaz A, Jaiswal R, Jain K, et al. Development of a new outcome prediction model in early-stage squamous cell carcinoma of the oral cavity based on histopathologic parameters with multivariate analysis: the Aditi-Nuzhat Lymph-node Prediction Score (ANLPS) system. Am J Surg Pathol. 2017;41(7):950–60.
9. Li C, Lin J, Men Y, Yang W, Mi F, Li L. Does medullary versus cortical invasion of the mandible affect prognosis in patients with oral squamous cell carcinoma? J Oral Maxillofac Surg. 2017;75(2):403–15.
10. Fives C, Nae A, Roche P, O'Leary G, Fitzgerald B, Feeley L, et al. Impact of mandibular invasion on prognosis in oral squamous cell carcinoma four centimeters or less in size. Laryngoscope. 2017;127(4):849–54.
11. Almulla A, Noel CW, Lu L, Xu W, O'Sullivan B, Goldstein DP, et al. Radiologic-pathologic correlation of extranodal extension in patients with squamous cell carcinoma of the oral cavity: implications for future editions of the TNM classification. Int J Radiat Oncol Biol Phys. 2018;102(4):698–708.
12. Carlton JA, Maxwell AW, Bauer LB, McElroy SM, Layfield LJ, Ahsan H, et al. Computed tomography detection of extracapsular spread of squamous cell carcinoma of the head and neck in metastatic cervical lymph nodes. Neuroradiol J. 2017;30(3):222–9.
13. Lewis JS Jr, Carpenter DH, Thorstad WL, Zhang Q, Haughey BH. Extracapsular extension is a poor predictor of disease recurrence in surgically treated oropharyngeal squamous cell carcinoma. Modern Pathol. 2011;24(11):1413–20.
14. Suton P, Salaric I, Granic M, Mueller D, Luksic I. Prognostic significance of extracapsular spread of lymph node metastasis from oral squamous cell carcinoma in the clinically negative neck. Int J Oral Maxillofac Surg. 2017;46(6):669–75.
15. Jose J, Coatesworth AP, Johnston C, MacLennan K. Cervical node metastases in squamous cell carcinoma of the upper aerodigestive tract: the significance of extracapsular spread and soft tissue deposits. Head Neck. 2003;25(6):451–6.
16. Ho AS, Kim S, Tighiouart M, Gudino C, Mita A, Scher KS, et al. Metastatic lymph node burden

and survival in oral cavity cancer. J Clin Oncol. 2017;35(31):3601–9.
17. Matos LL, Dedivitis RA, Kulcsar MAV, de Mello ES, Alves VAF, Cernea CR. External validation of the AJCC cancer staging manual, 8th edition, in an independent cohort of oral cancer patients. Oral Oncol. 2017;71:47–53.
18. Mermod M, Tolstonog G, Simon C, Monnier Y. Extracapsular spread in head and neck squamous cell carcinoma: a systematic review and meta-analysis. Oral Oncol. 2016;62:60–71.
19. Buchakjian MR, Tasche KK, Robinson RA, Pagedar NA, Sperry SM. Association of main specimen and tumor bed margin status with local recurrence and survival in oral cancer surgery. JAMA Otolaryngol Head Neck Surg. 2016;142(12):1191–8.
20. Maxwell JH, Thompson LD, Brandwein-Gensler MS, Weiss BG, Canis M, Purgina B, et al. Early oral tongue squamous cell carcinoma: sampling of margins from tumor bed and worse local control. JAMA Otolaryngol Head Neck Surg. 2015;141(12):1104–10.
21. Mair M, Nair D, Nair S, Dutta S, Garg A, Malik A, et al. Intraoperative gross examination vs frozen section for achievement of adequate margin in oral cancer surgery. Oral Surg Oral Med Oral Pathol Oral Radiol. 2017;123(5):544–9.
22. Nieberler M, Haussler P, Kesting MR, Kolk A, Deppe H, Weirich G, et al. Clinical impact of intraoperative cytological assessment of bone resection margins in patients with head and neck carcinoma. Ann Surg Oncol. 2016;23(11):3579–86.
23. Meier JD, Oliver DA, Varvares MA. Surgical margin determination in head and neck oncology: current clinical practice. the results of an International American Head and Neck Society Member Survey. Head Neck. 2005;27(11):952–8.
24. Ch'ng S, Corbett-Burns S, Stanton N, Gao K, Shannon K, Clifford A, et al. Close margin alone does not warrant postoperative adjuvant radiotherapy in oral squamous cell carcinoma. Cancer. 2013;119(13):2427–37.
25. Buchakjian MR, Ginader T, Tasche KK, Pagedar NA, Smith BJ, Sperry SM. Independent predictors of prognosis based on oral cavity squamous cell carcinoma surgical margins. Otolaryngol Head Neck Surg. 2018;2018:194599818773070.
26. Ross MI, Reintgen D, Balch CM. Selective lymphadenectomy: emerging role for lymphatic mapping and sentinel node biopsy in the management of early stage melanoma. Semin Surg Oncol. 1993;9(3):219–23.
27. Yang Y, Zhou J, Wu H. Diagnostic value of sentinel lymph node biopsy for cT1/T2N0 tongue squamous cell carcinoma: a meta-analysis. Eur Archiv Otorhino-laryngol. 2017;274(11):3843–52.
28. Lin R, Yan J, Liu W, Fan T, Tang L. The predictive value of cervical lymph node metastasis through sentinel lymph node biopsy in patients with oral cancer: a meta-analysis. J Cancer Res Ther. 2016;12(Suppl):C256–c9.
29. Schilling C, Stoeckli SJ, Haerle SK, Broglie MA, Huber GF, Sorensen JA, et al. Sentinel European Node Trial (SENT): 3-year results of sentinel node biopsy in oral cancer. Eur J Cancer. 2015;51(18):2777–84.
30. Civantos FJ, Zitsch RP, Schuller DE, Agrawal A, Smith RB, Nason R, et al. Sentinel lymph node biopsy accurately stages the regional lymph nodes for T1–T2 oral squamous cell carcinomas: results of a prospective multi-institutional trial. J Clin Oncol. 2010;28(8):1395–400.
31. Miura K, Hirakawa H, Uemura H, Yoshimoto S, Shiotani A, Sugasawa M, et al. Sentinel node biopsy for oral cancer: a prospective multicenter Phase II trial. Auris Nasus Larynx. 2017;44(3):319–26.
32. Liebig C, Ayala G, Wilks JA, Berger DH, Albo D. Perineural invasion in cancer: a review of the literature. Cancer. 2009;115(15):3379–91.
33. Tai SK, Li WY, Chu PY, Chang SY, Tsai TL, Wang YF, et al. Risks and clinical implications of perineural invasion in T1-2 oral tongue squamous cell carcinoma. Head Neck. 2012;34(7):994–1001.
34. Jardim JF, Francisco AL, Gondak R, Damascena A, Kowalski LP. Prognostic impact of perineural invasion and lymphovascular invasion in advanced stage oral squamous cell carcinoma. Int J Oral Maxillofac Surg. 2015;44(1):23–8.
35. Chatzistefanou I, Lubek J, Markou K, Ord RA. The role of neck dissection and postoperative adjuvant radiotherapy in cN0 patients with PNI-positive squamous cell carcinoma of the oral cavity. Oral Oncol. 2014;50(8):753–8.
36. Bur AM, Lin A, Weinstein GS. Adjuvant radiotherapy for early head and neck squamous cell carcinoma with perineural invasion: a systematic review. Head Neck. 2016;38(Suppl 1):E2350–7.
37. Liu T, Chua B, Batstone M. Postoperative radiotherapy for oral squamous cell carcinoma with histologic risk factors: are we over-treating? J Oral Maxillofac Surg. 2018;76(7):1565–70.
38. Cassidy RJ, Switchenko JM, Jegadeesh N, Sayan M, Ferris MJ, Eaton BR, et al. Association of lymphovascular space invasion with locoregional failure and survival in patients with node-negative oral tongue cancers. JAMA Otolaryngol Head Neck Surg. 2017;143(4):382–8.
39. Fives C, Feeley L, O'Leary G, Sheahan P. Importance of lymphovascular invasion and invasive front on survival in floor of mouth cancer. Head Neck. 2016;38(Suppl 1):E1528–34.
40. Hosni A, McMullen C, Huang SH, Xu W, Su J, Bayley A, et al. Lymph node ratio relationship to regional failure and distant metastases in oral cavity cancer. Radiother Oncol. 2017;124(2):225–31.
41. Bishop JA, Lewis JS Jr, Rocco JW, Faquin WC. HPV-related squamous cell carcinoma of the head and neck: An update on testing in routine pathology practice. Semin Diagn Pathol. 2015;32(5):344–51.
42. Ang KK, Harris J, Wheeler R, Weber R, Rosenthal DI, Nguyen-Tan PF, et al. Human papillomavirus and survival of patients with oropharyngeal cancer. N Engl J Med. 2010;363(1):24–35.

43. Wang F, Zhang H, Xue Y, Wen J, Zhou J, Yang X, et al. A systematic investigation of the association between HPV and the clinicopathological parameters and prognosis of oral and oropharyngeal squamous cell carcinomas. Cancer Med. 2017;6(5):910–7.
44. Westra WH. Detection of human papillomavirus (HPV) in clinical samples: evolving methods and strategies for the accurate determination of HPV status of head and neck carcinomas. Oral Oncol. 2014;50(9):771–9.
45. Mirghani H, Amen F, Moreau F, Lacau St Guily J. Do high-risk human papillomaviruses cause oral cavity squamous cell carcinoma? Oral Oncol. 2015;51(3):229–36.
46. Thomas J, Primeaux T. Is p16 immunohistochemistry a more cost-effective method for identification of human papilloma virus-associated head and neck squamous cell carcinoma? Ann Diagn Pathol. 2012;16(2):91–9.
47. Miller CS, Johnstone BM. Human papillomavirus as a risk factor for oral squamous cell carcinoma: a meta-analysis, 1982-1997. Oral Surg Oral Med Oral Pathol Oral Radiol Endod. 2001;91(6):622–35.
48. Kansy K, Thiele O, Freier K. The role of human papillomavirus in oral squamous cell carcinoma: myth and reality. Oral Maxillofac Surg. 2014;18(2):165–72.
49. Poling JS, Ma XJ, Bui S, Luo Y, Li R, Koch WM, et al. Human papillomavirus (HPV) status of non-tobacco related squamous cell carcinomas of the lateral tongue. Oral Oncol. 2014;50(4):306–10.
50. Harris SL, Thorne LB, Seaman WT, Hayes DN, Couch ME, Kimple RJ. Association of p16(INK4a) overexpression with improved outcomes in young patients with squamous cell cancers of the oral tongue. Head Neck. 2011;33(11):1622–7.
51. Lingen MW, Xiao W, Schmitt A, Jiang B, Pickard R, Kreinbrink P, et al. Low etiologic fraction for high-risk human papillomavirus in oral cavity squamous cell carcinomas. Oral Oncol. 2013;49(1):1–8.
52. Kruger M, Pabst AM, Walter C, Sagheb K, Gunther C, Blatt S, et al. The prevalence of human papilloma virus (HPV) infections in oral squamous cell carcinomas: a retrospective analysis of 88 patients and literature overview. J Cranio-maxillo-fac Surg. 2014;42(7):1506–14.
53. Bryne M, Koppang HS, Lilleng R, Kjaerheim A. Malignancy grading of the deep invasive margins of oral squamous cell carcinomas has high prognostic value. J Pathol. 1992;166(4):375–81.
54. Brandwein-Gensler M, Teixeira MS, Lewis CM, Lee B, Rolnitzky L, Hille JJ, et al. Oral squamous cell carcinoma: histologic risk assessment, but not margin status, is strongly predictive of local disease-free and overall survival. Am J Surg Pathol. 2005;29(2):167–78.
55. Safi AF, Grandoch A, Nickenig HJ, Zoller JE, Kreppel M. The importance of lymph node ratio for locoregional recurrence of squamous cell carcinoma of the tongue. J Cranio-maxillo-fac Surg. 2017;45(7):1058–61.
56. Safi AF, Grandoch A, Nickenig HJ, Zoller JE, Kreppel M. Importance of lymph node ratio for locoregional recurrence of squamous cell carcinoma of the buccal mucosa. Head Neck. 2017;39(12):2488–93.

5 Surgical Factors Affecting Outcomes in Oral Squamous Cell Carcinoma

Justine Moe, Andrew Baker, and Brent Ward

5.1 Introduction

Oral cancer is the 16th most common cancer worldwide with an estimated incidence of 350,000 new cases per year [1]. Oral cavity squamous cell carcinoma (OCSCC) is the most common type of oral cancer and a cause of significant morbidity and mortality worldwide. The treatment of OCSCC follows the clinical practice guidelines established by the National Comprehensive Cancer Network [2]. Surgery is the primary treatment modality when possible, although definitive radiotherapy may be used for a select group of early stage OCSCC or for patients unable to undergo surgery. Adjuvant radiation, with or without chemotherapy, has been shown to improve disease-free survival and overall survival in advanced stages and in the presence of high-risk histological features.

The treatment for OCSCC should be personalized to some degree for each patient. There are multiple determinants that affect surgical outcomes, as well as prognosis, including a patient's surgical candidacy, the type and extent of surgery required, the mode and timing of reconstruction, and the use of adjunct surgical tools. This chapter discusses the factors that can allow the surgeon to optimize outcomes in the surgical treatment of OCSCC.

5.2 Care Team Factors

Multidisciplinary care is essential in the management of patients with OCSCC. Multimodality therapy is integral to the restoration of function, quality of life, and survival of these patients. Multidisciplinary team composition varies between institutions but typically include ablative surgeons, reconstructive surgeons, and members of medical oncology, radiation oncology, radiology, pathology, dentistry, speech and language pathology, nutrition, rehabilitation therapy, palliative care, and social work. Multidisciplinary tumor board conference allows for a comprehensive discussion of the optimal treatment for individual patients.

In addition, the institution at which surgery is performed should be well equipped to manage head and neck cancer patients in all phases of care. The institution should have microvascular capability as well as intensive care, floor, and operating room staff trained to care for head and neck cancer patients. The treatment of oral cancer at high volume centers is associated with improved survival for all stages of cancer. A retrospective cohort study of 13,655 patients found a higher incidence of positive margins at nonaca-

J. Moe · A. Baker · B. Ward (✉)
Department of Oral and Maxillofacial Surgery, University of Michigan, Ann Arbor, MI, USA
e-mail: jusmoe@med.umich.edu; abakes@med.umich.edu; bward@med.umich.edu

D. Kademani (ed.), *Improving Outcomes in Oral Cancer*, https://doi.org/10.1007/978-3-030-30094-4_5

demic facilities and low volume centers [3]. Trends toward the regionalization of care of oral cancer patients may be a factor in improved prognosis.

5.3 Patient Factors

Patients with OCSCC often have significant medical comorbidities because smoking, excessive alcohol consumption, poor dietary habits, and decreased oral intake are common in this population. A preoperative assessment of the patient's functional status and comorbidities should be completed by using one of many comorbidity indexes available. The Adult Comorbidity Evaluation (ACE-27) is a validated instrument that grades the severity of comorbidities of patients with cancer at the time of diagnosis [4]. The American Society of Anesthesiologists (ASA) physical status classification predicts perioperative risk and may be used as a proxy to evaluate comorbidity [5, 6].

In head and neck cancer patients, age alone is not a predictor of complication rates in the surgical treatment of OCSCC [7, 8]. Rather, a high comorbid burden is associated with increased surgical and anesthesia complications, prolonged hospital stay, and reduced functional outcome following treatment [5]. Comorbidity is also associated with increased perioperative mortality, increased short-term mortality, and decreased overall survival [5]. In early years following curative-intent surgery, a reported 16–40% of deaths is secondary to comorbid conditions and non-cancer-related causes, particularly cardiovascular, respiratory, gastrointestinal comorbidity, and diabetes [5, 9]. Severe comorbidity has been found to have comparable survival impact to a T4 tumor or N2 neck [9].

While surgery is essential to cure in most cases of OCSCC, the perioperative risks associated with a patient's medical status need to be weighed. Patients with high comorbid burden or poor functional status may be poor candidates for free flap reconstruction, and an alternative reconstructive method may be considered. Predictors of poor postoperative functional status need to be considered as a prolonged recovery may delay or prevent a patient from receiving adjunctive therapy. Patients with severe comorbidities unable to tolerate general anesthesia may not be candidates for surgery, and primary radiation with or without chemotherapy may be indicated.

Patients with recurrent OCSCC pose challenges for surgical treatment. Recurrent OCSCC often heralds an aggressive tumor biology with an associated poor prognosis. Additionally, in patients with previous head and neck radiation, radiation-induced inflammation and fibrosis distort normal anatomy and tissue planes. Previous surgeries also alter anatomy, potentially limiting reconstructive options.

5.4 Surgical Principles

The primary goal of oncologic surgery is the complete tumor extirpation with a cuff of surrounding normal tissue and negative margins. The goal of reconstructive surgery is the restoration of form and function. The schema of the "reconstructive ladder" has traditionally been used to describe the spectrum of options for orofacial reconstruction, based on the principle of selecting the least complex treatment required for the defect (Fig. 5.1). The surgeon should instead consider the "reconstructive toolbox," in which complex procedures such as free flaps should not be thought of as a last resort, but as one of the tools to be used when necessary to restore both form and function (Fig. 5.2).

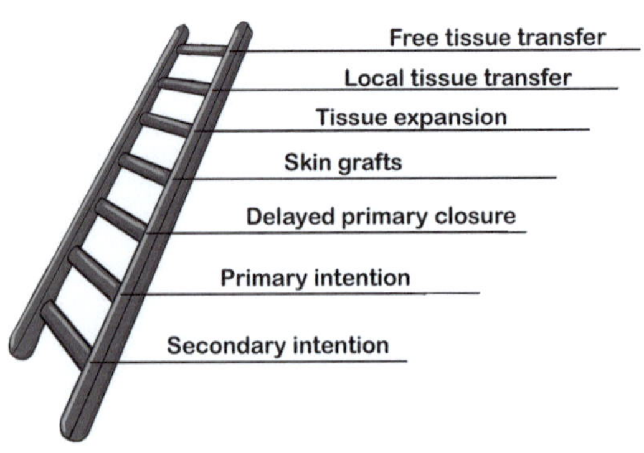

Fig. 5.1 Reconstructive ladder

When reconstructing orofacial defects, the component tissue types and structural subunits involved in the defect should be identified, and consideration should be made to reconstruct the critical components. The type of reconstruction should be chosen based on the size and composition of the defect. Soft tissue defects may be reconstructed using simple techniques or local, regional or free flaps; however, bony and composite defects most often require free flap reconstruction. Corticocancellous bone grafting is often not an option in the oncologic patient due to the need for primary reconstruction, the concomitant loss of soft tissue, large bony defects, the risk of graft loss with adjuvant therapy, or poor recipient bed vascularity following radiation. In addition, the success of corticocancellous bone grafts is associated with graft length. Failure rates have been reported as high as 17% for grafts 6 cm in length or less, increasing significantly for grafts greater than 9 cm to a failure rate of 75% for grafts greater than 12 cm [10].

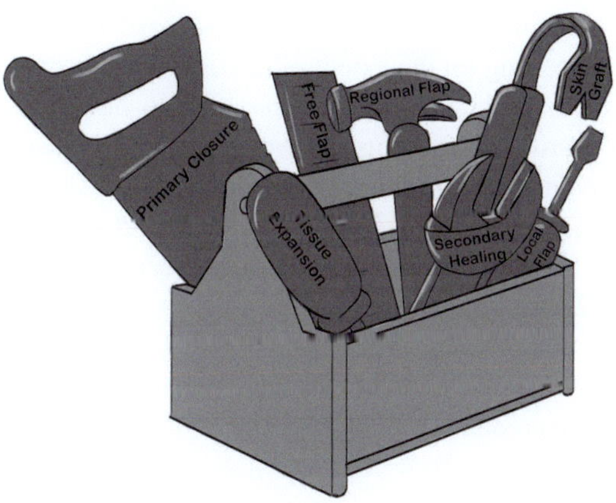

Fig. 5.2 Reconstructive toolbox

5.5 Management of the Primary Tumor

5.5.1 Mandible

OCSCC of the gingival, floor of mouth, buccal mucosa, and retromolar trigone can invade the mandible secondarily. Patterns of mandibular invasion include through periosteum, foramina, attached mucosa, cortical bone defects in the edentulous mandible, and periodontal ligament in the dentate mandible [11–13]. Mandibular involvement should be suspected in gingival SCC even in the absence of gross bone involvement clinically or on imaging.

For mandibular SCC with early bone involvement and in nonatrophic mandibles, a marginal mandibulectomy may be satisfactory to achieve negative margins while maintaining mandibular continuity. In such cases, prophylactic placement of a reconstruction plate may be required to prevent fracture. Segmental mandibulectomy is necessary for gross invasion of cancellous bone. Classification systems of mandibular defects

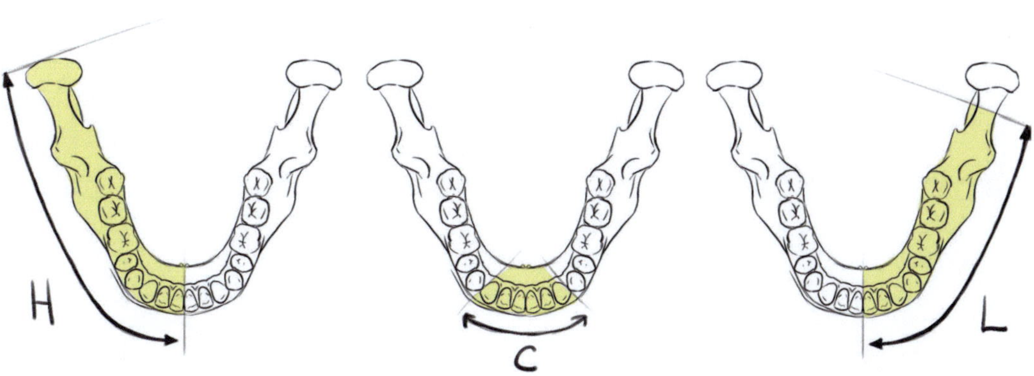

Fig. 5.3 H-C-L classification of mandibular defects. H implies a hemimandibulectomy defect including the condyle. C implies a central segment including both canines. L implies a lateral segment not inducing the condyle. (Adapted from Jewer et al. [14])

based on location and extent such as the HCL classification have been described to reflect the complexity of reconstruction (Fig. 5.3) [14].

When possible, immediate reconstruction with an osteocutaneous free flap is an optimal approach for the reconstruction of mandibular segmental defects. Corticocancellous grafts are often not amenable for use due to multiple reasons as listed above. The fibular free flap is the workhorse for mandibular reconstruction and has minimal donor site morbidity. Up to 25 cm of bone length may be harvested for the reconstruction of long-span mandibular defects and a reliable skin paddle allows for soft tissue reconstruction in composite defects.

The deep circumflex iliac artery (DCIA) free flap may be used to reconstruct the anterior or posterior mandible including the ramus, as the natural curvature of the iliac crest allows for a replication of the natural mandibular form often without osteotomies [15]. Internal oblique muscle may be harvested for soft tissue reconstruction. However, the poor reliability of the perforator skin paddle as well as the potential for significant donor site morbidity limits the utility of the DCIA flap. The scapular free flap provides 10–14 cm of bone length and large amount of soft tissue for the reconstruction of composite defects; however, limited bone stock and length often precludes mandibular reconstruction. The radial forearm (RF) osteocutaneous free flap provides poor-quality bone stock with significant donor site morbidity and is a poor choice for mandibular reconstruction.

While the restoration of mandibular continuity is ideal, soft tissue-only reconstruction in large composite defects has been described using pectoralis major myocutaneous (PMMC) pedicled flaps or anterolateral thigh (ALT) free flaps have been described with acceptable functional and cosmetic results [16].

5.5.2 Maxilla

OCSCC of the maxilla can involve the alveolus, palate, maxillary sinus, nasal cavity, orbit, ethmoid and sphenoid sinuses, and base of skull depending on the extent of disease. Various classification systems of maxillary defects have been described, including the Brown and Okay classification systems, which are used to assess the functional outcome of rehabilitation and to determine the extent and type of reconstruction (Figs. 5.4 and 5.5) [17, 18].

Approaches to the maxilla vary based on disease extent. Most Brown class I or II defects can be approached transorally. The midfacial deglov-

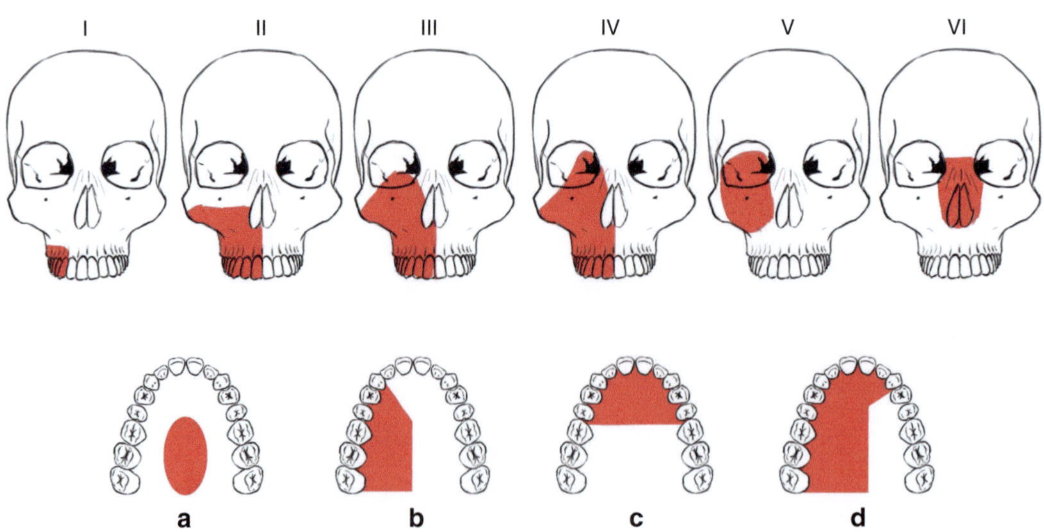

Fig. 5.4 Brown classification of maxillectomy defects. (Adapted from Brown et al. [17])

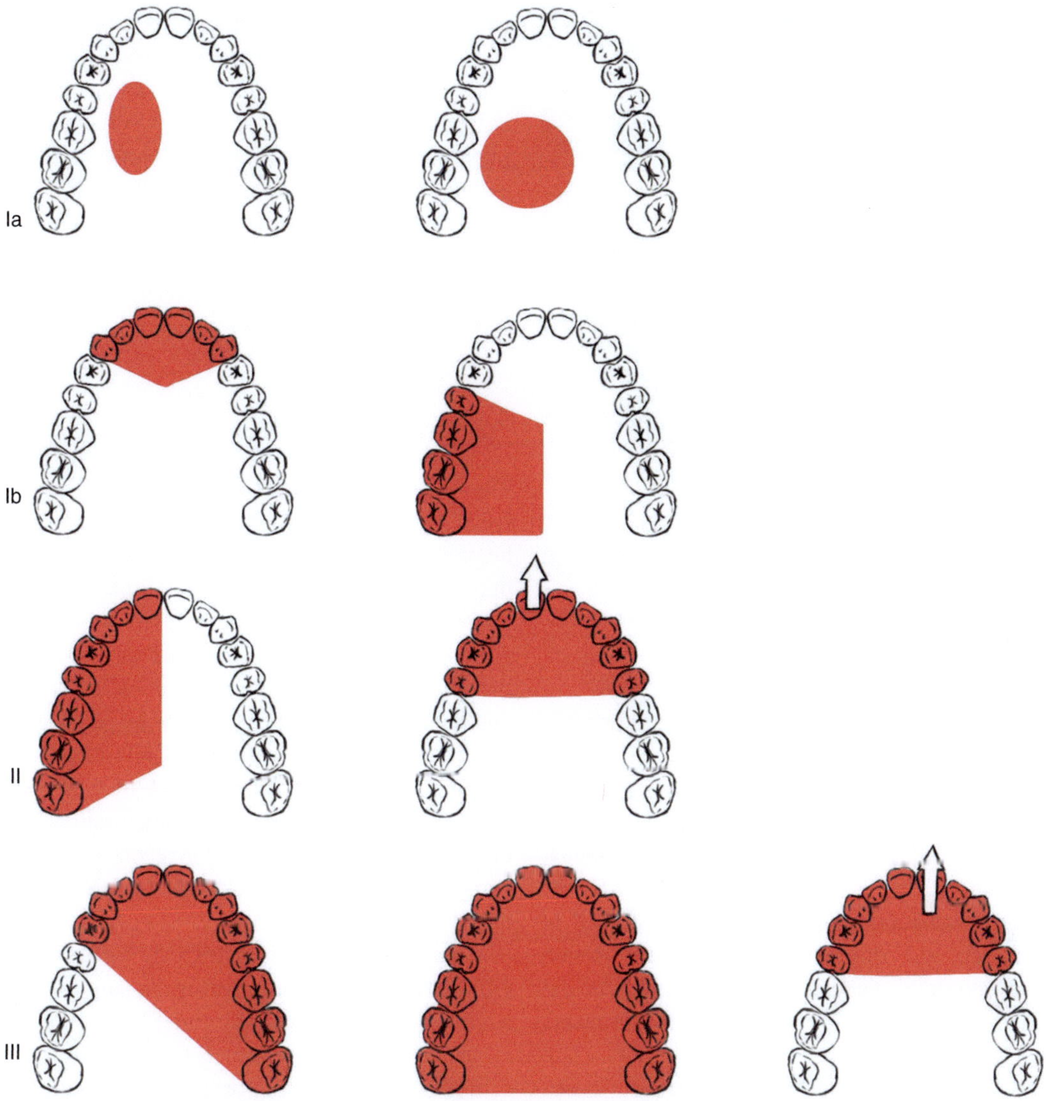

Fig. 5.5 Okay classification of maxillectomy defects. (Adapted from Okay et al. [18])

ing incision which includes sublabial and rhinoplasty incisions improves access to the bilateral anterior maxilla and paranasal sinuses without the need for facial incisions [19]. The Weber–Ferguson incision allows wide access to the entire maxilla and orbital floor. A lip split mandibulotomy improves access to tumors of the posterior maxilla with extension into the pterygoid plates or infratemporal fossa. Additional approaches to the pterygoid region and base of skull are described elsewhere.

Obturation has traditionally been the standard method of maxillary rehabilitation, with the primary goals of maxillectomy defect closure and separation of the oral cavity from the sinonasal cavities (Fig. 5.6) [18]. Obturation allows for shorter operative time, shorter hospital stay and direct visualization of the defect for oncologic surveillance [20]. However, maxillectomy site hygiene, placement and removal can be challenging, particularly in the setting of trismus, and frequent adjustments are required during the acute healing period. Poorly retentive or unstable obturators may be associated with hypernasal speech and regurgitation into the nasal cavity [21]. Endosseous and zygomatic implants can facili-

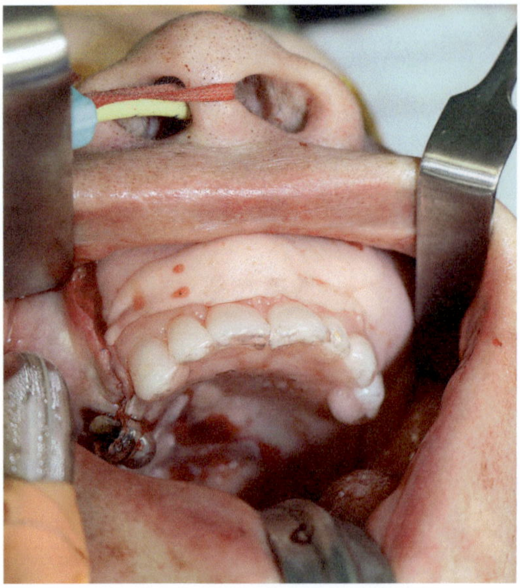

Fig. 5.6 Maxillectomy defect with a temporary maxillary obturator in place

tate retention and support of large obturators; this topic is discussed below.

In contrast, free tissue transfer allows for primary reconstruction with abundant tissue with relative freedom of orientation and shape. Fibula, scapula, DCIA, medial femoral condyle, RF, rectus, and ALT free flaps have been described in maxillary reconstruction. Fibula and DCIA free flaps provide adequate bone stock for dental rehabilitation with osseointegrated implants while scapula flaps often do not [22]. Disadvantages of free flaps in maxillary reconstruction include donor site morbidity, longer and more complex surgeries, and a prolonged hospital course. Immediate reconstruction with a free flap precludes direct inspection for cancer surveillance; however, no study to date has demonstrated a delay in the detection of local recurrence in patients with immediate reconstruction [23]. In these patients, computed tomography or magnetic resonance imaging as well as endoscopy allow for adequate assessment of recurrence without direct inspection [22].

Reconstruction of the palate and alveolar arch is critical to restore speech and swallowing, while the maxillary superstructure has little effect on these functional outcomes [24]. Okay Class I defects can be reconstructed using an obturator or soft tissue local or free flap; Class II defects can be reconstructed with an obturator or vascularized bone flap; and Class III defects have improved functional outcomes when reconstructed with a vascularized bone flap [24]. Orbital floor and zygomatic defects should be restored with bony reconstruction because obturators inadequately restore cosmesis to the midface in these instances [18].

5.5.3 Oral Tongue

The oral tongue is the most common site of OCSCC. Local excision, partial glossectomy, hemiglossectomy, subtotal, or total glossectomy may be required based on the disease extent. Early stage lesions can be excised transorally with the assistance of retraction sutures placed in the anterior tongue. The lip split mandibulotomy approach may facilitate access for larger or posterior tongue lesions or those involving the floor of mouth. A transcervical approach may be used for subtotal or total glossectomy defects, in which the resection and majority of the reconstruction is completed through the neck incision without the need for lip split [25].

Clear histological margins can be achieved with 95% confidence interval if the surgeon utilizes 1.5–2 cm surgical margins [26]. However, excess resection of normal tissue should be avoided on the tongue in order to preserve functional tissue, and therefore margins of 1.0–1.5 cm are standardly utilized.

Reconstruction of small tongue defects may be completed by primary closure, healing by secondary intention, split-thickness skin grafts, or similar substitutes. Larger tongue defects require reconstruction with regional pedicled flaps or free tissue transfer in order to restore tongue mobility, such as the PMMC flap, RF fasciocutaneous free flap and ALT free flap. Free flap reconstruction of the tongue has shown superior functional results related to swallowing and speech as compared to myocutaneous pedicled flaps and should thus be used over pedicled flaps when possible [27].

The utility of sensate flaps in tongue reconstruction remains a point of debate. Microsurgical reinnervation of flaps has been shown in small studies to improve sensory recovery [28]. However, there is insufficient evidence to discern any benefit from sensate flaps in improving speech and swallowing; these findings highlight the fact that functional recovery in these patients is complex and multifactorial [29].

Reconstruction of total glossectomy defects remains challenging, and functional outcomes are variable. The need for total laryngectomy with total glossectomy is controversial and may be advocated for the prevention of aspiration. However, total glossectomy with laryngeal preservation has been found to be associated with favorable swallowing and speech outcomes and meaningful long-term quality of life. Also, feeding tube dependence has not been found to be associated with laryngeal preservation or reconstructive technique [30, 31]. Laryngeal preservation is a valid option with total glossectomy, and postoperative rehabilitation is essential to optimize functional outcomes.

5.5.4 Buccal Mucosa

OCSCC of the buccal mucosa is an aggressive tumor, which may be due to an intrinsic aggressive biology, early invasion into the buccal fat pad, lack of a substantial anatomic barrier in this location, and the difficulty of achieving clear surgical margins without full-thickness resection of the cheek [32]. High incidence of regional metastasis have been reported, up to 28% in the clinically negative (cN0) neck [33], as have high locoregional recurrence rates, ranging from 30% to 80% [34–36]. Due to high recurrence rates, adjuvant radiotherapy should be considered in even early stage lesions [34].

Small buccal mucosal lesions may be excised with wide margins via a transoral approach with reconstruction by primary closure, healing by secondary intention, local rotational flaps, or with buccal fat advancement. Sialodochoplasty or stenting of Stenson's duct may be required if it lies within the resection margins. Free flap reconstruction of larger excisions of the buccal mucosa allows restoration of function and prevents trismus. The RF flap is often used to reconstruct the buccal mucosa as it is thin and pliable. More extensive lesions involving the skin of the cheek, mandible, maxilla, and infratemporal fossa require composite resections including a marginal or segmental mandibulectomy or partial maxillectomy and free flap reconstruction flap.

5.5.4.1 Retromolar Trigone

Tumors in the retromolar trigone may involve the lingual nerve, submandibular duct, and palatoglossus with the possible need to sacrifice these structures with tumor extirpation. Small superficial defects can be resected transorally with reconstruction by primary closure, skin grafts, local and regional flaps, and buccal fat. More extensive lesions may involve the mandible, maxilla, soft palate, and lateral pharyngeal wall, requiring a composite resection and free flap reconstruction with lateral, paramedian, or median mandibulotomy approaches.

5.5.5 Floor of Mouth

Tumors of the floor of mouth may involve the sublingual glands, submandibular duct, and lingual nerve. Early lesions of the floor of mouth are amenable to simple excisions. Sialodochoplasty and stenting of the submandibular duct is required if the duct lies within the resection margins and if the submandibular gland is not planned for removal such as with a neck dissection (Fig. 5.7) [37]. The stent is kept in place for 2–4 weeks and allows for formation of a neo-ostium in the floor of mouth. More extensive lesions may involve the tongue, mandible, and floor of mouth musculature and require composite resection and reconstruction of these structures. Floor of mouth tumors invading the lingual periosteum or lingual cortex may be managed with a lingual corticotomy. Midline or paramedian mandibulotomy can improve access to large floor of mouth lesions.

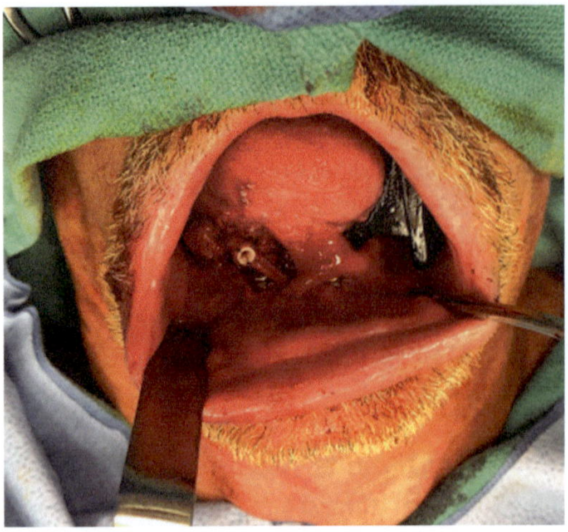

Fig. 5.7 Stent placed in right submandibular duct during resection of floor of mouth cancer. (*Courtesy of* Moe and Helman [37])

5.6 Evaluation of Margin Status

Complete tumor resection is a fundamental principle in oncologic surgery. Many studies have shown an improvement in both disease-free survival (DFS) and overall survival (OS) when negative margins are achieved [38–49]. A series of 148 patients with OCSCC found margin status to be an independent predictor of DFS with 5-year local control rates of 91.0% for clear margins, 80.4% for close margins, 81.8% for dysplasia at surgical margins, and 43.8% for positive margins [38].

The ablative head and neck surgeon strives for curative-intent surgery, as debulking procedures have not shown to be worthwhile. The surgeon should identify risk factors which make complete tumor extirpation more challenging. Late tumor stages involve more anatomic structures which increase the complexity of the tumor and relationship to its surrounding structures; in these cases, greater surgical complexity increases the risk of positive margins.

However, the prognostic significance of negative margins remains controversial, and a number of studies have not found an association between tumor margin status and prognosis. It is suggested that positive margin status may in fact be a function of tumor aggressiveness rather than inadequate surgical treatment, and highly aggressive tumors have a shorter time to recurrence regardless of margin status. In a series of 292 patients with OCSCC, margin status was not an independent predictor of local recurrence (LR) or OS but the histological features of worst pattern of invasion, perineural invasion, and lymphocytic response were [50]. Another study found advanced tumor stage to be a predictor of locoregional recurrence regardless of tumor margin status [38]. Both stage and histologic grade are independent factors on survival and should be considered when evaluating the need for adjuvant therapy regardless of surgical margins.

The definition of a negative margin in OCSCC in terms of the perpendicular distance from the tumor to the resection margin has not been standardized and remains a point of controversy. Tumor excision with a cuff of normal adjacent tissue is the standard of care, but excessive resection of normal anatomy should be avoided in order to preserve functionality. Pathologic negative margins are generally defined as greater than or equal to 5 mm, close margins are less than 5 mm, and a positive margin is defined as carcinoma in situ or invasive cancer at the margin [51]. More recently, this tenet has been questioned, with some evidence that maintaining a narrower margins of 2.2 mm is safe and confers a survival benefit [52]. The clinical margins should be greater than the anticipated pathologic margin to account for tumor shrinkage. Retraction of the mucosal margin following resection of OCSCC has been found to be 20–25% [53]. An additional 10% of tissue shrinkage occurs with formalin fixation and paraffin embedding [54]. Margin discrepancy following resection and processing has been reported to reach up to 75% in one study [55].

5.7 Margin Status on Frozen Section

Margin analysis on frozen section provides ablative surgeons the opportunity to assess the adequacy of resection in real time. Margin assessment with frozen sections have been shown to be highly accurate (96.7–98.4%), sensitive (72.0–88.8%), and specific (94.4–98.9%) with a positive predictive value ranging from 77.9% to 95.7% and a negative predictive value ranging from 96.0% to 99.2% [56–58]. Intraoperative margin analysis can be used to guide the adequacy of resection and allows for positive margins to be revised immediately to negative margins.

However, the prognostic and therapeutic implications of such revisions remain inconclusive [59–61]. The revision of positive to negative margins has been found in some studies to be a negative predictor of locoregional control. A cohort study of 156 patients with OCSCC found positive to negative revised margins to be an independent risk factor for local recurrence (LR), with a 42.2% rate of LR as compared to 16.2% in those with negative margins [59]. Other studies have found improved prognosis with re-resection of positive to negative margins. A retrospective review of 547 patients found that positive to negative revised margins in the presence of regional disease was associated with poorer local control but also found that revisions in the absence of regional disease lead to DSS similar to those with initially negative margins and no regional disease [60].

Errors in relocating the location of the positive margin on frozen section on the tumor bed may lead to sampling error during re-resection. A prospective study of one surgeon in 14 cases found a mean error in relocating a sample site of 9 mm for mucosal margins and 12 mm for deep margins [62]. This would suggest that re-resection to negative margins may be done in the erroneous location and may not necessarily treat the location of the positive margin. To prevent this sampling error, sites of frozen section should be marked with ink, suture or staple, and wide re-excisions should be completed [62]. Nevertheless, it is critical that a clear surgical resection with negative margins be completed on the initial attempt.

Margins on frozen section can be taken from the tumor bed in a defect-driven approach or from the resection specimen in a tumor-driven approach. Defect-driven margins obviate the need for the pathologist to orient the specimen

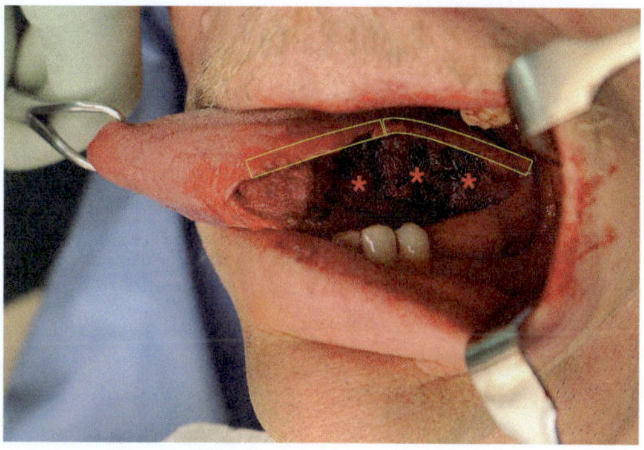

Fig. 5.8 Tumor bed margin assessment with mucosal shave margins (yellow) and deep margin sampling (red)

and to select the locations for sampling and allow the surgeon to sample multiple areas of the tumor bed quickly (Fig. 5.8). However, margins from the tumor bed do not assess distance of the margin to the tumor, and identification of small clusters of tumor cells can be difficult because the known position of tumor bulk is absent from the specimen [63]. In contrast, margins from the resected specimen allow for the evaluation of tumor distance to the specimen edge but require orientation of the specimen by the pathologist, which is often challenging with complex oral cavity tumors. Direct communication between the surgeon and pathologist is crucial to allow for an understanding of specimen orientation.

Margin assessment from the resected specimen has been shown to have improved accuracy and a better correlation with final margin status and patient survival [43, 64]. A retrospective study of 126 patients with oral tongue SCC found that specimen margin status was a predictor of local recurrence, while tumor bed margin status was not, and a positive specimen margin conferred a relative risk of 2.5 for local recurrence [43]. Tumor-driven specimens more accurately predict the completion of resection and local recurrence and should thus be taken whenever possible.

Two methods for retrieving sections to assess margins have been described (Fig. 5.9). A radial or perpendicular margin includes a portion of the tumor with the margin and is useful when the margin is clinically near the tumor. While it allows the distance between the tumor and mar-

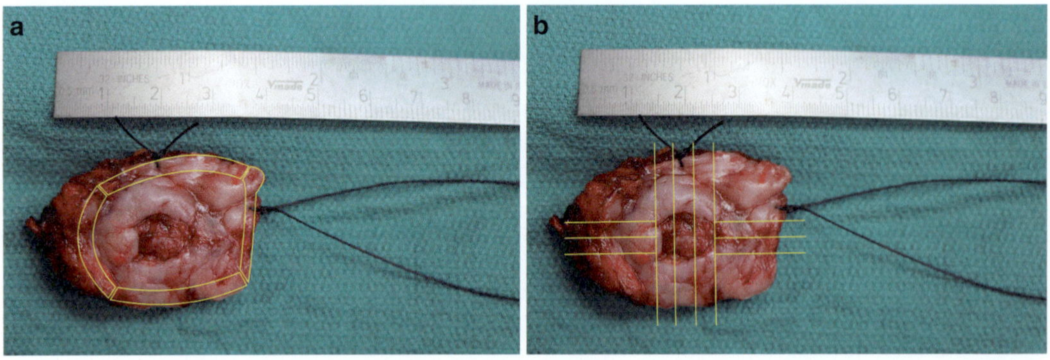

Fig. 5.9 Specimen margin assessment with (**a**) shave and (**b**) radial margins

gin to be measured, only a smaller amount of the margin is sampled. In comparison, shave margins include a large portion of the margin without the tumor and are useful for tumors far from the margin. While shave margins allow a larger area to be examined microscopically, the distance between the tumor and margin is not assessed. Shave and radial margins may both be inaccurate in tumors with discontinuous growth [65].

Three types of margins should be considered: mucosal margins, soft tissue or deep margins, and osseous margins. Deep margins include all connective tissue components including skeletal muscle, adipose tissue and neurovascular bundles. While bone is not amenable to rapid tissue analysis due to its high mineral content and need for decalcification, intraoperative bone margins assessment via cancellous bone sampling, marrow cytologic assessment, cortical bone osteotomy, and trephination have been described with high sensitivity (79–89%), specificity (98–100%), and accuracy (94–100%) [54, 66–69].

5.8 Management of the Clinically Negative Neck

Cervical node status is an independent predictor of survival in OCSCC, and nodal metastasis decreases 5-year survival by approximately 50%. Clinically overt nodal disease is present in 30% of all patients with OCSCC. However, in those with a clinically N0 neck, occult metastasis may be present in up to 34–44% of all stages and 20–30% of early stage OCSCC [70, 71]. T staging has been shown to be an independent risk factor of nodal involvement. Elective neck dissection (END) allows for both staging and treatment and is generally indicated in cN0 patients who are deemed to have a 15–20% risk of occult nodal disease based on features of the primary tumor.

Multiple studies have found improved overall survival and decreased relapse rates with END [72–78]. However, the current available evidence for END is not definitive as prospective trials have produced conflicting evidence [79–82]. The treatment of all cN0 patients with END would result in the overtreatment of a percentage of patients resulting in unnecessary cost and morbidity without evidence of a meaningful survival benefit. While END is accepted for late-stage tumors, management of the cN0 neck in early stage OCSCC remains an area of debate. Treatment options for T1T2N0 OCSCC include END, sentinel node biopsy (SNB), radiation, or watchful waiting with therapeutic neck dissection in the case of nodal relapse.

A 2015 randomized controlled clinical trial of 500 patients with T1T2N0 OCSCC found improved 3-year OS (80.0% vs. 67.5%) and DFS (69.5% vs. 45.9%) in patients that underwent an elective neck dissection versus those treated with surveillance and possible therapeutic neck dissection at a later date [83]. Multiple limitations of this study have been cited, including short follow-up duration, the omission of radiation as an option in the therapeutic neck dissection group,

Table 5.1 Cutoff DOI for oral cavity subsites over which neck dissection is indicated

Oral cavity subsite	Recommendation for neck dissection, mm
Tongue	2
Floor of mouth	2–3
Retromolar trigone	3–4
Alveolus/hard palate	3–4
All sites	2–4

Adapted from Brockhoff et al. [85]

and the inclusion of primarily high-risk patients [tongue tumors and primarily tumors with a depth of invasion (DOI) of greater than 3 mm] who would benefit from a neck dissection regardless. In addition, on multivariate analysis, while there was a survival benefit with END noted for T2 tumors, there was no survival benefit seen for T1 tumors or for tumors less than 3 mm in thickness. While END is generally indicated for T2 and above, the higher risk cohort of patients within the T1 N0 group has not yet been identified who would benefit from END.

Histologic features including DOI and tumor grade have been used to determine the need for END in early-stage SCC. DOI is an independent predictor of occult nodal metastasis; however, the cutoff DOI at which an END is indicated has not been standardized and ranges from 2 to 5 mm [84]. A retrospective review of 286 patients with OCSCC identified critical tumor depths at which the risk of occult metastasis exceeded 20% for various oral cavity subsites based on the correlation between tumor DOI and nodal positivity in surgical specimens [85]. The threshold DOIs at which END is indicated at various oral cavity subsites are shown in Table 5.1.

5.9 Extent of Neck Dissection

The extent and type of neck dissection required as a staging and therapeutic procedure remains a point of controversy (Table 5.2). The radical neck dissection (RND) described by Crile in 1906 has been traditionally used to treat nodal metastasis but is associated with significant morbidity [86].

Table 5.2 Classification of neck dissection

Type of neck dissection	Levels removed	Nonlymphatic structures removed
Radical	I, II, III, IV, V	SCM, IJV, SAN
Modified radical, type I	I, II, III, IV, V	SCM, IJV (SAN spared)
Modified radical, type II	I, II, III, IV, V	SCM (IJV, SAN spared)
Modified radical, type III (Functional)	I, II, III, IV, V	(SCM, IJV, SAN spared)
Selective neck dissection		
Supraomohyoid	I–III	
Lateral	II–IV	
Posterolateral	II–V	
Anterior	VI, VII	
Extended radical	I, II, III, IV, V, additional lymphatic groups (e.g., retropharyngeal, central compartment, mediastinal nodes)	Additional nonlymphatic structures (e.g., skin, platysma, digastric muscle, carotid artery, hypoglossal nerve, vagus nerve)

SCM sternocleidomastoid muscle, *IJV* internal jugular vein, *SAN* spinal accessory nerve

In the clinically negative neck, the selective neck dissection (SND) has been shown to be effective, but the extent of dissection has not been agreed upon. The goal of the SND is to achieve similar rates of regional control with less morbidity and operative time as compared with the RND.

The pattern of cervical node metastasis in OCSCC have been established. OCSCC typically follows a sequential metastatic pattern with the involvement of successive anatomic nodal levels from level I to V, with levels I, II, and III at greatest risk for nodal metastasis (Fig. 5.10). The risk of lower neck level metastasis and the risk of skip metastases, or the involvement of higher level nodes without the involvement of first echelon or intermediary node groups, threaten the efficacy of a selective neck dissection in regional control [87].

The reported incidence of skip metastasis past levels I and II is rare, ranging from 0% to 2%, with no skip metastasis to level V and an inci-

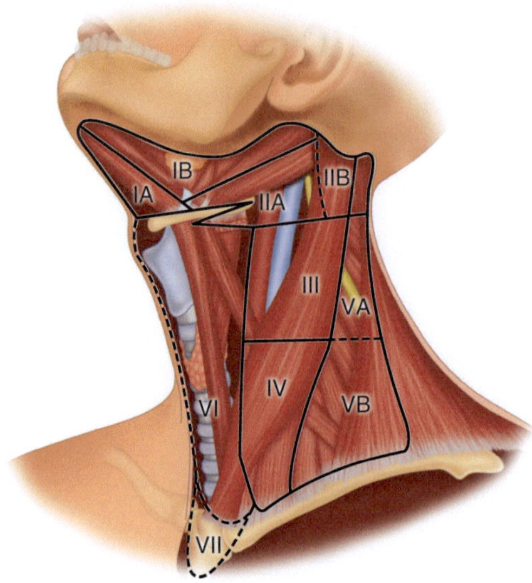

Fig. 5.10 Levels of the neck

dence of 0–1.9% to level IV [87]. A supraomohyoid neck dissection (levels I–III) is thus indicated for most N0 OCSCC. Some authors advocate for the inclusion of level IV in SND for all OCSCC as the procedure has minimal morbidity and does not significantly increase operating time [88]. In oral tongue cancer, while many studies have found no level IV involvement, up to 8% incidence of skip metastasis or subsequent recurrence in level IV has been reported. Many authors advocate for SND including levels I–IV for OCSCC of the tongue.

In the N+ neck, the incidence of level IV and V involvement ranges between 6.5% and 15% and between 2% and 6.9%, respectively [87, 89]. Therefore, modified radical neck dissection (MRND) or RND with removal of neck levels I to V is indicated in the N+ neck. When possible, the MRND has been shown to have similar oncological efficacy as compared to the RND, with comparable number of recovered lymph nodes and with less morbidity including shoulder dysfunction [90]. In a recent meta-analysis, SND was found to have similar locoregional control rates as compared to RND or MRND for select patients with limited N+ OCSCC, with adjuvant radiotherapy essential for disease control in these cases [91].

5.10 Sentinel Node Biopsy

SNB is an alternative management option of the neck in T1T2N0 OCSCC. The procedure relies on the theory that a primary oral cavity tumor drains first to a sentinel lymph node in the neck before subsequently spreading to the remaining lymph node basin. SNB has the advantages of being less invasive, more cost effective and results in a better patient quality of life; however, the diagnostic efficacy of SNB in early OCSCC is still debated [71].

Multiple techniques of SNB have been described. In general, a radioactive tracer is injected around the tumor preoperatively. Preoperative lymphoscintigraphy, intraoperative gamma probe, and/or blue dye are used for sentinel node localization. Following sentinel lymph node removal, serial sectioning and immunohistochemical staining are completed for the detection of micrometastasis. Superselection of the nodes most likely reflecting the disease status of the rest of the neck reduces the number of lymph nodes for pathologic evaluation and allows for more in-depth evaluation of the small number of sentinel nodes [92]. While pathologic evaluation of the sentinel node currently is done in a delayed fashion, early trials of intraoperative sentinel node evaluation techniques show promise [93, 94].

A meta-analysis of 66 studies of T1T2N0 OCDCC found that SNB had a pooled identification rate of 96.3%, a sensitivity of 87%, a negative predictive value of 94%, and an overall diagnostic efficacy of 94% [71]. The addition of immunohistochemistry was found to improve SNB diagnostic sensitivity. SNB has high diagnostic accuracy in T1T2N0 OCSCC and is an acceptable alternative to END. However, sentinel node analysis is currently completed by postoperative pathologic procedure, and the clinical applicability of SNB by frozen section has not yet been validated. Furthermore, the implementation of SNB requires protocolized co-ordination between surgery, pathology, and radiology departments, as well as hospital services; thus, SND has not been broadly adopted at present.

5.11 Dental Rehabilitation

Dental rehabilitation has become an integral aspect of the reconstructive plan following ablative and reconstructive surgery for patients with OCSCC. Dental implants are often necessary for prosthetic rehabilitation due to severe alterations of normal anatomy of the dental arches precluding traditional prosthetic options. In OCSCC, dental implants are used for both the retention of palatal obturators as well as for dental rehabilitation following bony reconstruction of the maxilla or mandible. Dental prosthetic design and fabrication are discussed elsewhere.

Palatal obturators are the traditional method of reconstructing maxillary defects, but retention and support by the remaining dentition, remaining palate, and maxillectomy cavity can be compromised in extensive defects. Implant-retained palatal obturators increase prosthetic retention and support, minimize unfavorable forces on the remaining dentition, and distribute force to the facial skeleton [95].

Dental implants may be placed in remaining alveolar bone or bone surrounding the maxillectomy site. Zygomatic implants are an effective alternative when conventional implant placement is not possible due to extensive bony resection, and they allow obturation in extensive defects otherwise only amenable to free flap reconstruction (Fig. 5.11). A retrospective review of 28 zygomatic implants in nine patients following maxillectomy found a 79% success rate of zygomatic implants, with failures attributed to radiation therapy [96]. Other studies have reported greater success rates of zygomatic implant rehabilitation in maxillectomy defects ranging from 94.1% to 100% [95–97].

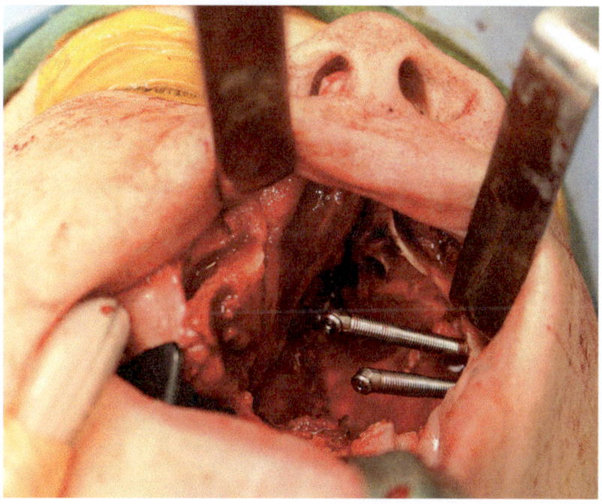

Fig. 5.11 Maxillectomy defect with zygomatic implants in place

Bony free flap reconstruction of the maxilla and mandible allows for dental rehabilitation with endosseous implants. Realistically, only a small percentage of patients will ultimately receive implant-supported prostheses due to several contributing factors including financial constraints, disease progression, flap complications, implant failure, trismus, and an inability to tolerate a prosthesis. The reported rates of dental rehabilitation following free flap reconstruction are low, ranging from 2% to 46% [98, 99]. The effect of irradiation on implant success is controversial. The success rate of endosseous implants in irradiated native bone ranges between 74% and 97% [100]. Implant success in osseous free flaps has not been shown to be significantly different with irradiation or with the timing of irradiation, with success rates ranging from 72.5% to 97.5% [101–103].

When implant restoration is planned, the prosthetic plan should be discussed with the restoring dentist or prosthodontist prior to surgery. The DCIA and fibula free flap both provide adequate bone stock for implant placement. The DCIA free flap provides adequate bone volume and height to restore the alveolus but has limited bone length, a shorter vascular pedicle, and higher risk of significant donor site morbidities. The fibula free flap provides a long bony seg-

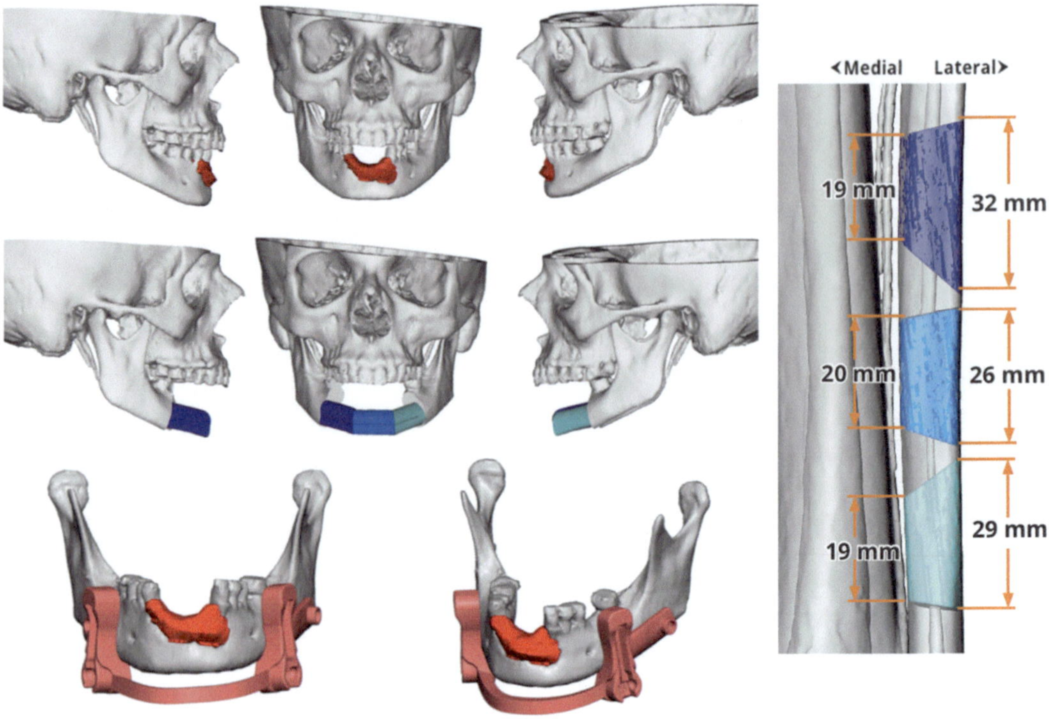

Fig. 5.12 Virtual surgery planning for resection of an anterior mandibular squamous cell carcinoma and reconstruction with fibular free flap

ment with a long pedicle, easy to harvest, but lacks vertical bone height with the fibula averaging 13–15 mm in height. To improve dental implant placement, discrepancies between the height of the dentate mandible and fibula may be overcome by fixating the fibula superiorly to the inferior mandibular border, distraction osteogenesis of fibular segments, or performing a double barrel technique [104].

5.12 Adjunct Surgical Tools

Virtual surgery planning (VSP) and guided surgery using three-dimensional printing technology have allowed for patient-specific, highly precise bony ablation, and reconstruction in OCSCC. VSP confers reproducible accuracy for maxillary and mandibular reconstructions, with a great benefit for reconstructions with multiple segments (Fig. 5.12) [105, 106]. The use of virtual planning and guided surgery have been shown to be financially favorable with costs offset by decreased operative time and subsequently decreased operating room cost [107].

Surgical navigation is a useful tool to guide oncologic resections and to improve the precision of reconstruction (Fig. 5.13) [108]. Image-guided resection has been described for resection of advanced tumors involving the skull base, sinuses, and infratemporal fossa. It has been suggested to improve the accuracy and safety in these cases, potentially leading to better local disease control [109]. Surgical navigation has also been described for the reconstruction of orbital floor defects with maxillectomy [110]. The utility of navigation in OCSCC has only started to be explored, and navigation may be a useful adjunct in the management of OCSCC in the future.

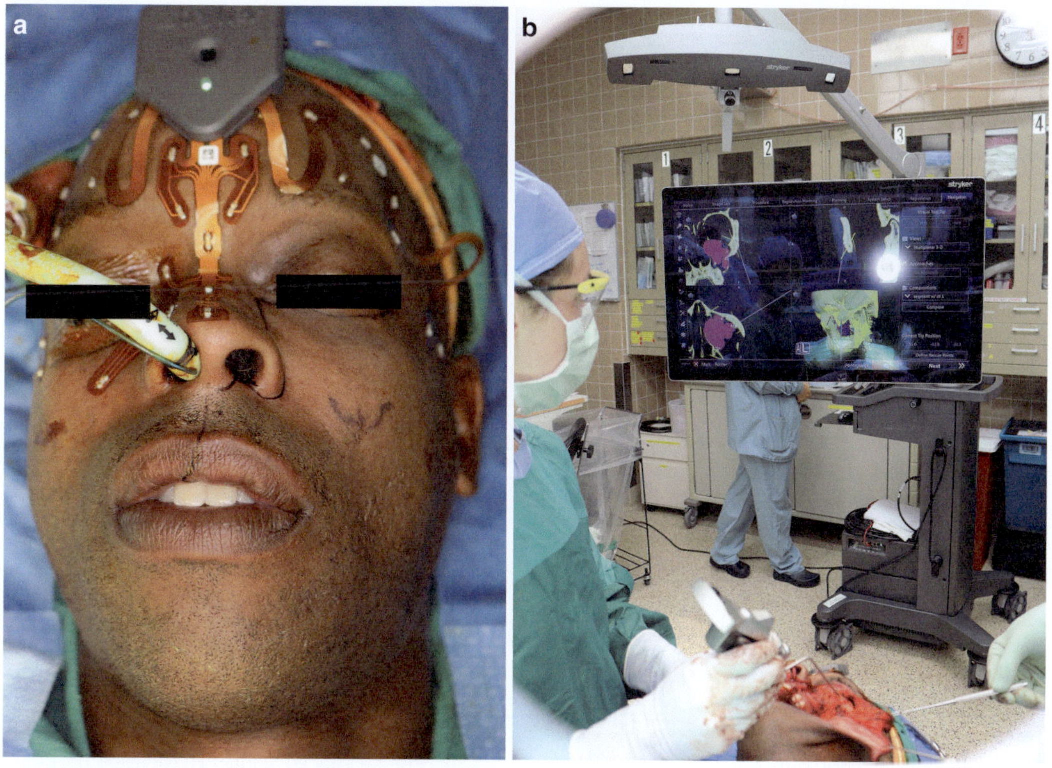

Fig. 5.13 Surgical navigation patient tracking system (**a**) and display (**b**) used in the resection of a maxillary tumor

5.13 Conclusion

Surgery remains the primary treatment modality for OCSCC, and as such, the role of the surgeon is pivotal in the management of patients with OCSCC. By considering complex patient-related, tumor-related, and procedure-related factors, the surgeon can optimize the surgical management of OCSCC and can improve surgical outcomes and overall prognosis.

Acknowledgements The authors would like to acknowledge Raea Bucher, illustrator, for providing Figs. 5.1–5.5 and 5.10 for this chapter.

References

1. Global Cancer Observatory. Cancer today. http://gco.iarc.fr/today/fact-sheets-populations. Accessed 23 Sep 2018.
2. National Comprehensive Cancer Network. NCCN clinical practice guidelines in oncology. https://www.nccn.org/professionals/physician_gls/default.aspx. Accessed 23 Sep 2018.
3. Schwam ZG, Judson BL. Improved prognosis for patients with oral cavity squamous cell carcinoma: analysis of the National Cancer Database 1998–2006. Oral Oncol. 2016;52:45.
4. Piccirillo JF. Importance of comorbidity in head and neck cancer. Laryngoscope. 2000;110:593.
5. Paleri V, Wight RG, Silver CE, Haigentz M, Takes RP, Bradley PJ, Rinaldo A, Sanabria A, Bień S, Ferlito A. Comorbidity in head and neck cancer: a critical appraisal and recommendations for practice. Oral Oncol. 2010;46:712.
6. Ferrier MB, Spuesens EB, Le Cessie S, Baatenburg de Jong RJ. Comorbidity as a major risk factor for mortality and complications in head and neck surgery. Arch Otolaryngol Head Neck Surg. 2005; 131:27.
7. Jun MY, Strong EW, Saltzman EI, Gerold FP. Head and neck cancer in the elderly. Head Neck. 1983;5:376.
8. Yamada S-I, Kurita H, Tomioka T, Ohta R, Yoshimura N, Nishimaki F, Koyama Y, Kondo E, Kamata T. Healthy life expectancy of oral squamous cell carcinoma patients aged 75 years and older. Oral Oncol. 2017;64:22.
9. Datema FR, Ferrier MB, van der Schroeff MP, de Jong RJB. Impact of comorbidity on short-term mortality

and overall survival of head and neck cancer patients. Head Neck. 2010;32:728.
10. Pogrel MA, Podlesh S, Anthony JP, Alexander J. A comparison of vascularized and nonvascularized bone grafts for reconstruction of mandibular continuity defects. J Oral Maxillofac Surg. 1997;55:1200.
11. McGregor AD, MacDonald DG. Patterns of spread of squamous cell carcinoma to the ramus of the mandible. Head Neck. 1993;15:440.
12. He Y, Zhang ZY, Zhu HG, Sader R, He J, Kovács AF. Free fibula osteocutaneous flap for primary reconstruction of T3–T4 gingival carcinoma. J Craniofac Surg. 2010;21:301.
13. Pandey M, Rao LP, Das SR, Mathews A, Chacko EM, Naik BR. Patterns of mandibular invasion in oral squamous cell carcinoma of the mandibular region. World J Surg Oncol. 2007;5:12.
14. Jewer DD, Boyd JB, Manktelow RT, Zuker RM, Rosen IB, Gullane PJ, Rotstein LE, Freeman JE. Orofacial and mandibular reconstruction with the iliac crest free flap: a review of 60 cases and a new method of classification. Plast Reconstr Surg. 1989;84:391.
15. Urken ML, Vickery C, Weinberg H, Buchbinder D, Lawson W, Biller HF. The internal oblique-iliac crest osseomyocutaneous free flap in oromandibular reconstruction: report of 20 cases. Arch Otolaryngol Head Neck Surg. 1989;115:339.
16. Kekatpure VD, Manjula BV, Mathias S, Trivedi NP, Selvam S, Kuriakose MA. Reconstruction of large composite buccal defects using single soft tissue flap—analysis of functional outcome. Microsurgery. 2013;33:184.
17. Brown JS, Rogers SN, McNally DN, Boyle M. A modified classification for the maxillectomy defect. Head Neck. 2000;22:17.
18. Okay DJ, Genden E, Buchbinder D, Urken M. Prosthodontic guidelines for surgical reconstruction of the maxilla: a classification system of defects. J Prosthet Dent. 2001;86:352.
19. Maniglia AJ. Indications and techniques of midfacial degloving: a 15-year experience. Arch Otolaryngol Head Neck Surg. 1986;112:750.
20. Davison SP, Sherris DA, Meland NB. An algorithm for maxillectomy defect reconstruction. Laryngoscope. 1998;108:215.
21. Sharaf MY, Ibrahim SI, Eskander AE, Shaker AF. Prosthetic versus surgical rehabilitation in patients with maxillary defect regarding the quality of life: systematic review. Oral Maxillofac Surg. 2018;22:1.
22. Futran ND, Wadsworth JT, Villaret D, Farwell DG. Midface reconstruction with the fibula free flap. Arch Otolaryngol Head Neck Surg. 2002;128:161.
23. Uglešić V, Virag M, Varga S, Knežević P, Milenović A. Reconstruction following radical maxillectomy with flaps supplied by the subscapular artery. J Cranio-Maxillofac Surg. 2000;28:153.
24. Moreno MA, Skoracki RJ, Hanna EY, Hanasono MM. Microvascular free flap reconstruction versus palatal obturation for maxillectomy defects. Head Neck. 2010;32:860.
25. Li W, Li R, Safdar J, Huang S, Xu Z, Tan X, Sun C. Modified visor approach applied to total or subtotal glossectomy and reconstruction: avoidance of lip splitting and mandibulotomy and cutting off mental nerve. Tumour Biol. 2014;35:7847.
26. Yuen PW, Lam KY, Chan AC, Wei WI, Lam LK. Clinicopathological analysis of local spread of carcinoma of the tongue. Am J Surg. 1998;175:242.
27. Guerin-Lebailly C, Mallet Y, Lambour V, Fournier C, Bedoui El S, Ton Van J, Lefebvre JL. Functional and sensitive outcomes after tongue reconstruction: about a series of 30 patients. Oral Oncol. 2012;48:272.
28. Kuriakose MA, Loree TR, Spies A, Meyers S, Hicks WL. Sensate radial forearm free flaps in tongue reconstruction. Arch Otolaryngol Head Neck Surg. 2001;127:1463.
29. Namin AW, Varvares MA. Functional outcomes of sensate versus insensate free flap reconstruction in oral and oropharyngeal reconstruction: a systematic review. Head Neck. 2016;38:1717.
30. Dziegielewski PT, Ho ML, Rieger J, Singh P, Langille M, Harris JR, Seikaly H. Total glossectomy with laryngeal preservation and free flap reconstruction: objective functional outcomes and systematic review of the literature. Laryngoscope. 2013;123:140.
31. Lin DT, Yarlagadda BB, Sethi RKV, Feng AL, Shnayder Y, Ledgerwood LG, Diaz JA, Sinha P, Hanasono MM, Yu P, Skoracki RJ, Lian TS, Patel UA, Leibowitz J, Purdy N, Starmer H, Richmon JD. Long-term functional outcomes of total glossectomy with or without total laryngectomy. JAMA Otolaryngol Head Neck Surg. 2015;141:797.
32. Lubek JE, Clayman L. An update on squamous carcinoma of the oral cavity, oropharynx, and maxillary sinus. Oral Maxillofac Surg Clin North Am. 2012;24:307.
33. Niu LX, Feng Z, Li JN, Li CZ, Peng X, Guo CB. Prognostic factors of squamous cell carcinoma of the buccal mucosa: a retrospective study of 168 cases in North China. J Oral Maxillofac Surg. 2014; 72:2344.
34. Lin C-S, Jen Y-M, Cheng M-F, Lin Y-S, Su W-F, Hwang J-M, Chang L-P, Chao H-L, Liu D-W, Lin H-Y, Shum W-Y. Squamous cell carcinoma of the buccal mucosa: an aggressive cancer requiring multimodality treatment. Head Neck. 2006;28:150.
35. Jan J-C, Hsu W-H, Liu S-A, Wong Y-K, Poon C-K, Jiang R-S, Jan J-S, Chen IF. Prognostic factors in patients with buccal squamous cell carcinoma: 10-year experience. J Oral Maxillofac Surg. 2011;69:396.
36. Chiou W-Y, Lin H-Y, Hsu F-C, Lee M-S, Ho H-C, Su Y-C, Lee C-C, Hsieh C-H, Wang Y-C, Hung S-K. Buccal mucosa carcinoma: surgical margin less than 3 mm, not 5 mm, predicts locoregional recurrence. Radiat Oncol. 2010;5:79.
37. Moe J, Helman JI. Surgical techniques for the management of submandibular salivary duct strictures. Atlas Oral Maxillofac Surg Clin. 2018;26:99.
38. Kurita H, Nakanishi Y, Nishizawa R, Xiao T, Kamata T, Koike T, Kobayashi H. Impact of different surgical

margin conditions on local recurrence of oral squamous cell carcinoma. Oral Oncol. 2010;46:814.
39. Loree TR, Strong EW. Significance of positive margins in oral cavity squamous carcinoma. Am J Surg. 1990;160:410.
40. Ravasz LA, Slootweg PJ, Hordijk GJ, Smit F, van der Tweel I. The status of the resection margin as a prognostic factor in the treatment of head and neck carcinoma. J Cranio-Maxillofac Surg. 1991;19:314.
41. Jacobs JR, Ahmad K, Casiano R, Schuller DE, Scott C, Laramore GE, Sarraf Al M. Implications of positive surgical margins. Laryngoscope. 1993;103:64.
42. Binahmed A, Nason RW, Abdoh AA. The clinical significance of the positive surgical margin in oral cancer. Oral Oncol. 2007;43:780.
43. Chang AMV, Kim SW, Duvvuri U, Johnson JT, Myers EN, Ferris RL, Gooding WE, Seethala RR, Chiosea SI. Early squamous cell carcinoma of the oral tongue: comparing margins obtained from the glossectomy specimen to margins from the tumor bed. Oral Oncol. 2013;49:1077.
44. Anderson CR, Sisson K, Moncrieff M. A meta-analysis of margin size and local recurrence in oral squamous cell carcinoma. Oral Oncol. 2015; 51:464.
45. Byers RM, Bland KI, Borlase B, Luna M. The prognostic and therapeutic value of frozen section determinations in the surgical treatment of squamous carcinoma of the head and neck. Am J Surg. 1978;136:525.
46. Chen TY, Emrich LJ, Driscoll DL. The clinical significance of pathological findings in surgically resected margins of the primary tumor in head and neck carcinoma. Int J Rad Oncol Biol Phys. 1987;13:833.
47. Jones AS. Prognosis in mouth cancer: tumour factors. Eur J Cancer B Oral Oncol. 1994;30:8.
48. Scholl P, Byers RM, Batsakis JG, Wolf P, Santini H. Microscopic cut-through of cancer in the surgical treatment of squamous carcinoma of the tongue: prognostic and therapeutic implications. Am J Surg. 1986;152:354.
49. Sieczka E, Datta R, Singh A, Loree T, Rigual N, Orner J, Hicks W Jr. Cancer of the buccal mucosa: are margins and T-stage accurate predictors of local control? Am J Otolaryngol. 2001;22:395.
50. Brandwein-Gensler M, Teixeira MS, Lewis CM, Lee B, Rolnitzky L, Hille JJ, Genden E, Urken ML, Wang BY. Oral squamous cell carcinoma: histologic risk assessment, but not margin status, is strongly predictive of local disease-free and overall survival. Am J Surg Pathol. 2005;29:167.
51. Colevas AD, Yom SS, Pfister DG, Spencer S, Adelstein D, Adkins D, Brizel DM, Burtness B, Busse PM, Caudell JJ, Cmelak AJ, Eisele DW, Fenton M, Foote RL, Gilbert J, Gillison ML, Haddad RI, Hicks WL, Hitchcock YJ, Jimeno A, Leizman D, Maghami E, Mell LK, Mittal BB, Pinto HA, Ridge JA, Rocco J, Rodriguez CP, Shah JP, Weber RS, Witek M, Worden F, Zhen W, Burns JL, Darlow SD. NCCN guidelines insights: head and neck cancers, version 1.2018. J Natl Compr Canc Netw. 2018;16:479.
52. Zanoni DK, Migliacci JC, Xu B, Katabi N, Montero PH, Ganly I, Shah JP, Wong RJ, Ghossein RA, Patel SG. A proposal to redefine close surgical margins in squamous cell carcinoma of the oral tongue. JAMA Otolaryngol Head Neck Surg. 2017;143:555.
53. Mistry RC, Qureshi SS, Kumaran C. Post-resection mucosal margin shrinkage in oral cancer: quantification and significance. J Surg Oncol. 2005;91:131.
54. Hinni ML, Ferlito A, Brandwein-Gensler MS, Takes RP, Silver CE, Westra WH, Seethala RR, Rodrigo JP, Corry J, Bradford CR, Hunt JL, Strojan P, Devaney KO, Gnepp DR, Hartl DM, Kowalski LP, Rinaldo A, Barnes L. Surgical margins in head and neck cancer: a contemporary review. Head Neck. 2013;35:1362.
55. Cheng A, Cox D, Schmidt BL. Oral squamous cell carcinoma margin discrepancy after resection and pathologic processing. J Oral Maxillofac Surg. 2008;66:523.
56. Du E, Ow TJ, Lo Y-T, Gersten A, Schiff BA, Tassler AB, Smith RV. Refining the utility and role of frozen section in head and neck squamous cell carcinoma resection. Laryngoscope. 2016;126:1768.
57. DiNardo LJ, Lin J, Karageorge LS, Powers CN. Accuracy, utility, and cost of frozen section margins in head and neck cancer surgery. Laryngoscope. 2000;110:1773.
58. Ord RA, Aisner S. Accuracy of frozen sections in assessing margins in oral cancer resection. J Oral Maxillofac Surg. 1997;55:663.
59. Ettl T, El-Gindi A, Hautmann M, Gosau M, Weber F, Rohrmeier C, Gerken M, Müller S, Reichert T, Klingelhöffer C. Positive frozen section margins predict local recurrence in R0-resected squamous cell carcinoma of the head and neck. Oral Oncol. 2016;55:17
60. Patel RS, Goldstein DP, Guillemaud J, Bruch GA, Brown D, Gilbert RW, Gullane PJ, Higgins KM, Irish J, Enepekides DJ. Impact of positive frozen section microscopic tumor cut-through revised to negative on oral carcinoma control and survival rates. Head Neck. 2010;32:1444.
61. Varvares MA, Poti S, Kenyon B, Christopher K, Walker RJ. Surgical margins and primary site resection in achieving local control in oral cancer resections. Laryngoscope. 2015;125:2298.
62. Kerawala CJ, Ong TK. Relocating the site of frozen sections? Is there room for improvement? Head Neck. 2001;23:230.
63. Shapiro M, Salama A. Margin analysis: squamous cell carcinoma of the oral cavity. Oral Maxillofac Surg Clin. 2017;29:259.
64. Yahalom R, Dobriyan A, Vered M, Talmi YP, Teicher S, Bedrin L. A prospective study of surgical margin status in oral squamous cell carcinoma: a preliminary report. J Surg Oncol. 2008;98:572.
65. Chiosea SI. Intraoperative margin assessment in early oral squamous cell carcinoma. Surg Pathol Clin. 2017;10:1.
66. Arick Forrest L, Schuller DE, Karanfilov B, Lucas JG. Update on intraoperative analysis of mandibular margins. Am J Otolaryngol. 1997;18:396.

67. Mahmood S, Conway D, Ramesar KCRB. Use of intraoperative cytologic assessment of mandibular marrow scrapings to predict resection margin status in patients with squamous cell carcinoma. J Oral Maxillofac Surg. 2001;59:1138.
68. Oxford LE, Ducic Y. Intraoperative evaluation of cortical bony margins with frozen-section analysis. Otolaryngol Head Neck Surg. 2016;134:138.
69. Wysluch A, Stricker I, Hölzle F, Wolff K-D, Maurer P. Intraoperative evaluation of bony margins with frozen-section analysis and trephine drill extraction technique: a preliminary study. Head Neck. 2010;32:1473.
70. Greenberg JS, Naggar El AK, Mo V, Roberts D, Myers JN. Disparity in pathologic and clinical lymph node staging in oral tongue carcinoma. Cancer. 2003;98:508.
71. Liu M, Wang SJ, Yang X, Peng H. Diagnostic efficacy of sentinel lymph node biopsy in early oral squamous cell carcinoma: a meta-analysis of 66 studies. PLoS ONE. 2017;12:e0170322.
72. Lydiatt DD, Robbins KT, Byers RM, Wolf PF. Treatment of stage I and II oral tongue cancer. Head Neck. 1993;15:308.
73. Yuen APW, Wei WI, Wong YM, Tang KC. Elective neck dissection versus observation in the treatment of early oral tongue carcinoma. Head Neck. 1997;19:583.
74. Haddadin KJ, Soutar DS, Oliver RJ, Webster MH, Robertson AG, MacDonald DG. Improved survival for patients with clinically T1/T2, N0 tongue tumors undergoing a prophylactic neck dissection. Head Neck. 1999;21:517.
75. Keski-Säntti H, Atula T, Törnwall J, Koivunen P, Mäkitie A. Elective neck treatment versus observation in patients with T1/T2 N0 squamous cell carcinoma of oral tongue. Oral Oncol. 2006;42:95.
76. Capote A, Escorial V, Guerra MFM, Campo FJR, Gamallo C, Naval L. Elective neck dissection in early-stage oral squamous cell carcinoma—does it influence recurrence and survival? Head Neck. 2007;29:3.
77. Huang SF, Kang C-J, Lin CY, Fan KH, Yen T-C, Wang H-M, Chen IH, Liao C-T, Cheng AJ, Chang JTC. Neck treatment of patients with early stage oral tongue cancer. Cancer. 2008;112:1066.
78. Huang SF, Tung-Chieh Chang J, Liao C-T, Kang C-J, Lin C-Y, Fan KH, Wang H-M, Chen IH. The role of elective neck dissection in early stage buccal cancer. Laryngoscope. 2014;125:128.
79. Vandenbrouck C, Garnier HS, Chassagne D, Saravane D, Cachin Y, Micheau C. Elective versus therapeutic radical neck dissection in epidermoid carcinoma of the oral. Cavity results of a randomized clinical trial. Cancer. 1980;46:386.
80. Fakih AR, Rao RS, Borges AM, Patel AR. Elective versus therapeutic neck dissection in early carcinoma of the oral tongue. Am J Surg. 1989;158:309.
81. Kligerman J, Lima RA, Soares JR, Prado L, Dias FL, Freitas EQ, Olivatto LO. Supraomohyoid neck dissection in the treatment of T1/T2 squamous cell carcinoma of oral cavity. Am J Surg. 1994;168:391.
82. Yuen APW, Ho CM, Chow TL, Tang LC, Cheung WY, Ng RWM, Wei WI, Kong CK, Book KS, Yuen WC, Lam AKY, Yuen NWF, Smith NJT, Chan YW, Wong BYH, Li GKH, Ho ACW, Ho WK, Wong SY, Yao TJ. Prospective randomized study of selective neck dissection versus observation for N0 neck of early tongue carcinoma. Head Neck. 2009;31:765.
83. D'Cruz AK, Vaish R, Kapre N, Dandekar M, Gupta S, Hawaldar R, Agarwal JP, Pantvaidya G, Chaukar D, Deshmukh A, Kane S, Arya S, Ghosh-Laskar S, Chaturvedi P, Pai P, Nair S, Nair D, Badwe R, Head and Neck Disease Management Group. Elective versus therapeutic neck dissection in node-negative oral cancer. N Engl J Med. 2015;373:521.
84. Pentenero M, Gandolfo S, Carrozzo M. Importance of tumor thickness and depth of invasion in nodal involvement and prognosis of oral squamous cell carcinoma: a review of the literature. Head Neck. 2005;27:1080.
85. Brockhoff HC, Kim RY, Braun TM, Skouteris C, Helman JI, Ward BB. Correlating the depth of invasion at specific anatomic locations with the risk for regional metastatic disease to lymph nodes in the neck for oral squamous cell carcinoma. Head Neck. 2017;39:974.
86. Crile G. Landmark article Dec 1, 1906: excision of cancer of the head and neck. With special reference to the plan of dissection based on one hundred and thirty-two operations. JAMA. 1987;258:3286–93.
87. Patel S, Sakthivel P, Singh I, Gulati A, Gupta D. Frequency of skip metastases in oral cancer: an overview. Int J Head Neck Surg. 2015;6:80.
88. Cariati P, Cabello Serrano A, Fernandez Solis J, Martinez Lara I. Distribution of cervical metastasis in tongue cancer: are occult metastases predictable? A retrospective study of 117 oral tongue carcinomas. J Craniomaxillofac Surg. 2018;46:155.
89. Feng Z, Li JN, Niu LX, Guo CB. Supraomohyoid neck dissection in the management of oral squamous cell carcinoma: special consideration for skip metastases at level IV or V. J Oral Maxillofac Surg. 2014;72:1203.
90. Kohler HF, Cunha IWD, Kowalski LP. Impact of modified radical neck dissections on the number of retrieved nodes, recurrence and survival. Braz J Otorhinolaryngol. 2010;76:374.
91. Rodrigo JP, Grilli G, Shah JP, Medina JE, Robbins KT, Takes RP, Hamoir M, Kowalski LP, Suárez C, López F, Quer M, Boedeker CC, de Bree R, Coskun H, Rinaldo A, Silver CE, Ferlito A. Selective neck dissection in surgically treated head and neck squamous cell carcinoma patients with a clinically positive neck: systematic review. Eur J Surg Oncol. 2018;44:395.
92. Alkureishi LWT, Ross GL, Shoaib T, Soutar DS, Robertson AG, Thompson R, Hunter KD, Sorensen JA, Thomsen J, Krogdahl A, Alvarez J, Barbier L, Santamaria J, Poli T, Sesenna E, Kovács AF, Grünwald F, Barzan L, Sulfaro S, Alberti F. Sentinel node biopsy in head and neck squamous cell cancer: 5-year follow-up of a European Multicenter Trial. Ann Surg Oncol. 2010;17:2459.
93. Ferris RL, Stefanika P, Xi L, Gooding W, Seethala RR, Godfrey TE. Rapid molecular detection of metastatic head and neck squamous cell carcinoma as an intraoperative adjunct to sentinel lymph node biopsy. Laryngoscope. 2012;122:1020.

94. Shaw R, Christensen A, Java K, Maddani El R, Liloglou T, Asterios T, Buchwald von C, Wessel I, Kiss K, Kjaer A, Lelkaitis G, Long A, Risk J, Robinson M. Intraoperative sentinel lymph node evaluation: implications of cytokeratin 19 expression for the adoption of OSNA in oral squamous cell carcinoma. Ann Surg Oncol. 2016;23:4042.
95. Boyes-Varley JG, Howes DG, Davidge-Pitts KD, Branemark I, McAlpine JA. A protocol for maxillary reconstruction following oncology resection using zygomatic implants. Int J Prosthodont. 2007;20:521.
96. Schmidt BL, Pogrel MA, Young CW, Sharma A. Reconstruction of extensive maxillary defects using zygomaticus implants. J Oral Maxillofac Surg. 2004;62:82.
97. Zwahlen RA, Grätz KW, Oechslin CK, Studer SP. Survival rate of zygomatic implants in atrophic or partially resected maxillae prior to functional loading: a retrospective clinical report. Int J Oral Maxillofac Implants. 2006;21:413.
98. van Gemert JTM, van Es RJJ, Rosenberg AJWP, van der Bilt A, Koole R, Van Cann EM. Free vascularized flaps for reconstruction of the mandible: complications, success, and dental rehabilitation. J Oral Maxillofac Surg. 2012;70:1692.
99. Barrowman RA, Wilson PR, Wiesenfeld D. Oral rehabilitation with dental implants after cancer treatment. Aust Dent J. 2011;56:160.
100. Shugaa-Addin B, Al-Shamiri H-M, Al-Maweri S, Tarakji B. The effect of radiotherapy on survival of dental implants in head and neck cancer patients. J Clin Exp Dent. 2016;8:e194.
101. Sclaroff A, Haughey B, Gay WD, Paniello R. Immediate mandibular reconstruction and placement of dental implants: at the time of ablative surgery. Oral Surg Oral Med Oral Pathol Oral Radiol. 1994;78:711.
102. Salinas TJ, Desa VP, Katsnelson A, Miloro M. Clinical evaluation of implants in radiated fibula flaps. J Oral Maxillofac Surg. 2010;68:524.
103. Jackson RS, Price DL, Arce K, Moore EJ. Evaluation of clinical outcomes of osseointegrated dental implantation of fibula free flaps for mandibular reconstruction. JAMA Facial Plast Surg. 2016;18:201.
104. He Y, Zhang ZY, Zhu HG, Wu YQ, Fu HH. Double-Barrel fibula vascularized free flap with dental rehabilitation for mandibular reconstruction. J Oral Maxillofac Surg. 2011;69:2663.
105. Zweifel DF, Simon C, Hoarau R, Pasche P, Broome M. Are virtual planning and guided surgery for head and neck reconstruction economically viable? J Oral Maxillofac Surg. 2015;73:170.
106. Metzler P, Geiger EJ, Alcon A, Ma X, Steinbacher DM. Three-dimensional virtual surgery accuracy for free fibula mandibular reconstruction: planned versus actual results. J Oral Maxillofac Surg. 2014;72:2601.
107. Roser SM, Ramachandra S, Blair H, Grist W, Carlson GW, Christensen AM, Weimer KA, Steed MB. The accuracy of virtual surgical planning in free fibula mandibular reconstruction: comparison of planned and final results. J Oral Maxillofac Surg. 2010;68:2824.
108. Azarmehr I, Stokbro K, Bell RB, Thygesen T. Surgical navigation: a systematic review of indications, treatments, and outcomes in oral and maxillofacial surgery. J Oral Maxillofac Surg. 2017;75:1987.
109. Feichtinger M, Pau M, Zemann W, Aigner RM, Kärcher H. Intraoperative control of resection margins in advanced head and neck cancer using a 3D-navigation system based on PET/CT image fusion. J Cranio-Maxillofac Surg. 2010;38:589.
110. Zhang W-B, Mao C, Liu X-J, Guo CB, Yu G-Y, Peng X. Outcomes of orbital floor reconstruction after extensive maxillectomy using the computer-assisted fabricated individual titanium mesh technique. J Oral Maxillofac Surg. 2015;73:20653.e1.

6 Pathological Factors Affecting Outcomes in Oral Cancer

Eric R. Carlson and J. Michael McCoy

It has been estimated that 300,000 new cases of oral cancer are diagnosed internationally on an annual basis [1]. These cancers represent the sixth most common cancer and account for approximately 140,000 deaths each year [1]. Squamous cell carcinoma accounts for 90% of oral cancer cases. The major risk factors associated with squamous cell carcinoma of the oral cavity include smoked and smokeless tobacco with a synergistic association with alcohol consumption and a clear dose–response relationship [2]. Human papillomavirus is noted in association with approximately 1–10% of cases of oral squamous cell carcinoma [3]. While impressive improvement has occurred in our comprehension of the molecular biology associated with the development of oral cancer and the staging of these malignancies, only modest improvements in outcomes have been realized over the past 50 years. In fact, patients with similar stages of disease may demonstrate very different clinical courses even when treated with identical regimens [1]. As such, the search for reliable and uniform prognostic indices is an important venture to elucidate our true understanding of these complex malignancies and to guide treatment accordingly. To this end, the poor prognosis of oral cavity squamous cell carcinoma is seen related to high-grade cancers, increased depth of invasion, perineural invasion, noncohesive patterns of invasion, high-grade dysplasia at the surgical margins, positive margins, and cervical lymph node metastases with or without extracapsular extension and soft tissue spread. It is the purpose of this chapter to discuss these and other unfavorable pathologic features of oral squamous cell carcinoma while citing the international literature that represents a great source of prognostic information. Where appropriate, adverse feature driven recommendations for the administration of adjuvant therapy will be discussed.

E. R. Carlson (✉)
Department of Oral and Maxillofacial Surgery, University of Tennessee Graduate School of Medicine, Knoxville, TN, USA

Oral/Head and Neck Oncologic Surgery Fellowship Program, University of Tennessee Cancer Institute, Knoxville, TN, USA

Oral and Maxillofacial Surgery Residency Program, Department of Oral and Maxillofacial Surgery, University of Tennessee Graduate School of Medicine, Knoxville, TN, USA
e-mail: ecarlson@mc.utmck.edu

J. M. McCoy
Department of Oral and Maxillofacial Surgery, University of Tennessee Graduate School of Medicine, Knoxville, TN, USA

Oral and Maxillofacial Surgery Residency Program, Department of Oral and Maxillofacial Surgery, University of Tennessee Graduate School of Medicine, Knoxville, TN, USA

Department of Pathology, University of Tennessee Graduate School of Medicine, Knoxville, TN, USA

Department of Radiology, University of Tennessee Graduate School of Medicine, Knoxville, TN, USA
e-mail: mmccoy@mc.utmck.edu

D. Kademani (ed.), *Improving Outcomes in Oral Cancer*,
https://doi.org/10.1007/978-3-030-30094-4_6

6.1 American Joint Committee on Cancer (AJCC)/Union Internationale Contre le Cancer (UICC) Tumor Node Metastasis (TNM) Staging System

The tumor node metastasis (TNM) staging for classification of human cancers was initially established and published by Pierre Denoix in 1952 [4], and the first edition of the Union Internationale Contre le Cancer (UICC) TNM classification of malignant tumors was published in 1953. The American Joint Committee on Cancer (AJCC) was established in 1959 and published its first cancer staging manual in 1977. The collaboration of the UICC and the AJCC resulted in the creation of a universal system for the classification of tumors of epithelial origin. The eighth edition was published in 2016 for use effective in 2017. Of note are the designations of tumor depth of invasion (DOI) in the T classification and extranodal extension (ENE) in the N classification (Table 6.1). It has been recognized for decades that the prognosis of oral cancer worsens when the tumor is thicker [5]. More recent data suggest that depth of invasion is a better prognostic index than tumor thickness and cancers demonstrating higher grade and depths of invasion of 5 mm or greater should be considered for adjuvant radiation therapy [6]. Depth of invasion will adjust the T category, emphasizing the distinction between superficial or exophytic tumors (Fig. 6.1) and those that are more invasive or endophytic (Fig. 6.2). Staging no longer depends solely upon greatest surface dimension. Since data reported from a large international collaborative study of oral cancer demonstrated a significant difference in outcomes between T1 tumors with more than 5 mm DOI and T2 through T4 tumors with greater than 10 mm DOI, the T category for OCC has been modified in the eighth edition to improve hazard discrimination [7]. Therein, for every 5-mm increase in DOI, both cT and pT categories will increase one level according to the following: 5 mm, >5 mm but <10 mm, and >10 mm. Pathologically, DOI is

Table 6.1 The eighth edition of the AJCC staging of oral cancer

TX	Primary tumor cannot be assessed
Tis:	Carcinoma in situ
T1:	Tumor <2 cm; less than or equal to 5 mm depth of invasion (DOI)
T2:	Tumor less than or equal to 2 cm, DOI > 5 mm and less than or equal to 10 mm, or tumor >2 cm but <4 cm, and less than or equal to 10 mm DOI
T3:	Tumor >4 cm or any tumor >10 mm DOI
T4:	Moderately advanced or very advanced local disease
T4a:	Moderately advanced local disease: (lip) tumor invades through cortical bone or involves the inferior alveolar nerve, floor of mouth, or skin of face (i.e., chin or nose); (oral cavity) tumor invades adjacent structures only (e.g., through cortical bone of the mandible or maxilla, or involves the maxillary sinus or skin of the face); note that superficial erosion of bone/tooth socket (alone) by a gingival primary is not sufficient to classify a tumor as T4
T4b:	Very advanced local disease; tumor invades masticator space, pterygoid plates, or skull base and/or encases the internal carotid artery
NX	Regional lymph nodes cannot be assessed
N0:	No regional lymph node metastasis
N1:	Metastasis in a single ipsilateral lymph node, 3 cm or less in greatest dimension and ENE-negative
N2:	Metastasis in a single ipsilateral lymph node, 3 cm or less in greatest dimension and ENE-positive; or more than 3 cm but not more than 6 cm in greatest dimension and ENE-negative; or metastases in multiple ipsilateral lymph nodes, none more than 6 cm in greatest dimension and ENE-negative; or metastasis in bilateral or contralateral lymph nodes, none more than 6 cm in greatest dimension, ENE-negative
N2a:	Metastasis in a single ipsilateral or contralateral lymph node 3 cm or less in greatest dimension and ENE-positive; or metastasis in a single ipsilateral lymph node more than 3 cm but not more than 6 cm in greatest dimension and ENE-negative
N2b:	Metastasis in multiple ipsilateral lymph nodes, none more than 6 cm in greatest dimension and ENE-negative
N2c:	Metastasis in bilateral or contralateral lymph nodes, none more than 6 cm in greatest dimension and ENE-negative
N3:	Metastasis in a lymph node more than 6 cm in greatest dimension and ENE-negative; or metastasis in a single ipsilateral lymph node more than 3 cm in greatest dimension and ENE-positive; or metastasis in multiple ipsilateral, contralateral, or bilateral lymph nodes, with any ENE-positive

Table 6.1 (continued)

N3a: Metastasis in a lymph node more than 6 cm in greatest dimension and ENE-negative
N3b: Metastasis in a single ipsilateral node more than 3 cm in greatest dimension and ENE-positive; or metastasis in multiple ipsilateral, contralateral, or bilateral lymph nodes, with any ENE-positive

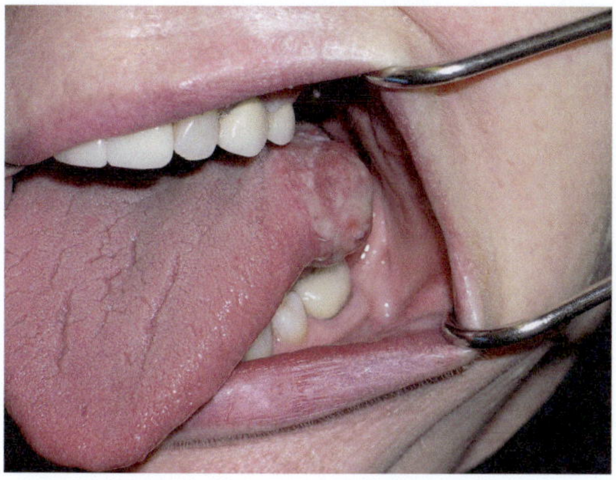

Fig. 6.1 An exophytic, stage II squamous cell carcinoma of the left tongue that exhibited a tumor thickness of approximately 1 cm and a depth of invasion of 3 mm

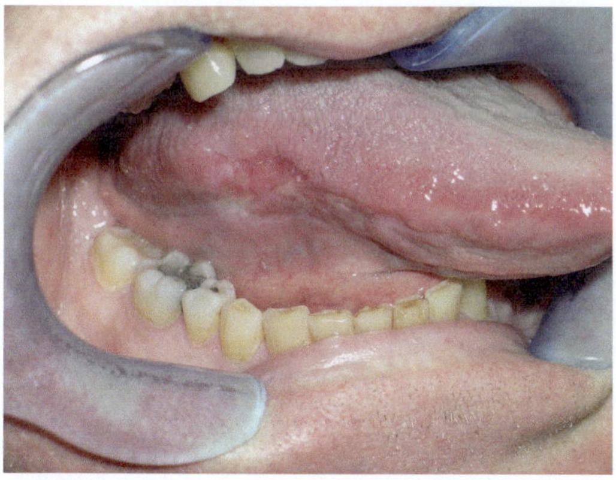

Fig. 6.2 An endophytic, stage II squamous cell carcinoma of the left tongue that exhibited a tumor thickness of approximately 1 cm and a depth of invasion of 8 mm. Compared to the tongue cancer illustrated in Fig. 6.1, this endophytic cancer with a larger depth of invasion has a more ominous prognosis, even with an identical tumor thickness

measured from the level of the basement membrane of the closest adjacent normal mucosa. The depth of invasion is measured as a perpendicular distance of the deepest point of tumor invasion from this line.

6.2 Grade

The grade of a human cancer has frequently been applied to a diagnosis to predict that cancer's prognosis. Grading systems are thought to represent practical prognostic indices that merely require tumor staining with hematoxylin and eosin (H&E) and a seasoned pathologist. Historical examples include the Nottingham histologic grade for breast cancer [8] and the Gleason grading scale for prostate cancer [9]. In terms of oral/head and neck cancer, Broders evaluated 537 cases of squamous cell carcinoma of the lip in 1920 and was the initial author to recommend a grading system that stratified patients based on the degree of differentiation of neoplastic cells and mitoses, with a special emphasis placed on differentiation [10]. The grading system was established with a score of 1–4. A grade of 1 was created for those tumors that showed three fourths of its structure to be differentiated epithelium and one fourth undifferentiated (Fig. 6.3). A grade of 2 was assigned to those tumors in which the differentiated and undifferentiated epithelium were essentially equivalent (Fig. 6.4). A grade of 3 was assigned to tumors in which the undifferentiated epithelium formed about three fourths and the differentiated tumor one fourth (Fig. 6.5), and a grade 4 tumor was one in which there was no tendency of the cells to differentiate (Fig. 6.6). The number of mitotic figures and cells with single large deeply staining nucleoli played an integral but secondary role in the grading of Broders' lip cancers. In terms of prognosis, 40 of 45 (88.88%) of patients with grade 1 tumors were alive, 128 of 192 (66.66%) patients with grade 2 tumors were alive, 16 of 65 (24.6%) of patients with grade 3 tumors were alive, and 0 patients with grade 4 tumors were alive during Broders' period of study.

The 2005 World Health Organization (WHO) classification [11] of oral squamous cell carcinoma places tumors into one of three categories, and the 2017 classification is unchanged in this regard [12]. Well-differentiated cancers resemble normal squamous epithelium (Fig. 6.7). Moderately differentiated cancers contain obvious nuclear pleomorphic and mitotic activity, including abnormal mitoses and less keratiniza-

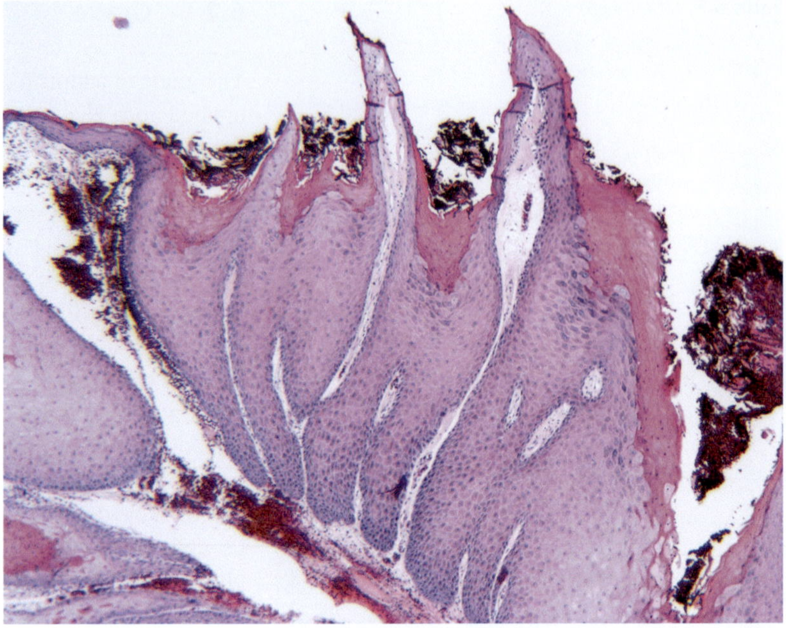

Fig. 6.3 Broders grade 1 squamous cell carcinoma. Near normal maturation of the epithelium is noted. (Hematoxylin & eosin, original magnification ×100)

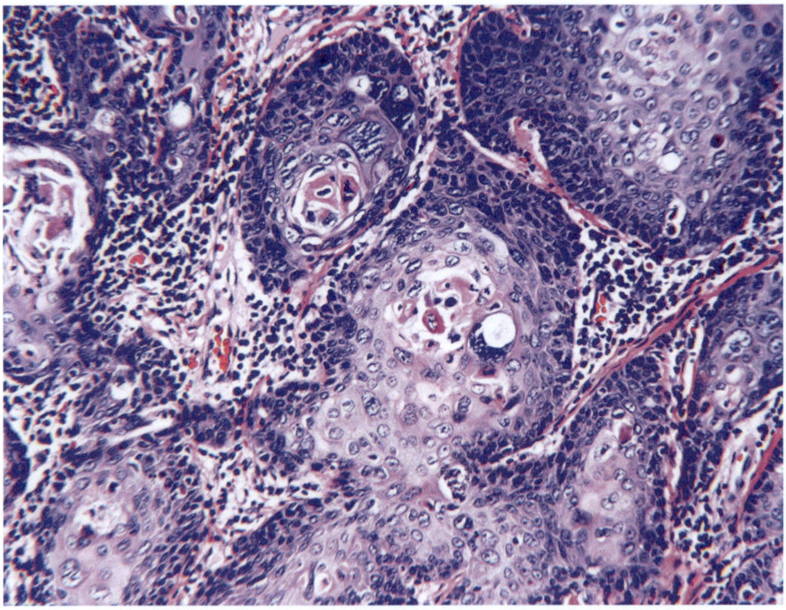

Fig. 6.4 Broders grade 2 squamous cell carcinoma. Multiple atypical cells exist, but some similarity of normal squamous maturation is noted in this specimen. (Hematoxylin & eosin, original magnification ×200)

tion (Fig. 6.8). In poorly differentiated tumors, immature cells are most common, and abundant typical and atypical mitoses are present with minimal or no keratinization (Fig. 6.9). The shortcoming of the Broders and WHO grading systems is that oral squamous cell carcinoma is most commonly a nonhomogenous tumor that presents in multiple stages of differentiation such that a lack of correlation between these classifications and prognosis exists and limits their prognostic utility [13]. As such, in 1973, Jacobsson et al. [14] and, in 1987, Anneroth et al. [15] developed a multifactorial grading system that assesses the histologic grading of the cancer based on three morphologic parameters of the tumor cells including the degree of keratinization,

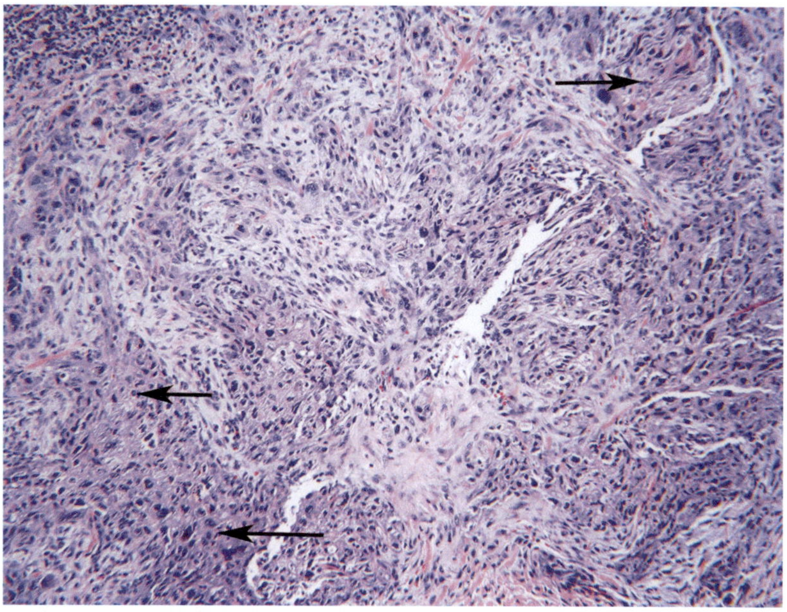

Fig. 6.5 Broders grade 3 squamous cell carcinoma. Only a few malignant cells (arrows) resemble their squamous origin. (Hematoxylin & eosin, original magnification ×100)

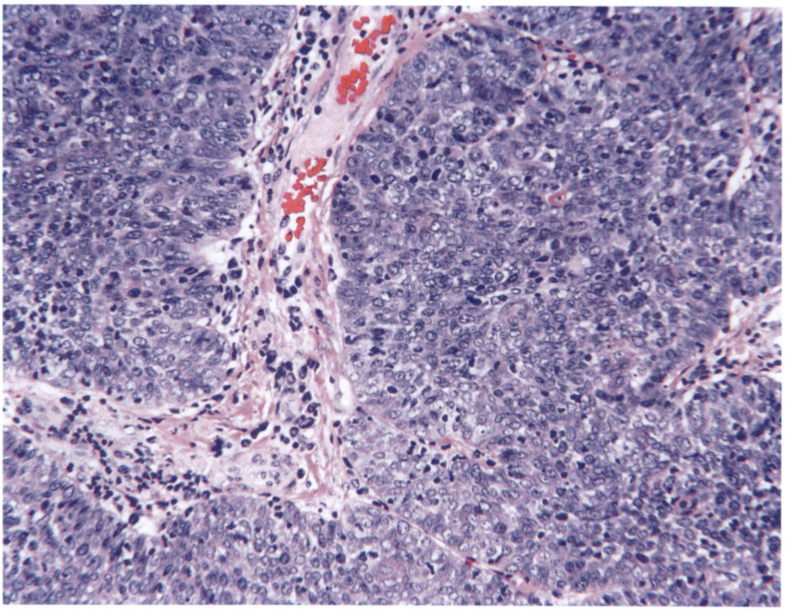

Fig. 6.6 Broders grade 4 squamous cell carcinoma. Tumor cells no longer appear squamous in origin. (Hematoxylin & eosin, original magnification ×100)

nuclear polymorphism, and number of mitoses per high-power field. In addition, the histologic grading of malignancy of the tumor–host relationship is assessed by three anatomic parameters including the pattern of invasion, the stage of invasion (depth), and lymphoplasmocytic infiltration (Table 6.2). Scores of 1–4 are assigned to each category, and the scores are subsequently added. A grade is assigned as follows: grade I (6–12), grade II (13–18), and grade III (19–24). In 1989 Bryne [13] introduced the concept that the more invasive front of the tumor should be examined since this area contains the part of the tumor that contains cells likely to determine the clinical behavior of the malignancy. The histologically invasive areas might be responsible for

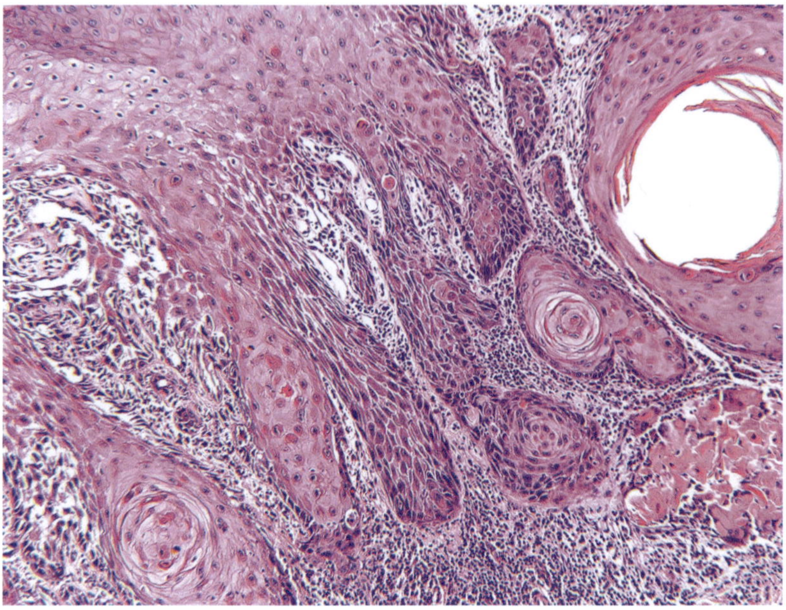

Fig. 6.7 Well-differentiated squamous cell carcinoma. Note the keratin-producing squamous cells that resemble normal squamous cell growth. (Hematoxylin & eosin, original magnification ×100)

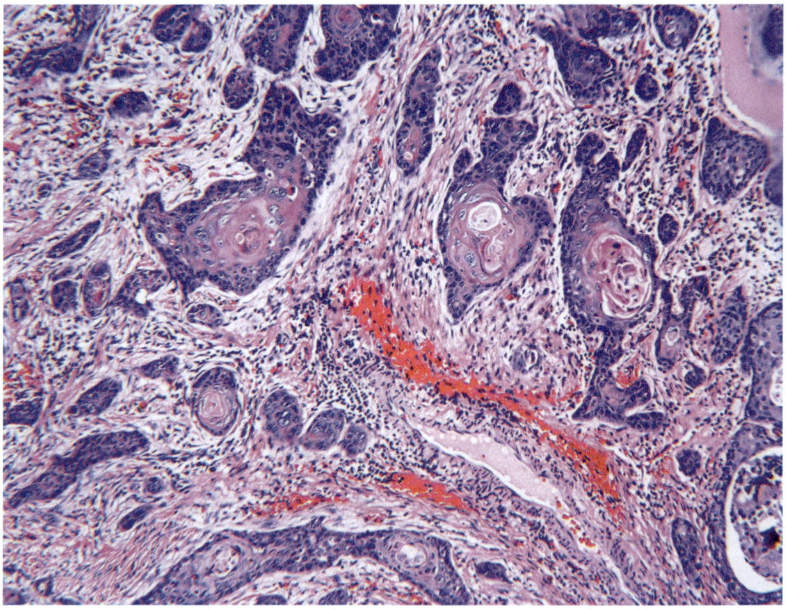

Fig. 6.8 Moderately differentiated squamous cell carcinoma. Each island of tumor still produces keratin but contains many more atypical cells. (Hematoxylin & eosin, original magnification ×100)

metastases, therefore being most prognostically significant, and therefore being of importance in terms of specific therapy for the malignancy. A small biopsy to merely establish the diagnosis of the tumor might not include the metastatic phenotype within the tumor such that the evaluation of definitively resected malignancies provides more accurate prognostic information than the corresponding incisional biopsy specimens. The dilemma is obviously seen in that the nonrepresentative nature of incisional biopsies forms the basis for surgical treatment that may introduce errors in surgical treatment under the circumstances. Bryne stated that this grading system

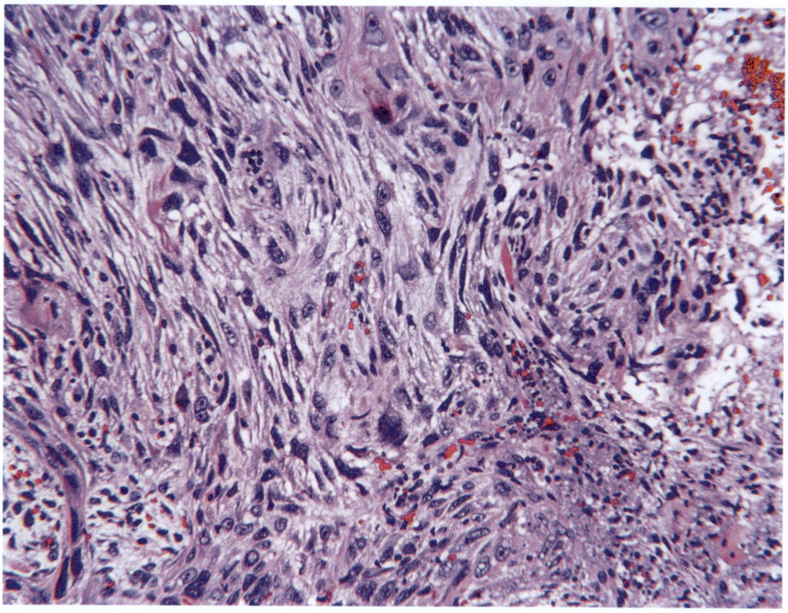

Fig. 6.9 Poorly differentiated squamous cell carcinoma. Each malignant spindle cell no longer has the microscopic appearance of its squamous origin. (Hematoxylin & eosin, original magnification ×200)

Table 6.2 Points attributed to each category of the different parameters used in Anneroth's and Bryne's grading systems

	Points			
Parameter	1	2	3	4
Degree of keratinization	Highly keratinized (>50% of the cells)	Moderately keratinized (20–50% of cells)	Minimal keratinization (5–20% of cells)	No keratinization (0–5% of cells)
Nuclear pleomorphism	Little nuclear pleomorphism (>75% of mature cells)	Moderately nuclear pleomorphism (50–75% of mature cells)	Abundant nuclear pleomorphism (25–50% of mature cells)	Extreme nuclear pleomorphism (0–25% of mature cells)
Number of mitosis/HPF[a]	0–1	2–3	4–5	>5
Pattern of invasion	Pushing, well-delineated infiltrating borders	Infiltrating solid cords	Small groups or cords of infiltrating cells ($n > 15$)	Marked and wide spread cellular dissociation in small groups ($n < 15$) and/or in single cells
Stage of invasion[b]	Carcinoma in situ and/or questionable invasion	Distinct invasion but involving lamina propria only	Invasion below lamina propria adjacent to muscles, salivary gland tissues, and periosteum	Extensive and deep invasion replacing most of the stromal tissue and infiltrating jaw bone
Lymphoplasmocytic infiltration	Marked	Moderate	Slight	None

HPF high-power field

Note: The score recorded for each morphologic feature was summed into a total malignancy score

[a]Excluded from Bryne [16] system

[b]Excluded from Bryne [13, 16] systems

was better than Broders' system for prognosticating oral squamous cell carcinoma, and that large and representative incisional biopsies should be procured to examine the underlying connective tissue as well as the tumor. In 1992, Bryne et al. [16] determined that the accuracy of the grading system could be improved by eliminating the mitotic count from grade designation while the prognostic value remained highly significant. This study retrospectively examined 61 cases of floor of mouth squamous cell carcinoma that were independently graded by two pathologists. The authors adopted their 1989 grading system and its five morphological features with scoring from 1 to 4 according to the definitions of Anneroth et al. [15]. These authors identified that the cancers were often less differentiated in the most invasive aspects of the tumor compared to their central parts. They confirmed their previous findings that invasive cell grading is highly prognostic while the conventional Broders grading of the entire tumor is not prognostically significant. The authors estimated that 15 percent of oral cancer biopsies cannot be assessed with invasive cell grading when clear invasion of tumor cells into the connective tissue is absent. They therefore recommended that larger incisional biopsies be taken from the tumors, and that a biopsy measuring 15 × 5 × 5 mm would be sufficient for invasive cell grading.

In 2017 Wagner et al. [1] performed a retrospective study of surgical specimens from 85 cases of primary oral squamous cell carcinoma diagnosed between 1996 and 2010 at the Pathology Laboratory of the Clinics Hospital of Porto Alegre, Brazil. Glass slides of the surgical specimens stained with H&E were acquired for histologic grading by three expert pathologists who were blinded to the clinicopathologic factors and patient outcomes. Specifically, the cases were graded by the criteria of the World Health Organization [11], Anneroth et al. [15], and Bryne's 1989 and 1992 classifications. The authors identified no association between the four grading systems and clinical features including alcohol consumption, the use of tobacco, the anatomic site of the cancer, the presence or absence of pain, TNM stage, the presence of absence of nodal metastases, and recurrence. The 1992 histologic grading system of Bryne et al. [16] was the only system predictive of patient survival ($p = 0.01$). A statistically significantly greater percentage of deceased patients were noted in Bryne [16] grade III cases ($p < 0.05$). Cox univariate survival analyses demonstrated that the 1992 Bryne grade III cases were significantly associated with poor survival rates ($p = 0.02$). This grading system was subjected to a multivariate analysis, including age, gender, the cancer's clinical stage, and the type of treatment. The results indicated that the 1992 Bryne grading system was an independent prognostic factor for squamous cell carcinoma of the oral cavity ($p = 0.03$) even after considering these factors. The multivariate analysis indicated that patients classified as grade III demonstrated a sixfold higher likelihood of dying in the follow-up period compared to patients classified as grade I. No association was noted between the grading systems of the World Health Organization [11], Anneroth et al. [15], and Bryne [13] and patient survival.

In 2015, Sawazaki-Calone et al. [17] evaluated the prognostic significance of additional histopathological grading systems including the histological risk (HR) system of Brandwein-Gensler [18] that evaluated tumor specimens utilizing three histopathological parameters including the worst pattern of invasion (WPOI), lymphocytic host response (LHR), and perineural invasion (PNI), and Almangush et al. [19] who first proposed the BD model based on tumor budding (B) and depth of tumor invasion (D). Sawazaki-Calone et al. evaluated 113 oral squamous cell carcinoma patients and assessed the outcomes of these patients as a function of the grading systems of the World Health Organization [11], Bryne [16], Brandwein-Gensler et al. [18], and Almangush et al. [19]. The 5-year disease-specific survival and disease-free survival were 46% and 62%, respectively. Disease-specific survival was directly influenced by T stage ($p = 0.001$), lymph node status ($p = 0.001$), WHO grading system ($p = 0.01$), and BD model ($p = 0.009$). The disease-free survival was only correlated with the BD model ($p = 0.005$). The adjusted multivariate analysis based on Cox proportion regression demonstrated that age and lymph node metastases were significantly correlated with disease-specific survival, whereas T stage and BD model were the features significantly associated with disease-free survival.

6.3 Perineural Invasion

Perineural invasion is a histopathologic feature of some squamous cell carcinomas of the oral/head and neck region associated with aggressive tumor behavior, disease recurrence, and increased morbidity and mortality. Squamous cell carcinoma of the oral cavity is a well-recognized neurotropic malignancy with perineural involvement by the tumor identified in 6–30% of cases [20]. Cruveilheir initially described perineural involvement in the head and neck region in 1835, and surgeons, medical oncologists, and radiation oncologists continue to discuss and debate the significance of this finding in terms of adjuvant treatment of oral squamous cell carcinoma [21]. Perineural invasion represents a distinct means of cancer cell dissemination in and along nerve bundles as noted by the development of disease beyond the extent of local invasion and can be noted without lymphatic or vascular invasion. In the case of a neurotropic squamous cell carcinoma of the oral cavity, perineural spread in a retrograde fashion toward the skull base or in an antegrade fashion along smaller peripheral branches can occur. Antegrade perineural spread is the more commonly observed pattern of spread in oral cancer patients [21]. Perineural invasion can also be classified as clinical or subclinical depending on the presence of absence of pain, hypesthesia, dysesthesia, or motor deficits. As many as 40% of patients with perineural invasion are without clinical symptoms as the onset of nerve dysfunction may be delayed [21].

While there is no internationally agreed upon definition of perineural invasion, the criteria proposed by Liebig et al. [22] is most widely utilized and referenced. According to these criteria, perineural invasion is diagnosed when tumor cells are noted in association with any of the three layers of the nerve sheath (endoneurium, epineurium, perineurium), and tumor is identified in close proximity to the nerve, involving greater than one-third of its circumference (Fig. 6.10). Involvement less than one-third is considered abutment rather than invasion (Fig. 6.11).

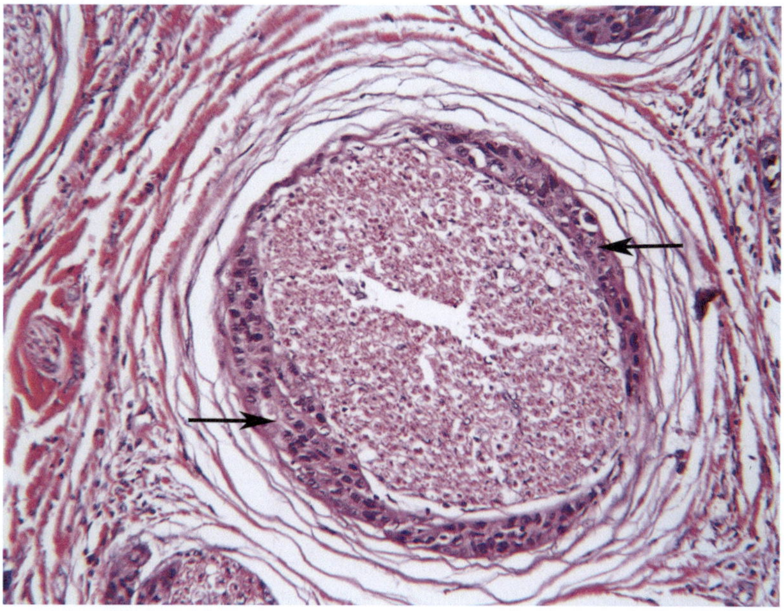

Fig. 6.10 Perineural invasion. Near total encasement of the nerve bundle (arrows) by tumor is present. (Hematoxylin & eosin, original magnification ×400)

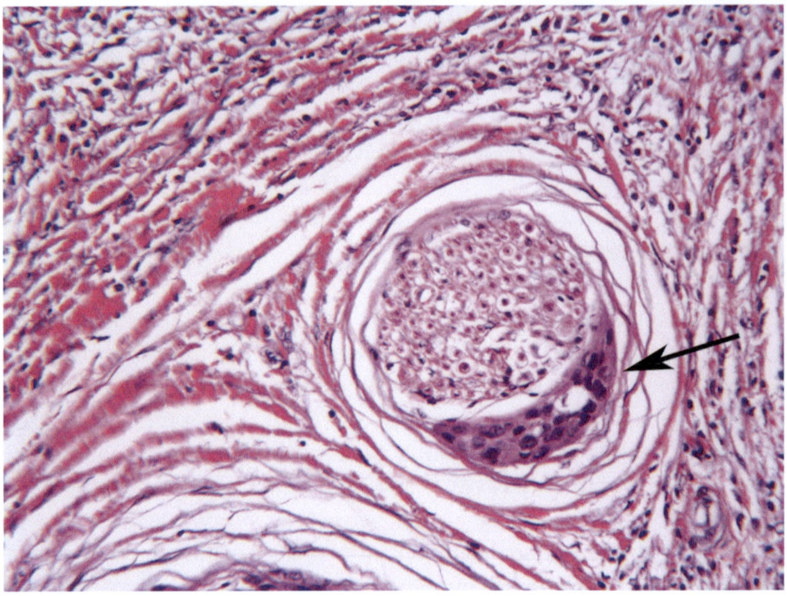

Fig. 6.11 Nerve abutment by tumor. Note that less than one-third of the nerve bundle (arrow) is involved by tumor. (Hematoxylin & eosin, original magnification ×400)

Tarsitano et al. [20] retrospectively studied 236 consecutive patients with oral squamous cell carcinoma and specifically investigated the impact of perineural invasion as an independent prognostic factor for local and regional failure. Extirpative surgery was the primary method of treatment offered to all patients with elective neck dissection (I–III) performed in 116 patients (49.1%), modified radical neck dissection performed in 48 patients (20.4%), and no neck dissection in 72 patients (30.5%). One hundred fifty-six patients (66.1%) were treated with surgery alone while 80 patients (33.9%) received postoperative radiation therapy. Fifty-one of the 236 patients' tumors (21.6%) demonstrated perineural invasion. Cancers of the tongue and floor of mouth were the most commonly associated with perineural invasion in 38% and 47% of cases, respectively. Overall failure was noted in 71 of the 236 patients (30%) and a significant difference ($p = 0.007$) in local failure was seen in patients with perineural invasion [31/51 (60.7%)] compared to patients without perineural invasion [22/185 (11.9%)]. A statistically significant difference ($p = 0.041$) was also noted in regional failures with perineural invasion [10/51 (19.6%)] compared to those without perineural invasion [7/185 (3.8%)] in this study. No statistically significant difference ($p = 1.0$) was noted in distant failures for perineural invasion [1/51 (1.9%)] vs. no perineural invasion [0/185 (0%)].

Cracchiolo et al. [23] retrospectively reviewed 381 patients treated with primary surgery for squamous cell carcinoma of the oral tongue over a 13-year period of time. One hundred five patients (28%) demonstrated perineural invasion in their primary cancer specimens. There were 96 deaths with 55 deaths related to disease. Recurrent disease was noted in 97 patients including 58 local recurrences, 53 regional recurrences, and 23 distant recurrences. Patients whose specimens identified perineural invasion were more likely to demonstrate a higher T classification and lymph node metastasis. Fifty patients with perineural invasion (13.1%) demonstrated microscopically positive lymph nodes compared to 35 patients (9.18%) without perineural invasion demonstrating microscopically positive lymph nodes. In this study, perineural invasion was associated with a worse disease-specific survival (DSS) on univariate analysis. On multivariate analysis, while adjusting for tumor size, adjuvant therapy, and lymph node status, patients with perineural invasion demonstrated a decreased DSS. Although perineural invasion predicted local and regional recurrence on univariate analysis, it was not predictive on multivariate analysis.

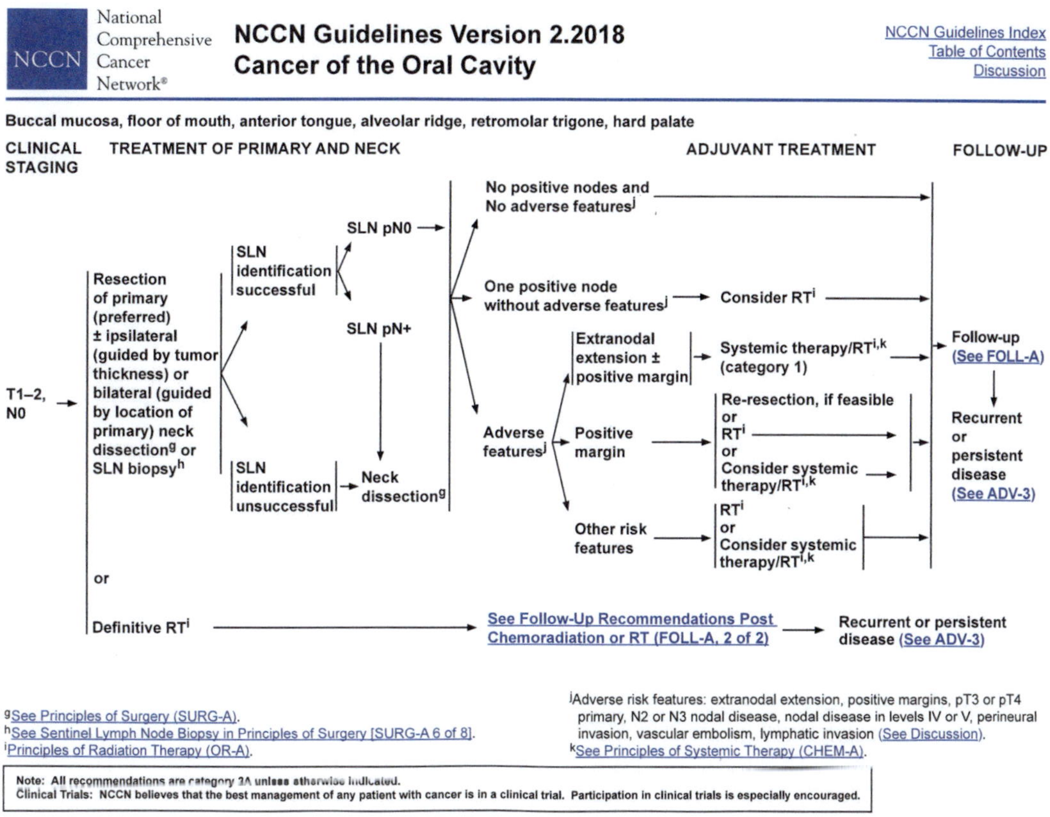

Fig. 6.12 Treatment recommendations for T1–2, N0 squamous cell carcinoma of the buccal mucosa, floor of mouth, anterior tongue, alveolar ridge, retromolar trigone, and hard palate according to the National Comprehensive Cancer Network (NCCN). Adjuvant treatment for the adverse features of extranodal extension, positive surgical margins, perineural invasion, and others are discussed. Reproduced with permission from the NCCN Clinical Practice Guidelines in Oncology (NCCN Guidelines®) for Head and Neck Cancer V.2.2018, page OR-2.

The microscopic presence of perineural invasion is well accepted as an adverse feature in oral squamous cell carcinoma and is associated with increased recurrence and a decrease in survival. The 2018 National Comprehensive Cancer Network (NCCN) guidelines (Figs. 6.12 and 6.13) recommend adjuvant radiation therapy when perineural invasion is identified in the cancer specimen [24]. In addition the NCCN guidelines recommend considering adjuvant chemoradiation therapy for patients with perineural invasion based on the results of the European Organization for Research and Treatment of Cancer 22,931, a prospective randomized study comparing postoperative radiation therapy alone vs. chemoradiation therapy in high-risk squamous cell carcinomas of the head and neck that showed a survival advantage for patients receiving adjuvant cisplatin concurrently with radiation therapy [25].

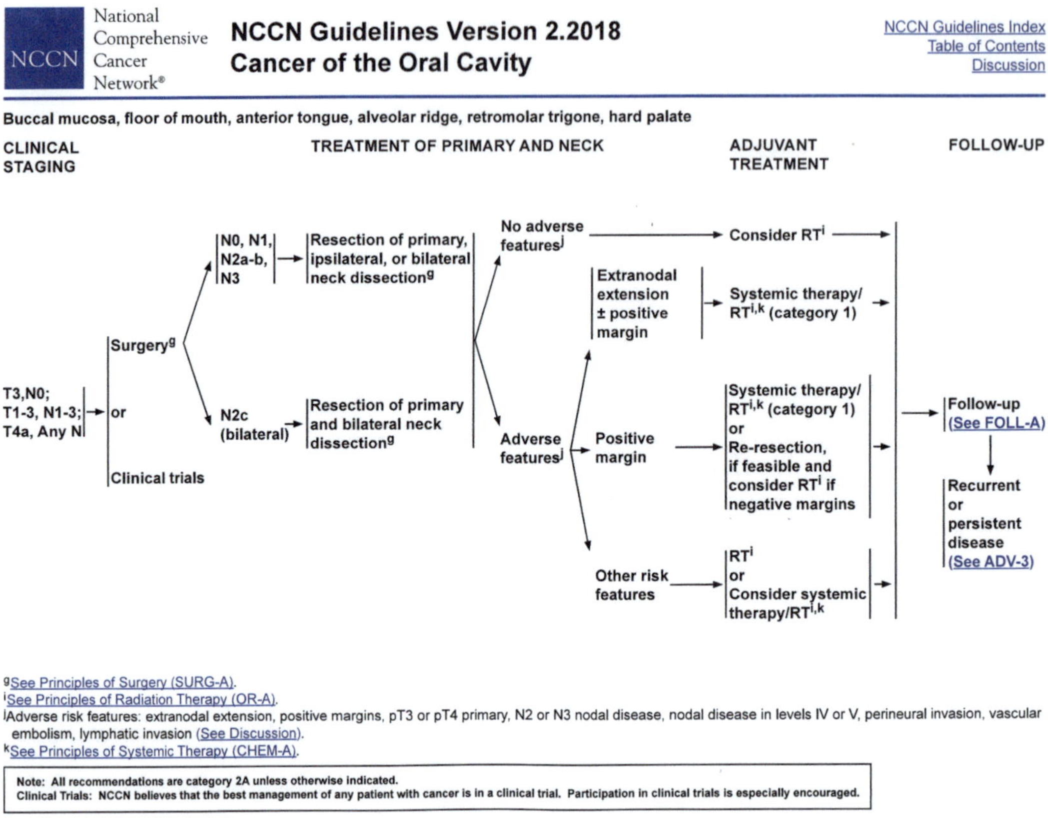

Fig. 6.13 Treatment recommendations for T3, N0; T1–3, N1–3; T4a, any N squamous cell carcinoma of the buccal mucosa, floor of mouth, anterior tongue, alveolar ridge, retromolar trigone, and hard palate. The same adverse features are considered for adjuvant therapy as the smaller, less advanced cancers. Reproduced with permission from the NCCN Clinical Practice Guidelines in Oncology (NCCN Guidelines®) for Head and Neck Cancer V.2.2018, page OR-3. © 2018 National Comprehensive Cancer Network, Inc. All rights reserved. The NCCN Guidelines® and illustrations herein may not be reproduced in any form for any purpose without the express written permission of NCCN. To view the most recent and complete version of the NCCN Guidelines, go online to NCCN.org. The NCCN Guidelines are a work in progress that may be refined as often as new significant data become available. NCCN makes no warranties of any kind whatsoever regarding their content, use, or application and disclaims any responsibility for their application or use in any way

6.4 Status of the Surgical Margins

The surgical margin is a clinical and quantified linear margin that separates the advancing tumor front from the inked margin on the specimen. The inclusion of this linear margin at the periphery of the specimen is with intentionality and recognizes the ability of neoplasms to spread beyond their clinical demarcations. The surgical margin therefore represents the only prognostic factor over which the ablative surgeon has influence when removing oral squamous cell carcinoma. To this end, therefore, the specimen handoff from surgeon to pathologist is paramount to the identification of true surgical margins, clinically concerning margins, and those margins that ought to be evaluated by frozen sections. The handoff procedure represents a specimen orientation that occurs in a face-to-face fashion. While this procedure has not been studied scientifically, experience indicates that the handoff process minimizes ambiguity in margin determination [26]. The discussion of anatomic landmarks in the specimen, oncologic levels of lymph nodes in a composite resection specimen, measurement of tumor in the unfixed state, gross assessment of margins, directionality of the surgical specimen, and the identification of areas of concern to the surgeon represent topics of discussion during the handoff orientation.

The traditionally accepted definition of an oncologic surgical margin is an anatomic clearance of all malignant cells in a three-dimensional orientation [27]. There is agreement by the National Comprehensive Cancer Network (NCCN), the American College of Pathologists (ACP), and the Royal College of Pathologists (RCP) that a negative margin is defined by the presence of at least 5 mm of normal tissue in the margin [28, 29] (Fig. 6.14). A close margin is defined as negative but one where the distance from the invasive tumor to the specimen's margin is less than 5 mm (Fig. 6.15), and a positive margin is variably defined. The ACP defines a positive margin as invasive cancer less than 1 mm from the surgical margin (Fig. 6.16) while both the RCP and the NCCN define a positive margin as invasive cancer, carcinoma-in-situ, or high-grade dysplasia present at the microscopic margins [28] (Fig. 6.17). Therein, a negative margin implies that the entirety of the malignancy is encased within the resection specimen. This notwithstanding, local tumor recurrences are noted to occur even when pathologists declare that all surgical margins are negative for cancer. Byers et al. [30] identified a 12% incidence of local recurrence of oral squamous cell carcinoma when surgical margins were noted to be negative and an 80% incidence of recurrence when margins were positive. Dillon et al. [29] performed a retrospective cohort study that examined 174 patients with oral squamous cell carcinoma of whom 54 met the study inclusion criteria. Of these 54 patients, 9 patients (17%) demonstrated greater than or equal to 5 mm (negative) surgical margins, 21 (39%) demonstrated 1–5 mm (close) surgical margins, and 24 (44%) demonstrated less than 1 mm (positive) surgical margins. In all, 83% of patients had close or positive margins that speak to the difficulty of obtaining negative margins in this patient population, despite good intentions. The 2-year survival rates were 78%, 62%, and 50%, respectively, for the negative, close, and positive margins. Seventy-nine percent of patients with positive margins received adjuvant chemotherapy, radiation therapy, or combined chemoradiation therapy, and 42% of patients developed locoregional recurrences at 2 years. Sixty-two percent of patients with close margins received adjuvant therapy, with 31% of patients develop-

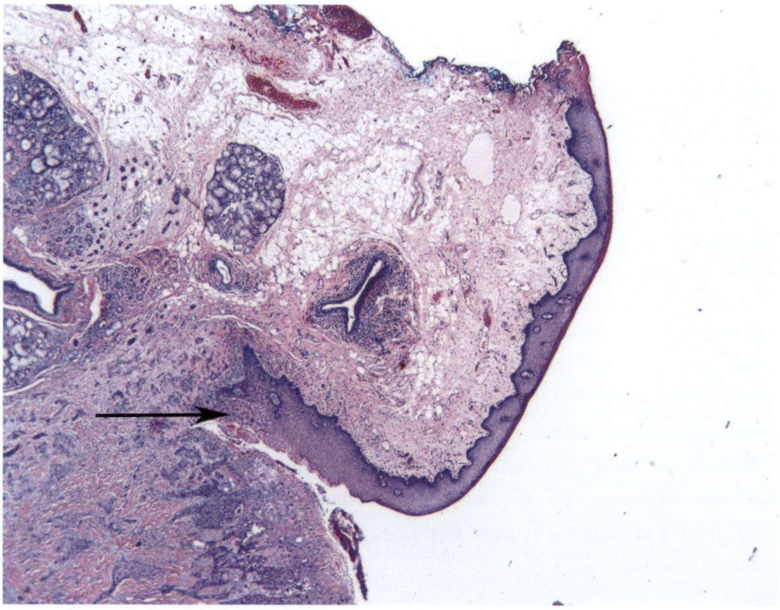

Fig. 6.14 Surgical margin greater than 5 mm. Note the discontinuance of tumor growth (arrow) far from the surgical margin that is unequivocally considered a negative margin. (Hematoxylin & eosin, original magnification ×40)

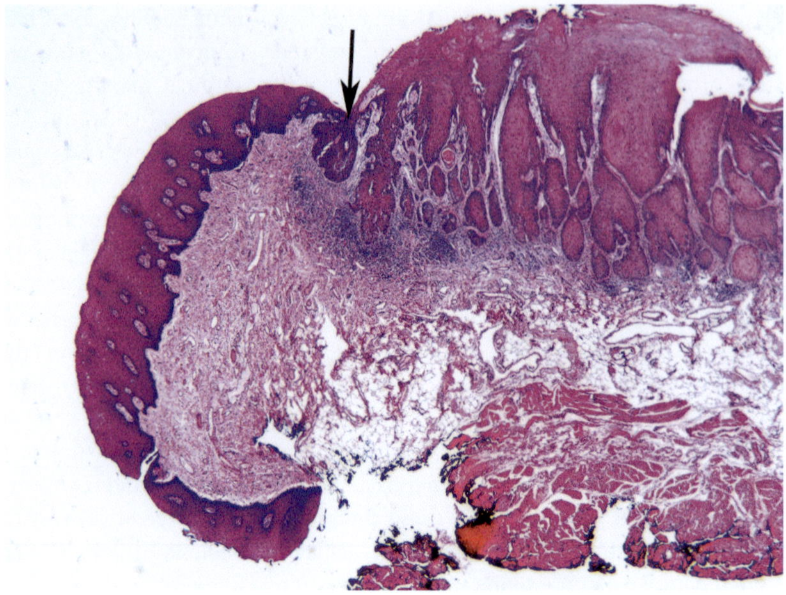

Fig. 6.15 Surgical margin less than 5 mm. The tumor (arrow) is within 3–4 mm of the surgical margin. This distance connotes a close margin. (Hematoxylin & eosin, original magnification ×100)

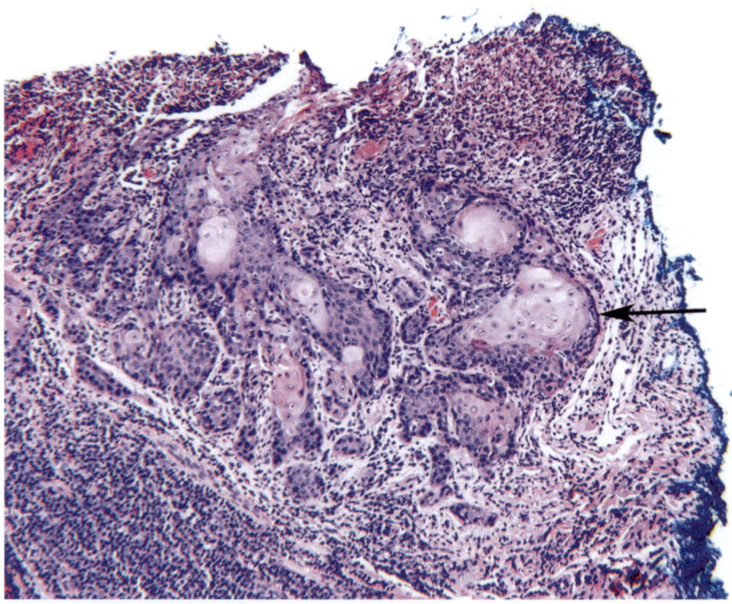

Fig. 6.16 Surgical margin 1 mm or less. Note the proximity of the tumor (arrow) to the surgical margin. (Hematoxylin & eosin, original magnification ×100)

ing locoregional recurrences at 2 years. Seventy-eight percent of patients with negative margins received adjuvant therapy with 29% of patients developing locoregional recurrences at 2 years. The authors concluded their study by indicating that the presence of close surgical margins (1–5 mm) is an adverse feature that is similar to a positive margin.

Tissue shrinkage associated with formalin fixation may falsely proclaim truly negative margins as close and close surgical margins as positive. In 1997, Johnson et al. [31] reviewed the shrinkage associated with margins in the oral mucosa in dogs. They indicated that a 30–50% discrepancy exists in margins measured in situ and following processing. They noted that most

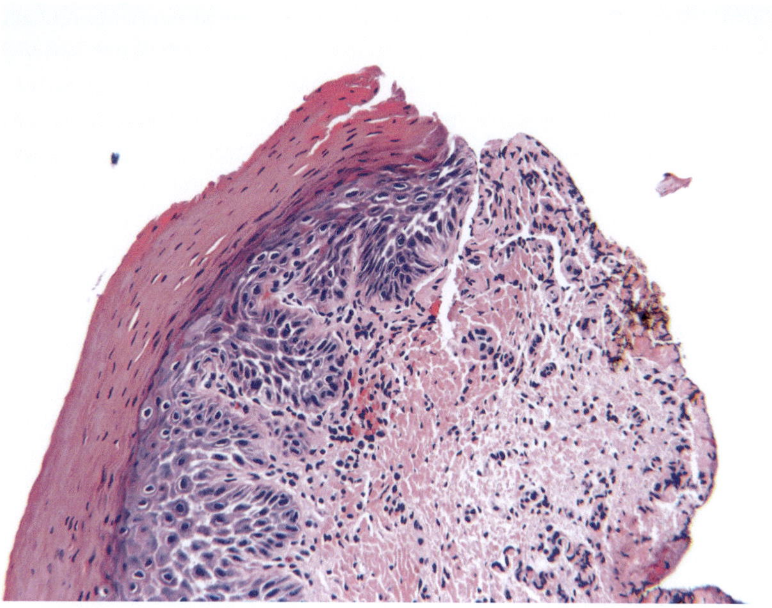

Fig. 6.17 High-grade dysplasia at the surgical margin. Note the atypical maturation of the epithelium at the surgical margin. (Hematoxylin & eosin, original magnification ×100)

of the shrinkage occurred immediately after excision. The labiobuccal margin demonstrated 38.3% loss after excision and an additional 10.5% loss following fixation. Tongue margins showed 24.8% loss after excision and an additional 7.6% loss after fixation. The authors attributed the shrinkage to unopposed contractility of the underlying muscles in the surgical specimen and the release from surrounding tissues. In 2005, Mistry et al. [32] determined that the mean shrinkage of tumor margins for buccal mucosal and tongue specimens were 21.1% and 23.5%, respectively. They also determined that tumor shrinkage was less for T3 and T4 tumors (9.2%) than T1 and T2 tumors (25.6%). The authors suggested that increased tumor burdens translate to less contractility of the margins. Cheng et al. [33] evaluated oral mucosal shrinkage as a function of anatomic site and noted that retromolar trigone, mandibular alveolar ridge, and buccal mucosa exhibited the greatest tissue shrinkage (71%) compared to hard palate and maxillary alveolar ridge (53%) and oral tongue mucosa (42%). All of these studies indicate the need for ablative surgeons to increase the width of the soft tissue linear margin on the specimen by 25–50% in order to avoid the dilemma of close or positive margins [27].

Intraoperative frozen sections represent one additional method to avoid the dilemma of close or positive margins, a technique employed by greater than 97% of ablative surgeons managing cancer of the oral cavity [28]. Frozen sections involve procuring tissue from the periphery of the excised specimen or the remaining tissue bed, embedding these soft tissue specimens in optimal cutting temperature compound, and freezing using a cryostat machine. Specimens are then thinly sectioned to an average thickness of approximately 7 μm, affixed to glass slides, stained with H&E, and microscopically evaluated by a pathologist. Ord et al. [34] retrospectively evaluated 49 consecutive patients with oral cancer. Arbitrary areas of anterior, posterior, medial, and lateral margins were subjected to frozen section analysis that yielded a total of 307 frozen sections, and an average of 6.2 frozen sections per patient. When compared to their permanently stained counterparts, 304 of the 307 sections showed a concordant accuracy of 99%. Two false-negative frozen sections were noted and one false-positive frozen section existed that resulted in a sensitivity of 86.6% and a specificity of 99.6%. The authors regarded the presence of dysplasia, carcinoma in situ, or invasive cancer within 5 mm of the margin as a positive margin.

Thirty-nine of the 49 patients (79.6%) showed clear surgical margins in the final analysis of their specimens. Thirty-eight of these patients had specimens with negative margins on initial frozen sections, whereas one patient had a specimen with an initial positive margin on frozen section that required additional excision that was negative for cancer. Four patients demonstrated cancer within 5 mm of the final surgical margin and one patient (25%) recurred. Four patients demonstrated dysplasia at the surgical margins and one patient (25%) recurred. Two patients demonstrated cancer at the surgical margins and both (100%) recurred. In all, seven patients (14.5%) did not benefit by the implementation of frozen sections. In addition, only one patient was benefitted by the use of frozen sections to clear a positive margin.

Ellis et al. [35] retrospectively evaluated a cohort of 250 patients with an analysis of five surgical and seven histologic variables to determine their effects on the surgical margins in oral cancer resections. The authors concluded six statistically meaningful study variables in terms of surgical margins. The results of the study indicated that surgeons who had resected higher volumes of oral cavity cancer had larger surgical margins than those with lower surgical volumes. High-volume surgeons were those who treated more than 40 patients, although the time period for this volume of work was not specified in the study. Low volume surgeons were defined as those who performed fewer than 40 cases, although this volume was similarly not categorized as to its time period. The variable of surgeon volume was statistically the most important variable of the study. The second variable was the cancer's location that demonstrated an association between shorter surgical margins and tumors located in the retromolar trigone. Thirdly, the study showed an association between smaller surgical margins and perineural invasion. Among the nonstatistically meaningful variables included free-flap reconstructive surgery of the ablative defect. The commitment to free-flap surgical reconstruction of ablative defects related to oral cancer at least theoretically reduces the likelihood of positive margins due to the ablative surgeon not being reticent to include a larger linear margin at the periphery of the specimen [36]. Ellis et al. [35] found no statistical difference in the surgical margin when a free-flap procedure was performed. Further, no statistically meaningful improvements in the surgical margins were identified using frozen sections, surgical access procedures, or tumor size. The authors concluded their study by emphasizing that improved patient outcomes are realized if ablative oral cancer surgery is performed at high-volume centers by high-volume surgeons.

Genetic analysis of surgical margins in head and neck cancer was introduced to the international literature by Brennan [37] in 1995. The presence of the p53 gene mutation in a histologically negative margin was associated with local recurrence in patients who had undergone surgical resection. Specifically, in their study, Brennan et al. [37] identified 30 of 69 patients with mutations of the p53 gene in their head and neck cancers. Seventy-eight surgical margins and 33 cervical lymph nodes were obtained from these 30 patients. Five patients had positive surgical margins on final histopathological analysis of their specimens and were eliminated from further analysis. Seventy-two margins containing no microscopic evidence of cancer in 25 patients therefore comprised the study group. These 72 negative margins were probed with the p53 mutant oligonucleotide derived from the primary tumors. In 13 of the 25 patients (52%), the amplified p53 region from at least one surgical margin hybridized to the tumor-specific probe, exhibiting the presence of mutated neoplastic cells within these negative margins. The estimated percentage of cells with mutations in the surgical margins was from 0.05% to 28%. The PCR products from the margins of the remaining 12 patients did not hybridize to the mutant-specific probes, indicating that those margins did not harbor neoplastic cells and were truly negative margins. Sections from 33 cervical lymph nodes in six patients identified metastatic squamous cell carcinoma in five lymph nodes (15%). However, molecular analysis identified mutant p53 genes in the PCR products of 11 nodes (33%). Of the 28 negative lymph nodes by light microscopy, 6

(21%) were identified to contain neoplastic cells. On follow-up, 5 of the 13 patients (38%) with positive margins by molecular analysis, yet negative surgical margins by light microscopy, developed biopsy-proven recurrences of carcinoma. None of the 12 patients whose surgical margins were negative for p53 mutations developed recurrent disease. The results of the lymph node examination by molecular analysis were felt to be noteworthy by the authors. Based on the discovery of p53 mutations in seemingly benign lymph nodes, four of these six patients would have been upstaged in terms of their N designation. This upstaging would have been significant in terms of the delivery of adjuvant therapy and would have been negatively impacting from a prognostic perspective.

Liu et al. [38] prospectively examined 168 patients with primary oral cavity cancer who underwent surgical ablation of their cancers. One hundred forty-five patients satisfied the author's study protocol including histologically negative margins of at least 5 mm. Six hundred fifty-one surgical margins were analyzed in the 145 study patients. Forty-two patients (29%) developed local recurrence, and seven patients (48%) developed distant metastatic disease. Six markers were utilized for microsatellite alteration analysis including D9S1748, THRB, D3S1300, IFNA. PCR2, D2S206, and D21S236. Microsatellite alteration was identified in 100 specimens from 145 patients. Fifty-five patients had microsatellite instability for one or more markers in the tumor specimen, and 85 patients had loss of heterozygosity for one or more markers in malignant tissues. Of the 55 patients with microsatellite instability in the specimen, 41 demonstrated microsatellite instability at the surgical margins and 14 showed no microsatellite instability at the margins. Recurrence was noted in 22 of the 41 (54%) patients in the former group and 4 of the 14 patients (29%) in the latter group. Those with microsatellite instability in the surgical margins demonstrated a higher rate of local recurrence than those without; 18 of 55 patients (33%) vs. 30 of 596 (5%), respectively. Patients with loss of heterozygosity in the surgical margin also demonstrated a higher rate of local recurrence than those without; 13 of 98 (13%), vs. 35 of 553 (6.3%), respectively.

de Carvalho et al. [39] retrospectively studied the specimens of 55 patients who underwent tumor ablation for head and neck squamous cell carcinoma with curative intent. Surgical margins that were histologically negative were evaluated from these patients and primary SCCA samples were obtained from a subset of 23 patients. The resected specimens demonstrated no invasive cancer or dysplasia at the surgical margins. Twenty-five oral mucosal tissue samples from healthy donors were included in the study. The conclusion of the study was that the identification of molecular factors in oral cancer specimens may provide useful prognostic information and influence the management of patients. Ferris et al. [40] demonstrated that PTHLH (parathyroid hormone-like hormone, also known as PTHrP) and EPCAM (epithelial cell adhesion molecule) expression could distinguish positive and negative lymph nodes with high accuracy. In addition, the immunohistochemical identification of MMP9 (matrix metalloproteinase-9) in surgical margins demonstrates a positive association with the risk of recurrence in head and neck squamous cell carcinoma patients. The study's goal was to identify the expression of PTHLH, EPCAM, MMP9, LGALS1 (lectin, galactoside-binding, soluble, 1), and MET (MET proto-oncogene, receptor tyrosine kinase) expression in histologically negative margins as a useful marker for the detection of molecular alterations associated with local disease control in these patients. Gene expression was assessed with quantitative reverse transcription polymerase chain reaction (qRT-PCR). MMP9 (91%), LGALS1 (83%), PTHLH (74%), MET (48%), and EPCAM (30%) were commonly overexpressed in the 23 SCCA samples (high sensitivity). MMP9, PTHLH, and EPCAM were rarely overexpressed in the 15 healthy oral mucosal samples (0%, 7%, 0%, respectively), confirming their overexpression as highly specific. MET and LGALS1 were overexpressed in 14% and 27%, respectively, of the normal controls, indicative of their lack of specificity. Based on the high specificity and sensitivity of MMP9, EPCAM, and

PTHLH, the expression of these genes was assessed in the 55 negative surgical margins. MMP9 was overexpressed in 23.6% (13/55) of the surgical margins evaluated, EPCAM in 10.9% (6/55), and PTHLH in 9.1% (5/55). Thirty-six percent of the negative margins demonstrated overexpression of at least one of the 3 selected genes, MMP9, EPAM, and PTHLH. Despite negative surgical margins, 11/55 (20%) patients in the study presented with local recurrences, suggesting that the molecular changes present in the margins, undetected by microscopic analysis, could directly be responsible for malignant transformation of this normal tissue and the poor outcomes realized by the patients in this study. In particular, the study indicated that the overexpression of PTHLH and MMP9 in negative SCCA margins is directly correlated with a high risk of local recurrence and the development of secondary primary tumors.

6.5 Depth of Invasion

Surgical decision-making regarding the clinically negative neck in patients with oral squamous cell carcinoma represents a formidable discipline, and assessment of tumor depth of invasion represents the greatest histologic predictor of occult cervical metastases [41]. To that end, tumor depth of invasion (Fig. 6.18) is distinguished from tumor thickness (Fig. 6.19), with depth of inva-

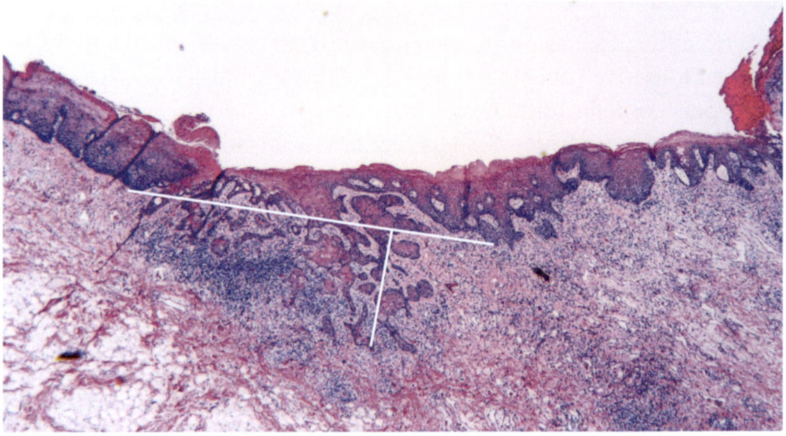

Fig. 6.18 Measuring depth of invasion (DOI). The horizontal line connects the basement membrane of the closest intact squamous mucosa on each side of the cancer. A "plumb" line is then dropped from the horizontal line to the deepest tumor cells. The measurement of this line represents the DOI. (Hematoxylin & eosin, original magnification ×40)

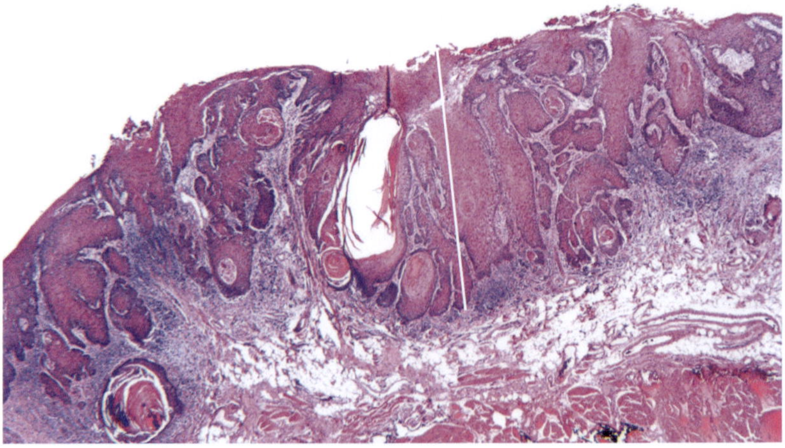

Fig. 6.19 The tumor thickness is measured from the most superior portion of the tumor to the deepest portion. This is often quite different than the DOI. (Hematoxylin & eosin, original magnification ×40)

sion being prognostically more reliable than tumor thickness. That said, some authors incorrectly equate or interchangeably utilize the terms depth of invasion and tumor thickness [5, 42]. Determining the exact metric for the depth of invasion that would dictate an elective neck dissection due to a threshold level of occult neck disease continues to represent a controversial issue in oral/head and neck oncologic surgery. An elective neck dissection is commonly performed in patients who demonstrate at least a 20% risk for occult cervical lymph node metastases [43]. Thin and superficially invasive squamous cell carcinomas of the oral cavity have a lower risk of regional lymph node metastases compared to thicker cancers that are deeply invasive of the underlying soft tissues. Although equating tumor thickness and depth of invasion, Spiro et al. [5] quantified the risk of occult neck disease for 105 T1 and T2 primary squamous cell carcinomas of the tongue and floor of mouth with no evidence of cervical metastases at the time of their primary surgical treatment. There were 43 patients in the group of patients with tumor thicknesses of 2 mm or less, 43 patients had a tumor thickness between 3 and 8 mm, and 19 patients had tumor thicknesses of 9 mm or greater. Univariate survival analysis indicated that tumor thickness and stage were the most important prognostic indices. Multivariate analysis confirmed that tumor thickness had the greatest impact on survival. Tumors 2 mm or less in thickness predicted a subthreshold risk of occult nodal metastases of 7.5%, overall incidence of nodal metastases of 13%, and 3% of patients died from their disease. Tumor thicknesses between 3 and 8 mm demonstrated a threshold risk of occult nodal metastases of 25.7%, 46% overall incidence of nodal metastases, and 17% of patients died from their disease. Tumors thicker than 9 mm show a threshold 41.2% risk of occult nodal metastases, 65% overall incidence of nodal metastases, and 35% of patients died from their disease. When treatment planning patients with oral squamous cell carcinoma, it would be ideal to know the approximate tumor thickness within these three categories. That said, it is not clinically or practically possible to possess that information prior to definitive surgical therapy of the primary cancer since biopsies are typically not representative of the entire thickness of an oral cancer. Nonetheless, palpation of the primary tumor may result in approximation of the thickness to determine the utility of elective neck dissection. In the Spiro et al. [5] study, treatment failure occurred in 32 determinate patients (35%). The primary site was involved in eight patients, the neck in 18 patients, and both sites in four patients. Neck recurrence was noted in 2 of the 29 patients who underwent elective neck dissection. Of the 63 patients whose necks were observed, metastases subsequently developed in 17 patients (27%) and 8 patients (47%) died of poorly controlled disease in the neck despite 15 patients undergoing radical neck dissection for salvage.

Brockhoff et al. [41] performed a retrospective review of their database at the University of Michigan and identified 286 patients who had undergone excisions of primary cancers and elective neck dissections. There were 105 cancers located in the oral tongue, 91 cancers of the alveolus/hard palate, 39 cancers of the floor of mouth, 25 cancers of the retromolar trigone, and 24 cancers located at other sites. Sixty-six patients had stage I disease, 54 patients had stage II disease, 39 patients had stage III disease, and 127 patients had stage IV disease. The shallowest depth of invasion where at least 20% of the neck dissections had histologically positive lymph nodes was 2 mm for tongue, 3 mm for floor of mouth, 3 mm for retromolar trigone, and 4 mm for alveolus/hard palate. This study therefore answered the question of threshold depth of invasion and its correlation with occult nodal metastases as a function of anatomic site of the primary cancer of the oral cavity.

Masood et al. [44] retrospectively analyzed 67 patients with T1 N0 ($n = 30$) and T2 N0 ($n = 37$) HPV-negative squamous cell carcinoma of the tongue. All patients underwent elective neck dissections. Thirty-five, twenty, and twelve patients demonstrated tumor thickness of less than or equal to 5 mm, between 5 and 10 mm, and greater than 10 mm, respectively. Thirty-seven, sixteen, and fourteen patients demonstrated primary tumor depth of invasion of less than or equal to

5 mm, between 5 and 10 mm, and greater than 10 mm, respectively. Five recurrences were noted among the 67 patients (7.46%). Two of the recurrences were local, two were regional, and one was distant. In the group with depth of invasion less than or equal to 5 mm ($n = 37$), there were two recurrences with one being local and one being regional. In the group with depth of invasion greater than 10 mm ($n = 14$), there were three recurrences, with one being local, one regional, and one distant. No recurrences were noted in the group with depth of invasion of between 5 and 10 mm. Depth of invasion was associated with occult nodal metastases and lymphovascular invasion. Tumor thickness was also a significant predictor of lymphovascular invasion, but not occult cervical metastases.

6.6 Status of the Cervical Lymph Nodes

In 1977, Kalnins et al. [45] retrospectively reported on the outcomes of 416 patients who had undergone radical neck dissection for squamous cell carcinoma of the oral cavity and tonsillar region. Three hundred forty determinate patients were followed for a minimum of 5 years. Histologic evaluation of the radical neck dissection specimens permitted the authors to categorize patients into four groups: group 1 consisted of patients with histologically negative neck dissection specimens; group 2 consisted of patients with one positive lymph node in the neck dissection specimen; group 3 consisted of patients with two positive lymph nodes; and group 4 consisted of patients with three or more positive lymph nodes. Of the 340 patients, 213 had histologically positive lymph nodes. Anatomic location of positive lymph nodes was determined for 108 patients demonstrating positive lymph nodes confined to the superior or suprahyoid region of the neck; 84 patients with positive lymph nodes in the middle third of the neck between the hyoid bone and the omohyoid muscle with or without involvement of the upper third of the neck; and 21 patients had positive lymph nodes in the lower third of the neck defined as inferior to the omohyoid muscle, with or without involvement of the middle or superior third of the neck. The 213 patients with histologically positive lymph nodes were again divided into three groups based on whether the lymph node capsule (Fig. 6.20) was intact, whether it was microscopically penetrated only (Fig. 6.21), and whether soft tissue spread had occurred (Fig. 6.22). Of the 160 patients with his-

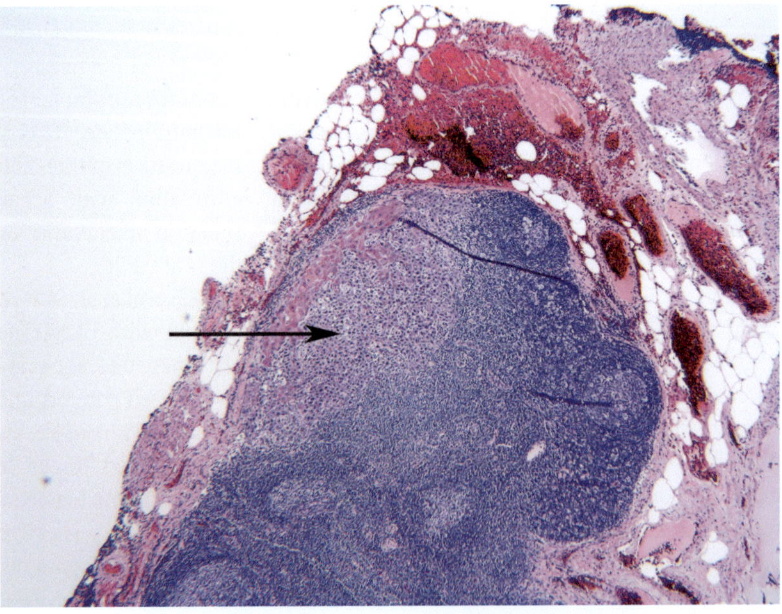

Fig. 6.20 Metastatic squamous cell carcinoma in a cervical lymph node. Well-defined metastatic squamous cell carcinoma (arrow) is noted within the confines of the lymph node and without involvement of the capsule. (Hematoxylin & eosin, original magnification ×40)

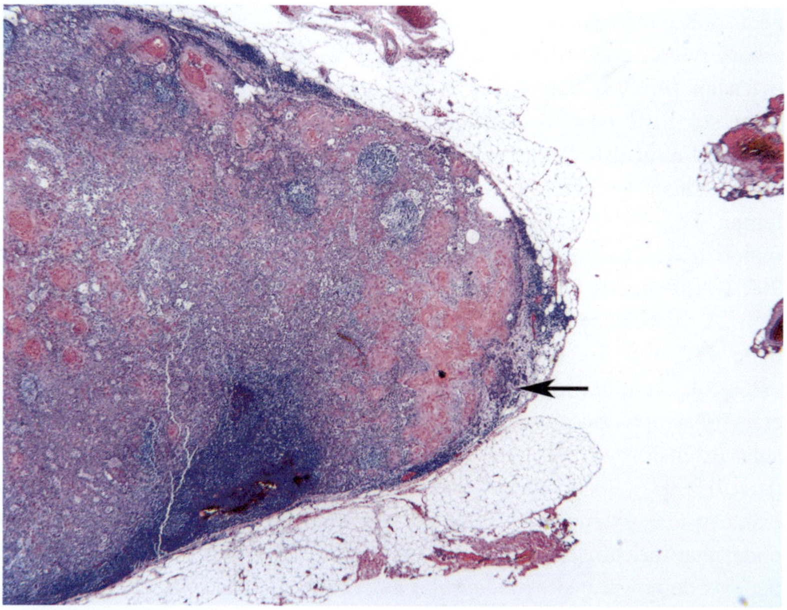

Fig. 6.21 Metastatic squamous cell carcinoma within a cervical lymph node with a focus of metastatic squamous cell carcinoma demonstrating minimal erosion of the lymph node capsule (arrow). (Hematoxylin & eosin, original magnification ×40)

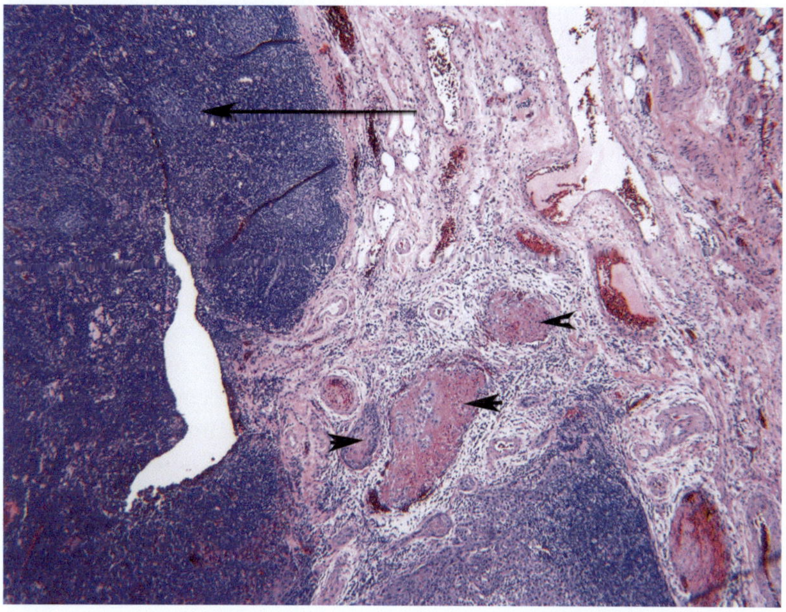

Fig. 6.22 Metastatic squamous cell carcinoma spreading from the lymph node into the surrounding soft tissues. Note the disrupted node (long arrow) and the spreading tumor cells (short arrow). (Hematoxylin & eosin, original magnification ×100)

tologically negative lymph nodes, disease-specific survival was 75% at 5 years. The disease-specific 5-year survival of patients with one positive lymph node, two positive lymph nodes, and three or more lymph nodes was 49%, 30%, 13%, respectively. The overall 5-year disease-specific survival was 29% for all patients with positive lymph nodes. When the lymph node capsule was intact, the disease-specific survival for all patients was 33%. The disease-specific survival for microscopic penetration of the lymph node capsule was 28%, and soft tissue spread led to a 5-year disease-specific survival rate of 11%.

Ghadjar et al. [46] retrospectively analyzed the neck dissection specimens of 133 patients with squamous cell carcinoma of the head and neck and preferentially studied those patients whose lymph nodes demonstrated extracapsular extension ($n = 98$). Four of the 98 patients underwent selective neck dissection, 37 underwent modified radical neck dissection, and 57 underwent radical neck dissection. A total of 431 lymph nodes were examined including 231 lymph nodes with extracapsular extension and 200 lymph nodes without extracapsular extension. A significant association between lymph node size and the incidence of extracapsular extension was noted in the study. The mean diameters for lymph nodes with and without extracapsular extension were 11 and 9 mm, respectively ($p = 0.0004$). Sixty-one patients demonstrated extracapsular extension in their positive lymph nodes that measured 10 mm or smaller while 22 patients demonstrated extracapsular extension in their positive lymph nodes that measured 5 mm or smaller. Overall, 48% of positive lymph nodes smaller than 10 mm exhibited extracapsular extension while 60% of positive lymph nodes between 10 and 30 mm exhibited extracapsular extension.

The utility of performing an elective neck dissection for clinically node-negative patients with oral squamous cell carcinoma is one of the most contentious issues in oral/head and neck oncologic surgery. Such patients may be thought to be acceptable candidates for exclusive surgical management of the primary cancer and watchful waiting of the neck since approximately 70% of these patients will demonstrate a histologically negative neck if the neck is dissected electively [47]. D'Cruz et al. [47] performed a prospective, randomized, controlled trial of 596 patients with T1 or T2 squamous cell carcinoma of the tongue, floor of mouth, or buccal mucosa. Patients were randomized to undergo either elective neck dissection (selective neck dissection I–III) or surgical ablation of the primary cancer with monitoring of the neck and therapeutic neck dissection only when cervical metastases became apparent. The authors designed the study in part to determine if a survival difference exists between the elective neck dissection and therapeutic neck dissection groups. Five hundred patients, 245 patients in the elective neck dissection group, and 255 patients in the therapeutic neck dissection group completed follow-up for at least 9 months and comprised the analysis. There were 81 recurrences (25 nodal, 23 local, 3 distant, 4 nodal and local, 16 second primary, 10 unknown) and 50 deaths in the elective neck dissection group and 146 recurrences (108 nodal, 7 local, 3 distant, 8 nodal and local, 11 second primary, and 9 not known) and 79 deaths in the therapeutic neck dissection group. The difference between nodal recurrences in the two groups is noteworthy; 114 of 253 patients (45.1%) in the therapeutic neck dissection group, and 72 of 243 patients (29.6%) in the elective neck dissection group. At 3 years postoperatively, elective neck dissection resulted in an improved rate of overall survival (80%) compared to the therapeutic neck dissection group (67.5%). At that time, patients in the elective neck dissection group had a higher rate of disease-free survival (69.5%) than the therapeutic neck dissection group (45.9%). The results of this study reveal the survival benefits of elective neck dissection compared to watchful waiting followed by therapeutic neck dissection for lymph node recurrence in patients with early stage, clinically node-negative oral squamous cell carcinoma. The results show an absolute overall survival benefit of elective neck dissection of 12.5% points and a disease-free survival benefit of 23.6% points. This fact translates to eight patients having to be treated with elective neck dissection to prevent one death, and four patients would need to be treated to prevent one recurrence.

Kuo et al. [48] addressed the issue of lymph node yield in oral cancer in recognition of prognostic lymph node yield thresholds that have been identified and incorporated into treatment guidelines for multiple human cancer sites including bladder, colorectal, and esophageal, but not for oral cancer. There are no guidelines, and there is no consensus regarding the number of lymph nodes removed, or lymph node yield, that indicates an acceptable neck dissection in patients with cancer of the oral cavity. In order to address this issue, patients with oral cancer in the National Cancer Database were accessed that included 13,143 cases. Higher lymph node yields in neck dissection specimens were noted in males, young patients, and those procedures performed in academic medical centers, in centers with higher case volumes, and certain geographic areas in the United States. Of the 6147 patients with known clinical lymph node status, 71.1% underwent neck dissection and 79% had clinically negative necks. The rate of neck dissection was 63.9% in the cN0 group and 98.3% in the cN+ group. Of the patients who underwent neck dissection, the median lymph node yield was 21 lymph nodes overall, 20 lymph nodes in the cN0 patients, and 25 lymph nodes in the cN+ patients. Multivariate analysis was performed on 3097 cN0 patients who underwent neck dissection in the cohort when controlling for patient age, sex, insurance status, year of diagnosis, pT and pN classification, tumor grade, surgical margin status, radiation status, and chemotherapy status. A threshold yield of 16 lymph nodes was validated in 2175 patients with N0 disease. For cN0 patients with fewer than 16 lymph nodes removed, the frequency of identifying at least one positive lymph node was 16.3% whereas the likelihood of identifying at least one positive lymph node in patients who had 16 or more lymph nodes removed was 27.2%. The identification of fewer than 16 lymph nodes in the cN0 patients resulted in significantly decreased survival rates. In cN+ patients, a threshold of 26 lymph nodes was validated in 1903 patients. Identification of fewer than 26 lymph nodes in the cN+ patients resulted in significantly decreased survival rates. The authors offered explanations for the observed survival benefit associated with more extensive lymph node dissections. In patients with cN0 disease, higher lymph node yields were associated with a greater likelihood of removing and identifying one positive lymph node. Removing more lymph nodes increases the likelihood, therefore, of a complete cancer surgery while also serving a role regarding the possibility of adjuvant therapy delivery, both advantages resulting in more favorable outcomes.

6.7 Human Papillomavirus

Approximately 25% of human cancer is caused by infection, and until recently, the major interest in head and neck squamous cell carcinoma has been the involvement of Epstein–Barr virus in nasopharyngeal cancer [49]. Recent attention has been drawn to the involvement of human papillo mavirus (HPV) in head and neck squamous cell carcinoma, particularly oropharyngeal cancer. Features distinguishing HPV-positive from HPV-negative oropharyngeal squamous cell carcinoma is the site predilection of tongue base and tonsil, basaloid histology (Fig. 6.23), younger age, high

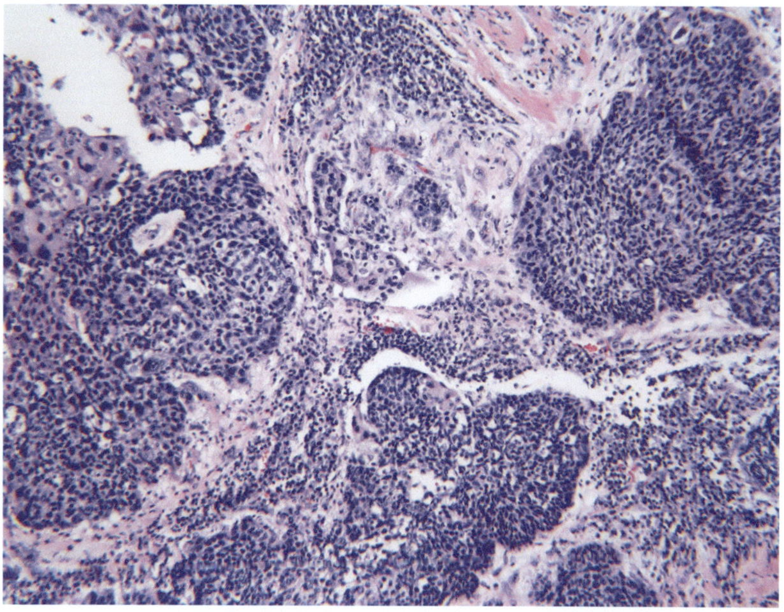

Fig. 6.23 Histopathology of HPV + base of tongue squamous cell carcinoma. Note the basal cell-like (basaloid) appearance of the tumor cells. (Hematoxylin & eosin, original magnification ×200)

socioeconomic status, sexual behavior risk factors, increasing incidence, and the distinct survival advantage of the HPV-positive cancers. Evidence also exists supporting the carcinogenic role of HPV in oral cavity sites, and sophisticated assays indicate that approximately 3–10% of oral squamous cell carcinoma is HPV-related. The number of cases is generally too small to establish meaningful and durable conclusions regarding the prognostic significance of HPV in oral squamous cell carcinoma. The detection of HPV in an oral cancer specimen is controversial, but most centers provide an initial screen with p16 immunohistochemistry (Fig. 6.24) that is relatively inexpensive to perform and is available in most pathology laboratories. The p16 immunohistochemistry tests for high-risk HPV, including HPV 16 and 18 that seem to be most often associated with HPV-related oral and oropharyngeal cancer. While the presence of HPV in the nucleus of the cancer cell is demonstrated by p16 immunohistochemistry, the genetic expression of the oncoproteins E6 and E7 must be demonstrated to establish a cause and effect relationship between HPV and oral squamous cell carcinoma. At least theoretically supporting the relationship between HPV and some oral cancers is the fact that approximately 7% of Americans harbor HPV in their saliva [50]. Extrapolating this data to the United States population suggests that in 2009–2010, there were approximately 15 million adult Americans with an oral HPV infection. Oral HPV infection seems to be affected by numerous behavioral and social factors including tobacco use, oral and conventional sexual practices, and immunosuppression, but not alcohol consumption [3]. In fact, the odds of HPV infection increase significantly in a dose-dependent fashion with increasing measure of current tobacco product use [3, 50] and are higher for women than men. Ever having performed oral sex, early oral and vaginal sexual debut, deep tongue kissing, increasing lifetime oral and vaginal sex partners, and ever having performed vaginal and anal sex are all significantly associated with oral HPV infection [3, 50, 51]. An observational study of oral HPV infection suggested that most oral infections with high-risk types are cleared within 1 year, with a median duration of infection of 6.9 months for any HPV, 6.3 months for oncogenic HPV, and 7.3 months for HPV 16, in particular [52]. Factors typically associated with persistence of oral HPV infection include current tobacco users, age above 44 years, CD4 count below 500 cells/mm, and increased incidence secondary to sexual behaviors and exposure frequency [53].

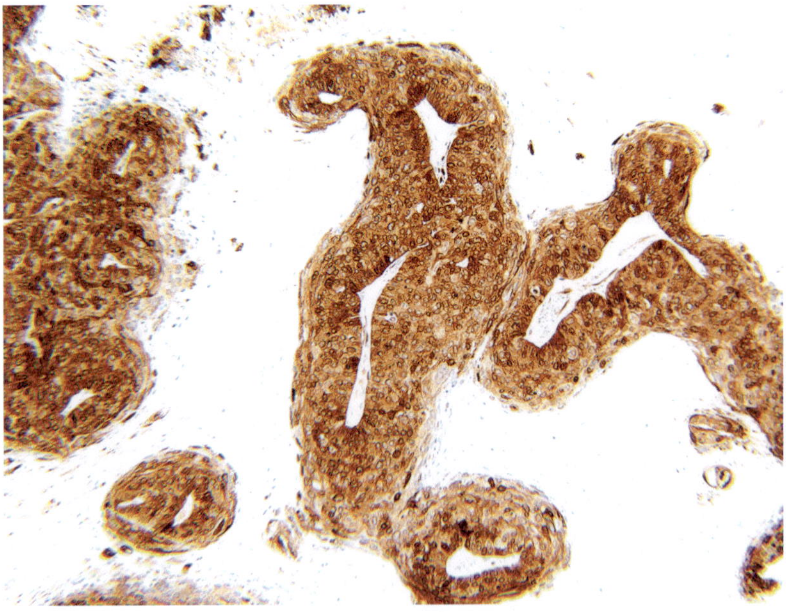

Fig. 6.24 3+ p16 immunohistochemistry of a squamous cell carcinoma of the tongue. The 3+ grading of the p16 indicates the presence of high-risk HPV in the cancer. (Original magnification ×200)

HPV-associated oral and oropharyngeal squamous cell carcinoma is a developing epidemic in the United States with distinctive demographic profiles, treatment responses, and inherent prognoses. Additional data are required regarding HPV-related oral squamous cell carcinoma to possibly offer support of a cause and effect relationship as seems to have been established with oropharyngeal squamous cell carcinoma.

6.8 Bone Invasion

The presence of mandibular invasion is a controversial issue in terms of whether it is an independent prognostic factor in patients with oral squamous cell carcinoma [54]. Prior editions of the staging manual of the AJCC have stated that all forms of mandibular bone invasion were to be designated as T4 tumors. The most recent edition of this manual reserves T4 designations to those cancers that invade beyond the cortex of the mandible (Table 6.1). Li et al. [54] performed a systematic review to determine if mandibular invasion, and cortical vs. medullary invasion specifically, could be considered an independent prognostic factor for patients with oral squamous cell carcinoma. Eighteen studies were included in Li et al.'s meta-analysis with a total of 3746 patients and 1444 patients with bone invasion. When all types of mandibular invasion were considered, the meta-analysis showed no statistical significance between disease-free survival and mandibular invasion ($p = 0.43$). Cortical invasion alone had no effect on disease-free survival ($p > 0.05$). When patients with medullary invasion were compared to patients with no bone invasion, adjusted data and unadjusted data indicated that medullary bone invasion of the mandible possessed statistically and clinically relevant effects on prognosis. The authors concluded that mandibular invasion cannot be considered a criterion for tumor staging, whereas medullary invasion can be considered a criterion for staging. Mandibular medullary invasion by oral squamous cell carcinoma, and not mandibular invasion or mandibular cortical invasion, could be an independent prognostic factor for patients with oral squamous cell carcinoma.

Surgical management of the mandible is an important strategy to consider in patients with squamous cell carcinoma of the mandibular gingiva (Fig. 6.25) as well as in many cases of squamous cell carcinoma of the floor of mouth and buccal mucosa, particularly when proximity of the cancer to the mandible exists with periosteal fixation. Advanced cases of squamous cell carcinoma of the tongue may also warrant mandibular resection. The decision-making process for marginal mandibular resection vs. segmental resection is an essential exercise for oral/head and neck ablative surgeons and is based on known outcomes according to the type of mandibular resection performed based on the type of invasion noted radiographically. This decision-making process is based on physical examination and radiographic assessment of the mandible. Precise analysis of the extent of invasion of the mandible is frequently difficult to determine clinically and often difficult to ascertain with plain film examination. Incipient bone invasion is typically manifested by mandibular cortical erosion with ultimate involvement of the medullary component of the mandible. Negative radiological studies may exist in the presence of microscopic bone invasion such that at least marginal resection of the mandible should be considered under such circumstances. It is generally accepted that marginal mandibular resection should not be performed in patients with gross destruction of cortical bone or extension of cancer to the medullary space of the mandible on radiographic evaluation. Invasion of the mandibular canal or a large soft tissue disease on the medial or lateral cortices of the mandible also represent contraindications to marginal resection. When tumor approximates the mandible, including with periosteal fixation yet without gross radiographic erosion, marginal mandibular resection may represent an oncologically safe procedure [55]. Petrovic et al. [55] retrospectively studied 1866 patients with oral cavity cancer of whom 332 patients (18%) were considered suitable for marginal mandibular resection. Three hundred twenty-six patients were included in the study. One hundred seven patients had gingival cancers, 113 patients had floor of mouth cancers, 50 patients had buccal mucosal cancers, 34 patients

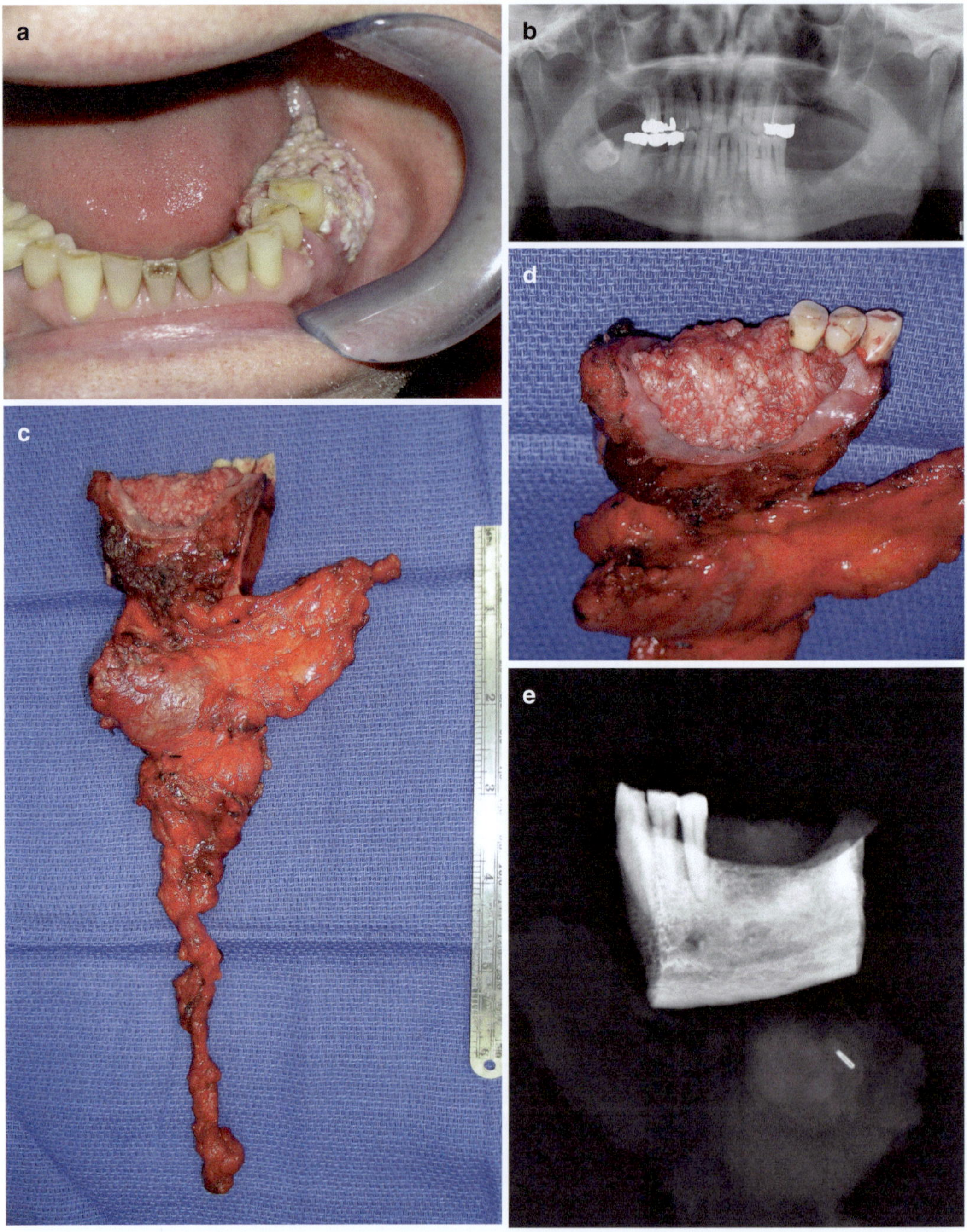

Fig. 6.25 A stage IV (cT4N0M0) squamous cell carcinoma of the left mandibular gingiva (**a**) that exhibited bone erosion on preoperative panoramic radiograph (**b**). The patient underwent composite resection of his left mandibular gingiva, mandible and selective neck dissection (I–III) (**c**). Close examination of the medial aspect of the primary cancer identifies significant involvement of the medial gingiva (**d**). Specimen radiograph (**e**) similarly identifies bone erosion. Final pathology of the composite resection specimen demonstrated negative soft tissue margins, infiltration of the medullary portion of the mandible by the cancer (arrow) (**f**) (Hematoxylin & eosin, original magnification ×100) with negative bone margins, and 1 of 31 lymph nodes positive for metastatic squamous cell carcinoma. A pathologic stage of pT4aN1 is offered

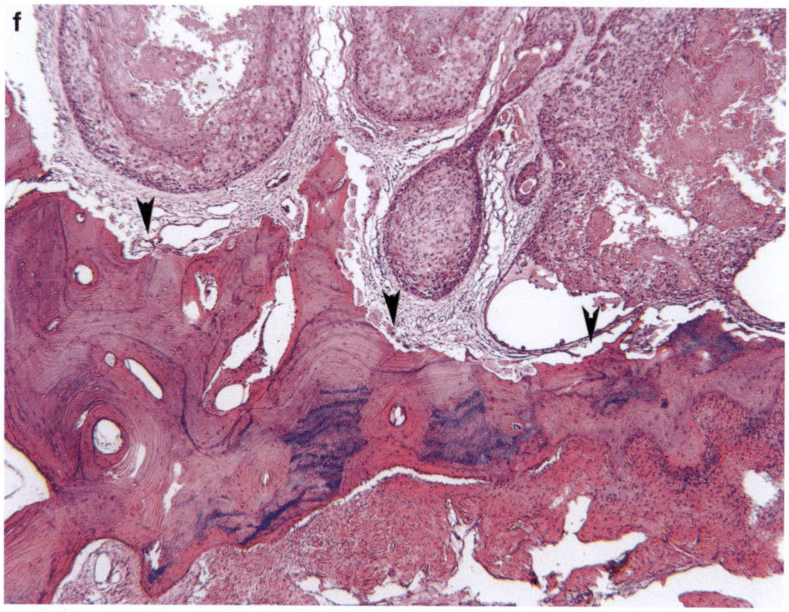

Fig. 6.25 (continued)

had retromolar cancers, and 22 patients had tongue cancers. Two hundred seventy-seven patients (85%) had no bone involvement and 49 patients (15%) had bone involvement. Thirty-two (65.3%) of the 49 patients with bone involvement demonstrated cortical bone erosion by the cancer and 13 patients (26.5%) demonstrated medullary bone erosion. In four patients, the type of bone involvement was not specified. Local recurrence-free survival in patients with and without bone invasion was 62.8% and 76.2%, respectively (p = 0.134). No patients demonstrating microscopic bone invasion required subsequent segmental resection of the mandible. Eight patients displayed positive bone margins, and five of these eight patients received adjuvant therapy; radiation therapy alone in four patients, and chemoradiation therapy in one patient. No patients developed local/regional recurrence; however, two of these patients died with distant metastases. The 5-year disease-specific survival was 78.1% for the entire cohort in this study with a disease-specific survival of 79.7% for patients without bone invasion compared to 66.0% for patients with bone invasion.

6.9 Lymphovascular Invasion

Invasion of the rich lymphatic (Fig. 6.26) and vascular channels (Fig. 6.27) surrounding a squamous cell carcinoma of the oral cavity at least theoretically represents an unfavorable prognostic index. Involvement of the local lymphatics and vasculature have long been considered histopathological features that promote locoregional recurrence or even distant metastases [56]. Adel et al. [56] assessed the outcomes of 571 consecutive patients who underwent primary surgical treatment of squamous cell carcinoma of the oral cavity. In particular, the authors assessed the independent influence of vascular invasion and lymphatic invasion on the development of locoregional recurrence and distant metastases in these patients. The tumor subsites were tongue (n = 211 patients), buccal mucosa (n = 209 patients), gingiva (n = 83 patients), hard palate (n = 15 patients), lip (n = 18 patients), and floor of mouth (n = 35 patients). Lymphatic invasion was noted in 28 patients (4.9%) and vascular invasion was noted in 16 (2.8%) patients. There were significant associations between lymphatic invasion

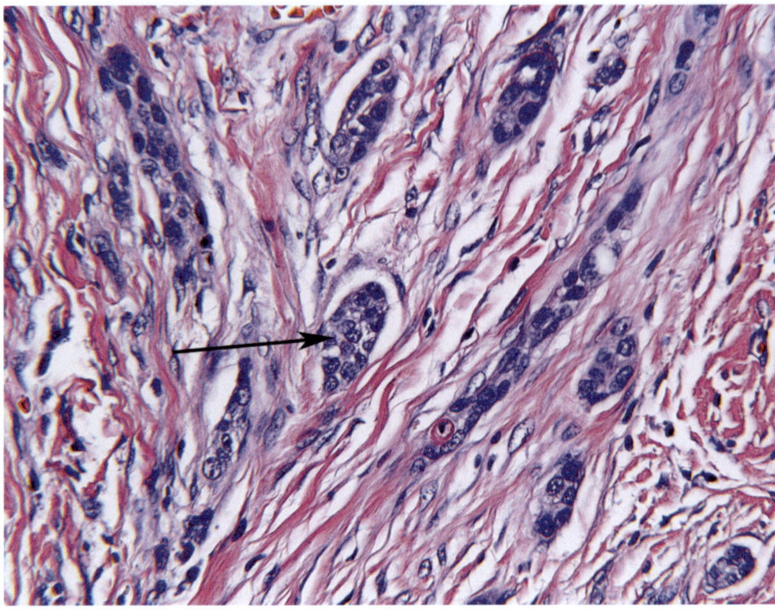

Fig. 6.26 An embolus of squamous cell carcinoma located within a lymphatic channel (arrow). (Hematoxylin & eosin, original magnification ×400)

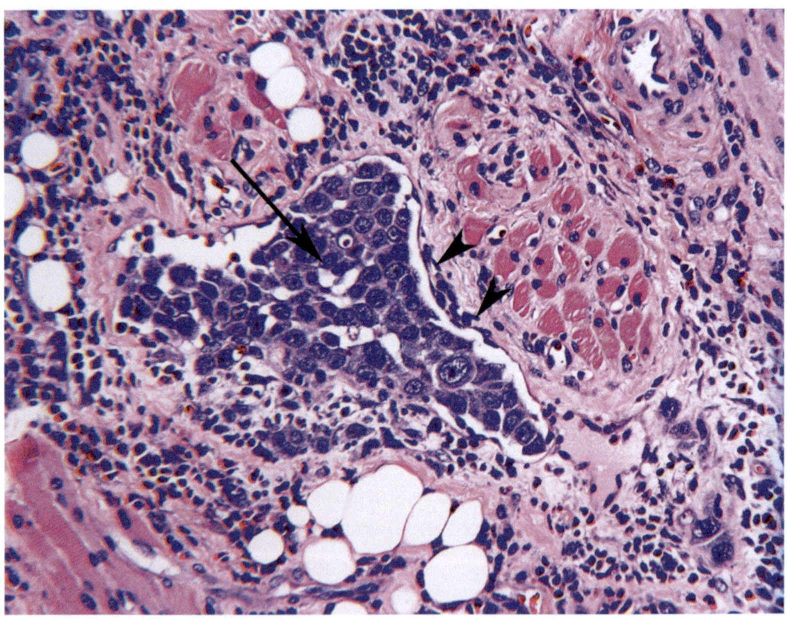

Fig. 6.27 An embolus of squamous cell carcinoma (large arrow) located within a small vein (small arrows). (Hematoxylin & eosin, original magnification ×200)

and T classification of the tumor ($p = 0.009$), nodal metastasis ($p < 0.001$), extracapsular spread ($p < 0.001$), perineural invasion ($p < 0.001$), bone invasion ($p = 0.004$), depth of invasion ($p < 0.001$), and pathologic differentiation ($p = 0.002$). There were significant associations between vascular invasion and T classification ($p = 0.025$), nodal metastasis ($p < 0.001$), extracapsular spread ($p < 0.001$), perineural invasion ($p < 0.001$), depth of invasion ($p = 0.001$), and pathologic differentiation ($p < 0.001$), while no significant association was observed with bone invasion ($p = 0.327$). These associations indicated that the histopathological findings of lymphatic and vascular invasion in the primary cancers were associated with positivity for cervical metastases, extracapsular spread, perineural invasion, poor differentiation, and deeper tumor depth. The presence of lymphatic and vascular invasion was not found to correlate with the variables of local recurrence, regional recurrence, or distant metastasis. Survival analysis indicated that the 5-year overall survival rates for patients with and without lymphatic invasion were statistically significant at 49.3% and 70.3%, respectively ($p < 0.001$). Overall survival of patients with vascular invasion were not significantly different ($p = 0.511$). In disease-specific survival analyses, the 5-year DSS rates for patients with and without lymphatic invasion were statistically significant at 51.6% and 76%, respectively ($p < 0.001$). The difference in DSS according to vascular invasion was not significantly different between those patients with and without vascular invasion in their specimens ($p = 0.247$). The disease-free survival rates for patients with and without lymphatic invasion were 51.6% and 64.4%, respectively ($p = 0.001$). The difference in disease-free survival according to vascular invasion was not statistically significant between those patients with and without vascular invasion in their cancer specimens ($p = 0.452$). In summary, the authors found that lymphatic and vascular invasion did not impact locoregional recurrence or distant metastases after treatment. That said, vascular invasion was not found to adversely affect patient survival, but lymphatic invasion was associated with worse overall survival, disease-specific survival, and disease-free survival. Based on these results, the authors indicated that the histopathologic demonstration of either lymphatic or vascular invasion might not be an indicator for adjuvant therapy in patients treated for squamous cell carcinoma of the oral cavity.

6.10 Conclusion

Oral squamous cell carcinoma is associated with numerous histopathologic factors that affect the patient's prognosis. As per the NCCN guidelines, these factors dictate the administration of adjuvant therapy. The molecular advances in the diagnosis of oral squamous cell carcinoma will further elucidate the significance of these histopathologic factors in the future.

References

1. Wagner VP, Webber LP, Curra M, Klein IP, Meurer L, Carrad VC, Martins MD. Bryne's grading system predicts poor disease-specific survival of oral squamous cell carcinoma: a comparative study among different histologic grading system. Oral Surg Oral Med Oral Pathol Oral Radiol. 2017;123:688–96.
2. Johnson NW, Amarashinghe HK, Qualliotine JR, Fakhry C. Epidemiology. In: Bell RB, Fernandes RP, Andersen PE, editors. Oral, head and neck oncology and reconstructive surgery. St. Louis, MO: Elsevier; 2018. p. 2–56.
3. Duncan LD, Winkler M, Carlson ER, Heidel RE, Kang E, Webb DE. Prevalence of human papillomavirus in squamous cell carcinoma of the oral cavity with correlation of p16 immunohistochemistry and human papillomavirus polymerase chain reaction. J Oral Maxillofac Surg. 2013;71:1367–75.
4. Vuity D, McMahon J, Takhiuddin S, Slinger C, McLellan D, Wales C, MacIver C, Thomson E, McCaul J, Hislop S, Lamb C, Stalker E, Young D. Is the 8th edition of the Union for International Cancer Control staging of oral cancer good enough? Br J Oral Maxillofac Surg. 2018;56:272–7.
5. Spiro RH, Huvos AG, Wong GY, Spiro JD, Gnecco CA, Strong EW. Predictive value of tumor thickness in squamous carcinoma of the tongue and floor of mouth. Am J Surg. 1986;152:345–50.
6. Shim SJ, Cha J, Koom WS, Kim GE, Lee CG, Choi EC, Keum KC. Clinical outcomes for T1-2 N0-1 oral tongue cancer patients underwent surgery with and without postoperative radiotherapy. Radiat Oncol. 2010;5:1–7.
7. Lydiatt WM, Patel SG, O'Sullivan B, Brandwein MS, Ridge JA, Migliacci JC, Loomis AM, Shah JP. Head and neck cancers – major changes in the American Joint Committee on Cancer eighth edition cancer staging manual. CA Cancer J Clin. 2017;67:122–37.
8. Elston CW, Ellis IOI. Pathological prognostic factors in breast cancer. I. The value of histological grade in breast cancer: experience from a large study with long-term follow-up. Histopathology. 1991;19:403–10.
9. Gleason DF. Classification of prostatic carcinoma. Cancer Chemother Rep. 1966;50:125–8.
10. Broders AC. Squamous cell epithelioma of the lip. JAMA. 1920;74:656–64.
11. Barnes L, Eveson JW, Reichart P, Sidransky D. WHO classification of tumors, vol. 9. Lyon: IARC; 2005.
12. Muller S. Update from the 4th edition of the World Health Organization of head and neck tumours: tumours of the oral cavity and mobile tongue. Head Neck Pathol. 2017;11:33–40.

13. Bryne M, Koppang HS, Lilleng R, Stene T, Bang G, Dabelsteen E. New malignancy grading is a better prognostic indicator than Broders' grading in oral squamous cell carcinomas. J Oral Pathol Med. 1989;18:432–7.
14. Jacobsson PA, Eneroth CM, Killander D, Moberger G, Martenson B. Histologic classification and grading of malignancy in carcinoma of the larynx (a pilot study). Acta Radiol Ther Phys Biol. 1973;12:1–8.
15. Anneroth G, Batsakis J, Luna M. Review of the literature and a recommended system of malignancy grading in oral squamous cell carcinoma. J Dent Res. 1987;95:229–49.
16. Bryne M, Koppang HS, Lilleng R, Kjaerheim A. Malignancy grading of the deep invasive margins of oral squamous cell carcinomas has high prognostic value. J Pathol. 1992;166:375–81.
17. Sawazaki-Calone I, Rangel ALCA, Bueno AG, Morais CF, Nagai HM, Kunz RP, Souza RL, Rutkauskis L, Salo T, Almangush A, Coletta RD. The prognostic value of histopathological grading systems in oral squamous cell carcinomas. Oral Dis. 2015;21:755–61.
18. Brandwein-Gensler M, Teixeira MS, Lewis CM, Lee B, Rolnitzky L, Hille JJ, Genden E, Urken M, Wang BY. Oral squamous cell carcinoma: histologic risk assessment, but not margin status, is strongly predictive of local disease-free and overall survival. Am J Surg Pathol. 2005;29:167–78.
19. Almangush A, Coletta RD, Bello IO, Bitu C, Keski-Santii H, Makinen LK, Kauppila JH, Pukkila M, Hagstrom J, Laranne J, Tommola S, Soini Y, Kosma VM, Koivunen P, Kawalski LP, Nieminen P, Grenman R, Leivo I, Salo T. A simple novel prognostic model for early stage oral tongue cancer. Int J Oral Maxillofac Surg. 2015;44:143–50.
20. Tarsitano A, Tardio ML, Marchetti C. Impact of perineural invasion as independent prognostic factor for local and regional failure in oral squamous cell carcinoma. Oral Surg Oral Med Oral Pathol Oral Radiol. 2015;119:221–8.
21. Chatzistefanou I, Lubek J, Markou K, Ord RA. The role of perineural invasion in treatment decisions for oral cancer patients: a review of the literature. J Cranio-Maxillofac Surg. 2017;45:821–5.
22. Liebig C, Ayala G, Wilks JA, Berger DH, Albo D. Perineural invasion in cancer: a review of the literature. Cancer. 2009;115:3379–91.
23. Cracchiolo JR, Xu B, Migliacci JC, Katabi N, Pfister DG, Lee NY, Patel SG, Ghossein RA, Wong RJ. Patterns of recurrence in oral tongue cancer with perineural invasion. Head Neck. 2018;40:1287–95.
24. National Comprehensive Cancer Network. NCCN clinical practice guidelines in oncology (NCCN guidelines). Head and neck cancers. Version 2.2018 – 20 Jun 2018. www.nccn.org. Accessed 14 Jul 2018.
25. Bernier J, Domenge C, Ozsahin M, Matuszewska K, Lefebvre JL, Greiner RH, Giralt J, Maingon P, Rolland F, Bolla M, Cognetti F, Bourhis J, Kirkpatrick A, van Glabbeke M. Postoperative irradiation with or without concomitant chemotherapy for locally advanced head and neck cancer. New Engl J Med. 2004;350:1945–52.
26. Magliocca KR. Surgical margins. The perspective of pathology. Oral Maxillofac Surg Clin North Am. 2017;29:367–75.
27. Weinstock YE, Allava I, Dierks EJ. Ptifalls in determining head and neck surgical margins. Oral Maxillofac Surg Clin North Am. 2014;26:151–62.
28. Shapiro M, Salama A. Margin analysis. Squamous cell carcinoma of the oral cavity. Oral Maxillofac Surg Clin North Am. 2017;29:259–67.
29. Dillon JK, Brown CB, McDonald TM, Ludwig DC, Clark PJ, Leroux BG, Futran ND. How does the close surgical margin impact recurrence and survival when treating oral squamous cell carcinoma? J Oral Maxillofac Surg. 2015;73:1182–8.
30. Byers RM, Bland KI, Borlase B, Luna M. The prognostic and therapeutic value of frozen section determinations in the surgical treatment of squamous cell carcinoma of the head and neck. Am J Surg. 1978;136:525–8.
31. Johnson RE, Sigman JD, Funk GF, Robinson RA, Hoffman HT. Quantification of surgical margin shrinkage in the oral cavity. Head Neck. 1997;19:281–6.
32. Mistry RC, Qureshi SS, Kumaran C. Post-resection mucosal margin shrinkage in oral cancer: quantification and significance. J Surg Oncol. 2005;91:131–3.
33. Cheng A, Cox D, Schmidt BL. Oral squamous cell carcinoma margin discrepancy after resection and pathologic processing. J Oral Maxillofac Surg. 2008;66:523–9.
34. Ord RA, Aisner S. Accuracy of frozen sections in assessing margins in oral cancer resection. J Oral Maxillofac Surg. 1997;55:663–9.
35. Ellis OG, David MC, Park DJ, Batstone MD. High-volume surgeons deliver larger surgical margins in oral cavity cancer. J Oral Maxillofac Surg. 2016;74:1466–72.
36. Edwards SP. Margin analysis – has free tissue transfer improved oncologic outcomes for oral squamous cell carcinoma? Oral Maxillofac Surg Clin North Am. 2017;29:377–81.
37. Brennan JA, Mao L, Hruban RH, Boyle JO, Eby YJ, Koch WM, et al. Molecular assessment of histopathological staging in squamous cell carcinoma of the head and neck. N Engl J Med. 1995;332:429–35.
38. Liu SA, Wang CC, Jiang RS, Wang WY, Lin JC. Genetic analysis of surgical margins in oral cavity cancer. Br J Surg. 2018;105:e142–9.
39. de Carvalho AC, Kowalski LP, Campos AHJF, Soares FA, Carvalho AL, Vettore AL. Clinical significance of molecular alterations in histologically negative surgical margins of head and neck cancer patients. Oral Oncol. 2012;48:240–8.
40. Ferris RL, Xi L, Raja S, Hung JL, Wang J, Gooding WE, Kelly L, Ching J, Luketich JD, Godfrey TE. Molecular staging of cervical lymph nodes in squamous cell carcinoma of the head and neck. Cancer Res. 2005;65:2147–56.
41. Brockhoff HC, Kim RY, Braun TM, Skouteris C, Helman JI, Ward BB. Correlating the depth of inva-

sion at specific anatomic locations with the risk for regional metastatic disease to lymph nodes in the neck for oral squamous cell carcinoma. Head Neck. 2017;39:974–9.

42. de Matos LL, Manfro G, dos Santos RV, Stabenow E, de Mello ES, Alves VAF, Pinto FR, Kulesar MAV, Brandao LG, Cernea CR. Tumor thickness as a predictive factor of lymph node metastasis and disease recurrence in T1N0 and T2N0 squamous cell carcinoma of the oral tongue. Oral Surg Oral Med Oral Pathol Oral Radiol. 2014;118:209–17.
43. Weiss MH, Harrison LB, Isaacs RS. Use of decision analysis in planning a management strategy for the stage N0 neck. Arch Otolaryngol Head Neck Surg. 1994;120:699–702.
44. Masood MH, Farquhar DR, Vanleer JP, Patel SN, Hackman TG. Depth of invasion on pathological outcomes in clinical low-stage oral tongue cancer patients. Oral Dis. 2018;24:1198–203.
45. Kalnins IK, Leonard AG, Sako K, Razack MS, Shedd DP. Correlation between prognosis and degree of lymph node involvement in carcinoma of the oral cavity. Am J Surg. 1977;134:450–4.
46. Ghadjar P, Schreier-Facklam H, Grater R, Evers C, Simcock M, Geretschlager A, Blumstein NM, Zbaren P, Zimmer Y, Wilkens L, Aebersold DM. Quantitative analysis of extracapsular extension of metastatic lymph nodes and its significance in radiotherapy planning in head and neck squamous cell carcinoma. Int J Radiat Oncol Biol Phys. 2010;76:1127–32.
47. D'Cruz AK, Vaish R, Kapre N, Dandekar M, Gupta S, Hawaldar R, Agarwal JP, Pantvaidya G, Chaukar D, Deshmukh A, Kane S, Arya S, Ghosh-Laskar S, Chaturvedi P, Pai P, Nair S, Nair D, Badwe R. Elective versus therapeutic neck dissection in node-negative oral cancer. N Engl J Med. 2015;373:521–9.
48. Kuo P, Mehra S, Sosa JA, Roman SA, Husain ZA, Burtness BA, Tate JP, Yarbrough WG, Judson BL. Proposing prognostic thresholds for lymph node yield in clinically lymph node-negative and lymph node-positive cancers of the oral cavity. Cancer. 2016;122:3624–31.
49. Shaw RJ, Brown J, Etti T, Risk JM. Prognostic factors in oral, oropharyngeal, and salivary gland cancer. In: Brennan PA, Schliephake H, Ghali GE, Cascarini L, editors. Maxillofacial surgery. 3rd ed. St. Louis, MO: Elsevier; 2017. p. 257–74.
50. Gillison ML, Broutian T, Pickard RK, Tong ZY, Xiao W, Kahle L, Graubard BI, Chaturvedi AK. Prevalence of oral HPV infection in the United States 2009–2010. JAMA. 2012;307:693–703.
51. Beachler DC, Weber KM, Margolick JB, Strickler HD, Cranston RD, Burk RD, Wiley DJ, Minkoff H, Reddy S, Stammer EE, Gillison ML, D'Souza G. Risk factors for oral HPV infection among a high prevalence population of HIV-positive and at risk HIV-negative adults. Cancer Epidemiol Biomark Prev. 2012;21:122–33.
52. Kreimer AR, Pierce Campbell CM, Lin HY, Fulp W, Papenfuss MR, Abrahamsen M, Hildesheim A, Villa LL, Salmeron JJ, Lazcano-Ponce E, Giulliano AR. Incidence and clearance of oral human papillomavirus infection in men: the HIM cohort study. Lancet. 2013;382:877–87.
53. Kreimer AR, Clifford GM, Boyle P, Franceschi S. Human papillomavirus types in head and neck squamous cell carcinomas worldwide: a systematic review. Cancer Epidemiol Biomark Prev. 2005;14:467–75.
54. Li C, Lin J, Men Y, Yang W, Mi F, Li L. Does medullary versus cortical invasion of the mandible affect prognosis in patients with oral squamous cell carcinoma? J Oral Maxillofac Surg. 2017;75:403–15.
55. Petrovic I, Montero PH, Migilacci MC, Palmer FL, Ganly I, Patel SG, Shah JP. Influence of bone invasion on outcomes after marginal mandibulectomy in squamous cell carcinoma of the oral cavity. J Craniomaxillofac Surg. 2017;45:252–7.
56. Adel M, Kao HK, Hsu CL, Huang JJ, Lee LY, Huang Y, Browne T, Tsang NM, Chang YL, Chang KP. Evaluation of lymphatic and vascular invasion in relation to clinicopathological factors and treatment outcome in oral cavity squamous cell carcinoma. Medicine. 2015;94:e1510.

7 Genetics of Oral Cancer

Anthony Morlandt and Hope Amm

Oral and oropharyngeal cancers affect as many as 275,000 individuals worldwide, including 53,000 in the United States in 2019 representing about 11 cases per 100,000 per year. Survival for all stages has demonstrated a modest increase over the past 40 years, from 50% to 65% disease-specific survival over 5 years [1]. Over 90% of the cancers occurring in the oral cavity arise from lining gingiva and mucosa and arise from the rapidly dividing squamous epithelial cells. Classically, these oral squamous cell carcinomas (OSCC) were observed to occur mainly in men, strike in the sixth and seventh decades of life, and were caused by tobacco and alcohol consumption. In the past decade, an increase in the number of cases affecting young people, in particular, white women less than 50 years old without identifiable risk factors, has fueled curiosity regarding the genetic basis of these tumors [2]. There are other cases which should respond to treatment with surgery, radiotherapy, and/or chemotherapy, but do not. Head and neck oncologists struggle with the patient who, after highly toxic and difficult treatments, recur either locally or in a distant fashion and as such suffer a shortened lifespan. Contemporary understanding of head and neck malignancy has shifted in recent decades: from treatment consisting of radical surgical extirpation espoused by Halsted, Conley, and Martin, to an attempt to understand the molecular basis of tumors and develop novel therapies directed toward specific tumor types. The genetics of oral cancer is a very broad topic and includes carcinogenesis via initiation, promotion, and progression, field cancerization, the host immune response, and regulatory genes associated with malignant transformation and metastasis.

Carcinogenesis is theorized as a multistep progression beginning with initiation, resulting from environmental injury such as cigarette smoke, oncogenic viruses such as HPV, or alcohol consumption [3]. In other cases, regulatory genes including proto-oncogenes and tumor suppressor genes contain inherited defects which initiate of carcinogenesis. Regardless of the cause of the defect, initiation represents a mutation which is self-perpetuating and irreversible, leading to malignant transformation of normal cells. The promotion phase follows and is characterized by unchecked cell growth, invasion, and metastasis. The role of chronic inflammation has been investigated in oral carcinogenesis and is being investigated with respect to MMP

A. Morlandt (✉)
Section of Oral Oncology, Department of Oral and Maxillofacial Surgery, University of Alabama at Birmingham, Birmingham, AL, USA
e-mail: morlandt@uab.edu

H. Amm
Department of Oral and Maxillofacial Surgery, University of Alabama at Birmingham, Birmingham, AL, USA
e-mail: hopeamm@uab.edu

D. Kademani (ed.), *Improving Outcomes in Oral Cancer*,
https://doi.org/10.1007/978-3-030-30094-4_7

expression in periodontal disease (see below). Progression is the final stage of carcinogenesis and follows a stepwise pattern. Knudson described the "two-hit hypothesis", where initial irreversible injury to one allele of a tumor suppressor gene does not result in phenotypic change (tumor formation). Loss of heterozygosity describes this phenomenon, where the normally functioning copy of the tumor suppressor gene inhibits cancer growth. The "second hit" by mutagenic agents permanently disrupts the gene's function, resulting in potential tumor cell growth, leading to invasion and metastasis [4].

With the increase in affordability and accessibility of sequencing technologies, the ability to examine changes in DNA, RNA, and microRNA (miRNA) has greatly expanded. Many of these technologies have been used to study genomic variations and changes in gene expression in head and neck cancer, including oral cancer, and can serve as biomarkers of carcinogenesis. Many mutations and single nucleotide polymorphisms (SNPs) in genes associated with carcinogenesis have been suggested to play a role in susceptibility and prognosis of OSCC. The Cancer Genome Network used a multiplatform approach to characterize the genomic alterations in 279 cases of HNSCC, including 172 cases of OSCC [5]. This study collected fresh, flash-frozen tumors from newly diagnosed HNSCC patients with either adjacent normal tissue or DNA from blood as normal controls. Along with the collection of clinical data, they isolated DNA and RNA for whole exome, RNA, and miRNA sequencing; methylation arrays; and DNA SNP arrays. The study confirmed P53 and CDKN2A loss-of-function mutations in many cases of smoking-related HNSCC. HPV(−) tumors tended to have amplification of oncogenes (CCND1, MYC), growth factor receptor tyrosine kinases (EGFR, FGFR1), and amplifications or mutations in PI3KCA. Mutations in FAT1 (23%) and NOTCH1 (19%) were also significantly prevalent in HNSCC. A subtype of OSCC with favorable prognosis was identified with wild-type P53, but mutations in HRAS and CASP8. As the number of patients evaluated with multiomic platforms increases, better definition of prognostic and predictive biomarkers may be available.

Regulation of the immune response is complicated and just beginning to be understood in cancer. Many molecules involved in immune regulation have shown genetic variation in OSCC, including interleukins, chemokines, and programmed cell death ligand 1 (PD-L1). The role of interleukins in tumor promotion and progression is a complicated story, with certain interleukins having either tumor promoting or tumor suppressive effects depending on the tumor origin and tumor microenvironment. However, in OSCC, particular interleukin (IL) SNPs have been associated with higher risk of OSCC or certain stages of OSCC. Correlative studies have shown a strong association between susceptibility to OSCC and SNPs in the genes for IL-4, IL-6, IL-8, IL-10, and TNFα [6]. In IL-10, a SNP in the promoter region was correlated with higher serum levels of IL-10 and increased risk of OSCC in an Indian population [7]. Another study of Indian populations showed that a polymorphism in IL-18 was associated with OSCC risk compared to healthy controls [8]. This IL-18 SNP was associated with other cancer types in different populations, but did not associate with HNSCC in Iranian or Greek populations. Therefore, the relative risk associated with SNPs may be dependent on ethnic background as well as cancer type. In a European population, IL-4 promoter polymorphisms were associated with increased OSCC risk and early-stage disease [9]. An IL-17A SNP was associated with late clinical stages and poor tumor differentiation [10]. A Taiwanese study found an IL-6 SNP (rs1800796) combined with poor dental care was significantly associated with high-risk of OSCC [11]. In a study of stage I/II OSCC patients, low serum levels of IL-6 correlated with longer disease-free survival [12]. In another study, high tumor stroma expression of S100A9 was shown to increase IL-6 expression in OSCC cells in vitro and in vivo [13]. High S100A9 expression in early-stage OSCC was correlated with shorter recurrence-free survival. This highlights how interleukins and upstream pathways, which regulate them, may play a role in the susceptibility to OSCC.

Another area of recent interest is the effect of miRNA on gene expression and tumorigenesis.

miRNAs are small noncoding RNAs that silence gene expression by binding to complimentary regions on mRNAs and interrupting their expression [14]. These miRNAs are known to regulate many targets including interleukins. In a study of esophageal squamous cell carcinoma, plasma levels of IL-6 correlated with overall survival and an increased incidence in recurrence [15]. They discovered patients with a SNP in mir608, a miRNA, had higher plasma levels of IL-6, and analytical studies showed this variant was less effective in regulating IL-6 expression. Another study showed that miRNA let-7c was decreased in OSCC patient samples, and that let-7c regulates IL-8 in a tumor-suppressing manner [14]. miRNAs are also being used to help develop oral diagnostics for OSCC. Yap et al. [16] used patient samples to identify a pattern of miRNA expression in OSCC. They showed increased miR-31 and miR-21 and decreased miR-99a, let-7c, miR-125b, and miR-100 in OSCC samples. They used this panel to differentiate between oral swirls (sterile water used to wash the mouth) from OSCC and control patients. They correctly identified 100% of the OSCC patients and 67% of controls. More work is required for effective and noninvasive diagnostics, but further definition of OSCC genetics will allow refinement of ongoing attempts.

Chemokines play an important role in regulating the immune system by attracting cells to particular locations. SNPs in CCL4, a monocyte/macrophage attractant, were associated with OSCC in a Taiwanese population. One particular SNP was associated with susceptibility to OSCC (increased presence in OSCC patients compared to healthy controls) but correlated with smaller tumor size [17]. Another immune modulatory molecule, programmed cell death protein 1 (PD-1) is the target of a promising therapeutics designed to activate tumor-specific T-cells [18]. PD-1 binds to programmed death ligand-1 (PD-L1) expressed by tumor cells, which suppresses the T-cell. Monoclonal antibodies bind to PD-1 to inhibit the suppression and activate T-cell-mediated cytotoxicity. Heineman et al. [18] showed HNSCC patients express high levels of PD-L1 relative to other tumor types. Another study showed increased expression of PD-L1 in OSCC tumor tissue as well as the peripheral blood of patients [19]. As immune checkpoint inhibitors continue to advance, HNSCC patients, including OSCC, may benefit from these therapies.

Tumor microenvironment regulation has been implicated in the progression and invasion of many human cancers [20]. Matrix metalloproteinases (MMP) are implicated in the degrading the extracellular matrix that encapsulate tumors allowing for invasion and promoting angiogenesis within tumors. In the promoter region of MMP-1, a particular SNP (2G allele) has been associated with OSCC in Japanese, Taiwanese, Chinese, and Indian populations [21–25]. A MMP-2 promoter SNP correlates with OSCC in Thai, Taiwanese, and Chinese populations [21, 22, 26, 27]. Additional studies have identified SNP in the promoters of MMP-3 and MMP-9 [28]. Additionally MMP-11 polymorphisms showed increased susceptibility for OSCC, and patients with a certain MMP-11 allele (rs738792) had increased lymph node metastasis [29]. When considering expression of MMP genes, an analysis of microarray data from OSCC samples originating from the tongue showed increased expression of MMP-9 compared to normal tissue [30]. In the future, detection of MMPs and related SNPs may be valuable in determining the relative risk for developing OSCC and the risk of OSCC progression.

Genetics may also play a role in racial disparities observed in OSCC. Ancestry-related SNPs in DNA polymerase B (POLB) were detected in African American patients with HNSCC from The Cancer Genome Network databases and were confirmed in additional patient databases [31]. The POLB SNPs correlated with significantly increased expression on POLB and worse overall survival and disease-free survival. As databases expand, include additional demographic information, and a wider variety of patients; our ability to detect molecular differences between types of tumors and markers of prognosis will increase.

Several studies have taken the approach of identifying genetic signatures or candidate genes as prognostic indicators. In a study of 311 patients, particular SNPs in cyclin D1 (rs9344) and retinoblastoma (rs427686) were related to disease-free survival [32]. Another study compared node-positive (LN+) versus node-negative (LN-) patients and identified six immune-related genes (APOE, C3AR1, CD163, CXCR4, FN1, TNFRSF9), which were increased in LN+ samples and correlated with significantly worse 5-year node-free survival [33]. In node-positive patients, a signature of 11 genes differentiated between patients with extracapsular spread and those without [34]. A meta-analysis of SNPs in case-controlled studies associated nine SNPs in eight genes with increased risk of OSCC (IL-10, TGFb, HIF, COX2, XRCC3, CYP1A1, GSTM1, MTHFR) by comparing OSCC patients to normal controls [35]. miRNA sequencing of Danish patients and healthy controls identified three up-regulated miRNAs and three down-regulated miRNAs [36]. Three of these miRNAs (miR-486-5p, miR-375, miR92b-3p) were detected in plasma and correlated with OSCC recurrence in Chinese patients with and without recurrence 9–12 months post surgical treatment. Expression of five miRNAs was linked to OSCC compared to normal oral mucosa [37]. Evaluation of plasma samples showed miR-30a-5p and miR-796-5p were detectable in patients with OSCC compared to healthy controls. These studies emphasize the diagnostic and prognostic possibilities that come with analyzed the molecular profile of OSCC.

Oral cancers are particularly difficult to diagnose for the general medical or dental practitioner. With no widely available screening assay using imaging (e.g., mammography, colonoscopy) or serum markers (e.g., PSA, CA 19-9), astute clinical examination is necessary and relies on patient access to specialists in many cases. In addition to standard white light visual examination and scalpel biopsy, novel detection modalities such as fluorescence imaging using antibody-based optical imaging are currently being investigated [38]. Antibody-based optical imaging offers a minimally invasive, antibody-specific approach to tumor detection and could enhance traditional approaches to screening in the general practitioners' office. Because EGFR is over-expressed in many tumors, especially OSCCs, a fluorophore can be annealed to the Fc segment of cetuximab which, when excited by a source light at the appropriate wavelength, can be visualized using an optical scanner, delineating the tumor. A significant advantage of this technology is the opportunity to assess surgical margins in real time, both macro- and microscopically, during ablative tumor surgery [39]. The surgeon may thereby use the probe to see a tumor's actual margins in the operating room, relying less on palpation and plain white light visualization, and the pathologist can use is for real-time immunohistochemistry in the frozen section room.

Non-antibody-based autofluorescence and tissue reflectance involves an extrinsic light source to excite fluorophores which are naturally occurring within the tissues and does not require an infusion with cetuximab or panitumumab. Increased histone protein concentration, cross-linked collagen, and hypervascular zones within a lesion (potentially resulting from angiogenesis) result in a difference between the excitation and emission wavelengths, and may be visible to the observer. Many general dental practitioners use these technologies in the dental office for screening purposes. A Cochrane review including 4002 patients with premalignant and malignant oral epithelial lesions suggested autofluorescence light systems may aid the surgeon already planning a biopsy by identifying the area of the lesion with the greatest metabolic activity but do not possess the sensitivity or specificity to be used for widespread population screening [40]. In the high-risk population of patients with previous OSCC who had undergone surgery, radiotherapy, or both, handheld light-based technology offered no benefit to tumor or dysplasia detection over plain white light visualization by a trained practitioner [41].

As precision medicine continues to gain in popularity, increasing the efficacy and safety of treatments for patients is key to long-term outcomes. Currently, the only FDA-approved first-line targeted therapy for OSCC is the epidermal growth factor receptor (EGFR) antagonist cetuximab [5, 42]. In 2016, the PDL-1 inhibitor pembrolizumab was approved for use in recurrent or metastatic disease. The success of clinically available biomarkers for tumor characterization is key to understanding the therapeutic profile and treatment effect of immunotherapies. Chia et al. [43] validated ex vivo models of HNSCC to determine therapeutic response of tumors. They used patient-derived primary cultures to screen for sensitivity to several drugs. Next, patient-derived xenografts (PDX) from the same patient were treated with drug; the cell culture indicated they were sensitive too. In each case shown, the drug produced a significant decrease in tumor volume. For one OSCC patient, cells and PDX models from both the primary site and metastatic site showed different genomic profiles and drug sensitivities. The patient was treated with gefitinib, an EGFR inhibitor, and showed significant regression within 6 weeks of treatment. The patient unfortunately progressed after 6 months of therapy, which was shown to a subpopulation of resistant tumor cells that expressed higher levels of YAP1. This study demonstrates the utility of patient-matched ex vivo studies to guide therapy selection and identify treatment response biomarkers. Many new therapies based on the expression of tumor markers or the presence of particular mutations are under development. Based on genomic information, the design of clinical trials is advancing. New basket and umbrella trials assign patients to treatment arms based on the presence of specific genetic alterations rather than tumor type [44]. These trials aim to leverage the tumor genetic profiles to match actionable mutations with the proper drug, improve patient outcomes, and streamline clinical development.

References

1. American Cancer Society Cancer Statistics Center. 2019. https://cancerstatisticscenter.cancer.org/?_ga=2.40982882.1193585586.1552078980-1333190596.1551989886#!/cancer-site/Oral%20cavity%20and%20pharynx.
2. Tota JE, Anderson WF, Coffey C, Califano J, Cozen W, Ferris R, St. John M, Cohen E, Chaturvedi A. Rising incidence of oral tongue cancer among white men and women in the United States, 1973–2012. Oral Oncol. 2017;67:146–52. https://doi.org/10.1016/j.oraloncology.2017.02.019.
3. Farah CS, Jessri M, Currie S, Alnuaimi A, Yap T, McCullough M. Aetiology of oral cavity cancer. In: Kuriakose MA, editor. Contemporary oral oncology: biology, epidemiology, etiology, and prevention. New York, NY: Springer; 2017.
4. Suresh A, Kuriakose M, Mohanta S, Siddapa G. Carcinogenesis and field cancerization in oral squamous cell carcinoma. In: Kuriakose MA, editor. Contemporary oral oncology: biology, epidemiology, etiology, and prevention. New York, NY: Springer; 2017.
5. Cancer Genome Atlas Network. Comprehensive genomic characterization of head and neck squamous cell carcinomas. Nature. 2015;517:576. https://doi.org/10.1038/nature14129.
6. Serefoglou Z, Yapijakis C, Nkenke E, Vairaktaris E. Genetic association of cytokine DNA polymorphisms with head and neck cancer. Oral Oncol. 2008;44:1093–9. https://doi.org/10.1016/j.oraloncology.2008.02.012.
7. Sharma U, Singhal P, Bandil K, Kumar A, Bose S, Ahuja P, et al. Genetic variations of IL-10: Identification of novel variations and evaluation of the impact of the SNPs/haplotype in the promoter region with the progression of oral squamous cell carcinoma in indian population. Cytokine. 2018;103:99–108. https://doi.org/10.1016/j.cyto.2017.09.016.
8. Singh PK, Ahmad MK, Kumar V, Hussain SR, Gupta R, Jain A, et al. Effects of interleukin 18 promoter (C607A and G137C) gene polymorphisms and their association with oral squamous cell carcinoma (OSCC) in northern India. Tumour Biol. 2014;35:12275–84. https://doi.org/10.1007/s13277-014-2538-0.
9. Vairaktaris E, Yannopoulos A, Vassiliou S, Serefoglou Z, Vylliotis A, Nkenke E, et al. Strong association of interleukin-4 (−590 C/T) polymorphism with increased risk for oral squamous cell carcinoma in Europeans. Oral Surg Oral Med Oral Pathol Oral Radiol Endod. 2007;104:796–802. https://doi.org/10.1016/j.tripleo.2006.12.029.
10. Li N, Zhang C, Chen Z, Bai L, Nie M, Zhou B, et al. Interleukin 17A and interleukin 17F polymorphisms are associated with oral squamous cell carcinoma susceptibility in a Chinese population. J Oral Maxillofac Surg. 2015;73:267–73. https://doi.org/10.1016/j.joms.2014.09.009.
11. Chang JS, Lo HI, Wong TY, Huang CC, Lee WT, Tsai ST, Chen KC, Yen CJ, Wu YH, Hsueh WT, Yang MW, Wu SY, Chang KY, Chang JY, Ou CY, Wang YH, Weng YL, Yang HC, Wang FT, Lin CL, Huang JS, Hsiao JR. Investigating the association between oral hygiene and head and neck cancer. Oral Oncol. 2013;49:1010–7. https://doi.org/10.1016/j.oraloncology.2013.07.004.
12. Goda H, Okamoto M, Nakashiro KI, Hino S, Murase R, Hamakawa H. Prognostic impact of preoperative serum interleukin-6 levels in patients with early-stage oral squamous cell carcinoma, defined by sentinel node biopsy. Oncol Lett. 2017;14:7965–9. https://doi.org/10.3892/ol.2017.7183.

13. Fang WY, Chen YW, Hsiao JR, Liu CS, Kuo YZ, Wang YC, et al. Elevated S100A9 expression in tumor stroma functions as an early recurrence marker for early-stage oral cancer patients through increased tumor cell invasion, angiogenesis, macrophage recruitment and interleukin-6 production. Oncotarget. 2015;6:28401–24. https://doi.org/10.18632/oncotarget.4951.
14. Peng CY, Wang TY, Lee SS, Hsieh PL, Liao YW, Tsai LL, et al. Let-7c restores radiosensitivity and chemosensitivity and impairs stemness in oral cancer cells through inhibiting interleukin-8. J Oral Pathol Med. 2018;47:590–7. https://doi.org/10.1111/jop.12711.
15. Yang PW, Huang PM, Yong LS, Chang YH, Wu CW, Hua KT, et al. Circulating interleukin-6 is associated with prognosis and genetic polymorphisms of MIR608 in patients with esophageal squamous cell carcinoma. Ann Surg Oncol. 2018;25:2449–56. https://doi.org/10.1245/s10434-018-6532-4.
16. Yap T, Koo K, Cheng L, Vella LJ, Hill AF, Reynolds E, et al. Predicting the presence of oral squamous cell carcinoma using commonly dysregulated microRNA in oral swirls. Cancer Prev Res (Phila). 2018;11:491–502. https://doi.org/10.1158/1940-6207.CAPR-17-0409.
17. Lien MY, Lin CW, Tsai HC, Chen YT, Tsai MH, Hua CH, et al. Impact of CCL4 gene polymorphisms and environmental factors on oral cancer development and clinical characteristics. Oncotarget. 2017;8:31424–34. https://doi.org/10.18632/oncotarget.15615.
18. Heineman TE, Widman A, Kuan EC, St John M. The genetic landscape of programmed death ligand-1 (PD-L1) alterations in head and neck cancer. Laryngosc Investig Otolaryngol. 2017;2:99–103. https://doi.org/10.1002/lio2.79.
19. Weber M, Wehrhan F, Baran C, Agaimy A, Buttner-Herold M, Preidl R, Neukam FW, Ries J. Pd-l1 expression in tumor tissue and peripheral blood of patients with oral squamous cell carcinoma. Oncotarget. 2017;8:112584–97. https://doi.org/10.18632/oncotarget.22576.
20. Kessenbrock K, Plaks V, Werb Z. Matrix metalloproteinases: regulators of the tumor microenvironment. Cell. 2010;141:52. https://doi.org/10.1016/j.cell.2010.03.015.
21. Lin SC, Chung MY, Huang JW, Shieh TM, Liu CJ, Chang KW. Correlation between functional genotypes in the matrix metalloproteinases-1 promoter and risk of oral squamous cell carcinomas. J Oral Pathol Med. 2004a;33:323–6. https://doi.org/10.1111/j.1600-0714.2004.00214.x.
22. Lin SC, Lo SS, Liu CJ, Chung MY, Huang JW, Chang KW. Functional genotype in matrix metalloproteinases-2 promoter is a risk factor for oral carcinogenesis. J Oral Pathol Med. 2004b;33:405–9. https://doi.org/10.1111/j.1600-0714.2004.00231.x.
23. Nishizawa R, Nagata M, Noman AA, Kitamura N, Fujita H, Hoshina H, et al. The 2G allele of promoter region of matrix metalloproteinase-1 as an essential pre-condition for the early onset of oral squamous cell carcinoma. BMC Cancer. 2007;7:187. https://doi.org/10.1186/1471-2407-7-187.
24. Chaudhary AK, Singh M, Bharti AC, Singh M, Shukla S, Singh AK, et al. Synergistic effect of stromelysin-1 (matrix metalloproteinase-3) promoter (−1171 5A->6A) polymorphism in oral submucous fibrosis and head and neck lesions. BMC Cancer. 2010;10:369. https://doi.org/10.1186/1471-2407-10-369.
25. Cao ZG, Li CZ. A single nucleotide polymorphism in the matrix metalloproteinase-1 promoter enhances oral squamous cell carcinoma susceptibility in a Chinese population. Oral Oncol. 2006;42:32. https://doi.org/10.1016/j.oraloncology.2004.08.015.
26. Chaudhary AK, Pandya S, Mehrotra R, Singh M, Singh M. Role of functional polymorphism of matrix metalloproteinase-2 (−1306 C/T and −168 G/T) and MMP-9 (−1562 C/T) promoter in oral submucous fibrosis and head and neck squamous cell carcinoma in an Indian population. Biomarkers. 2011;16:577–86. https://doi.org/10.3109/1354750X.2011.609602.
27. O-Charoenrat P, Khantapura P. The role of genetic polymorphisms in the promoters of the matrix metalloproteinase-2 and tissue inhibitor of metalloproteinase-2 genes in head and neck cancer. Oral Oncol. 2006;42:257–67. https://doi.org/10.1016/j.oraloncology.2005.07.008.
28. Pereira AC, Dias do Carmo E, Dias da Silva MA, Blumer Rosa LE. Matrix metalloproteinase gene polymorphisms and oral cancer. J Clin Exp Dent. 2012;4:e297–301. https://doi.org/10.4317/jced.50859.
29. Lin CW, Yang SF, Chuang CY, Lin HP, Hsin CH. Association of matrix metalloproteinase-11 polymorphisms with susceptibility and clinicopathologic characteristics for oral squamous cell carcinoma. Head Neck. 2015;37:1425–31. https://doi.org/10.1002/hed.23771.
30. Thangaraj SV, Shyamsundar V, Krishnamurthy A, Ramani P, Ganesan K, Muthuswami M, et al. Molecular portrait of oral tongue squamous cell carcinoma shown by integrative meta-analysis of expression profiles with validations. PLoS One. 2016;11:e0156582. https://doi.org/10.1371/journal.pone.0156582.
31. Ramakodi MP, Devarajan K, Blackman E, Gibbs D, Luce D, Deloumeaux J, et al. Integrative genomic analysis identifies ancestry-related expression quantitative trait loci on DNA polymerase beta and supports the association of genetic ancestry with survival disparities in head and neck squamous cell carcinoma. Cancer. 2017;123:849–60. https://doi.org/10.1002/cncr.30457.
32. Murali A, Varghese BT, Kumar RR, Kannan S. Combination of genetic variants in cyclin D1 and retinoblastoma genes predict clinical outcome in oral cancer patients. Tumour Biol. 2016;37:3609–17. https://doi.org/10.1007/s13277-015-4179-3.
33. Liu KYP, Lu XJD, Zhu Y, Yip S, Poh CF. Altered immune-related gene expressions indicate oral cancer nodal disease. J Dent Res. 2018;97:709–16. https://doi.org/10.1177/0022034518758045.

34. Wang W, Lim WK, Leong HS, Chong FT, Lim TK, Tan DS, et al. An eleven gene molecular signature for extra-capsular spread in oral squamous cell carcinoma serves as a prognosticator of outcome in patients without nodal metastases. Oral Oncol. 2015;51:355–62. https://doi.org/10.1016/j.oraloncology.2014.12.012.
35. Multani S, Saranath D. Genotypic distribution of single nucleotide polymorphisms in oral cancer: global scene. Tumour Biol. 2016;37:14501–12. https://doi.org/10.1007/s13277-016-5322-5.
36. Yan Y, Wang X, Veno MT, Bakholdt V, Sorensen JA, Krogdahl A, Sun Z, Gao S, Kjems J. Circulating miRNAs as biomarkers for oral squamous cell carcinoma recurrence in operated patients. Oncotarget. 2017;8:8206. https://doi.org/10.18632/oncotarget.14143.
37. Pedersen NJ, Jensen DH, Lelkaitis G, Kiss K, Charabi BW, Ullum H, Specht L, Schmidt AY, Nielsen FC, von Buchwald C. MicroRNA-based classifiers for diagnosis of oral cavity squamous cell carcinoma in tissue and plasma. Oral Oncol. 2018;83:46. https://doi.org/10.1016/j.oraloncology.2018.05.020.
38. Tipirneni KE, Rosenthal EL, Moore LS, Haskins AD, Udayakumar N, Jani AH, Carroll WR, Morlandt AB, Bogyo M, Rao J, Warram J. Fluorescence imaging for cancer screening and surveillance. Mol Imaging Biol. 2017;19:645–55.. https://do.org/10.1007/s11307-017-1050-5
39. Moore LS, Rosenthal EL, Chung TK, de Boer E, Patel N, Prince AC, Korb ML, Walsh EM, Young ES, Stevens TM, Withrow KP, Morlandt AB, Richman JS, Carroll WR, Zinn KR, Warram JM. Characterizing the utility and limitations of repurposing an open-field optical imaging device for fluorescence-guided surgery in head and neck cancer patients. J Nucl Med. 2017;58(2):246–51. https://doi.org/10.2967/jnumed.115.171413.
40. Macey R, Walsh T, Brocklehurst P, Kerr AR, Liu JLY, Lingen M, Ogden G, Warnakulasuriya S, Scully C. Diagnostic tests for oral cancer and potentially malignant disorders in patients presenting with clinically evident lesions. Cochrane Database Syst Rev. 2015;5:CD010276. https://doi.org/10.1002/14651858.CD010276.pub2.
41. Sweeny L, Dean NR, Agnuson JS, Carroll WR, Clemons L, Rosenthal EL. Assessment of tissue autofluorescence and reflectance for oral cavity cancer screening. Otolaryngol Head Neck Surg. 2011;145(6):956–60. https://doi.org/10.1177/0194599811416773.
42. Polverini PJ, D'Silva NJ, Lei YL. Precision therapy of head and neck squamous cell carcinoma. J Dent Res. 2018;97:614–21. https://doi.org/10.1177/0022034518769645.
43. Chia S, Low JL, Zhang X, Kwang XL, Chong FT, Sharma A, et al. Phenotype-driven precision oncology as a guide for clinical decisions one patient at a time. Nat Commun. 2017;8:435. https://doi.org/10.1038/s41467-017-00451-5.
44. Slosberg ED, Kang BP, Peguero J, Taylor M, Bauer TM, Berry DA, Braiteh F, Spira A, Meric Bernstam F, Stein S, Piha-Paul SA, Salvado A. Signature program: a platform of basket trials. Oncotarget. 2018;9:21383. https://doi.org/10.18632/oncotarget.25109.

8 Factors Affecting Response and Survival in Radiotherapy

Michael Awadallah, Kurt Nisi, and Ketan J. Patel

8.1 Introduction

Oral squamous cell carcinoma (OSCC) compromises a group of cancers with a prognosis that is inferior to other head and neck cancer sites. *Management of OSCC can comprise three different modalities including surgery, radiation therapy, and chemotherapy. These management modalities can be used in combination or independently. Although not typically used as a primary cure for oral squamous cell carcinomas, radiation therapy remains the primary mainstay of management for oropharyngeal cancers in combination with chemotherapy. If surgery is used primarily for curative intent, radiation could be used as an adjuvant for advance stage disease, positive margins not amenable to re-resection, multinodal disease, and other adverse features including perivascular or perineural disease*. The concept behind administrating postoperative radiation therapy is to eliminate any residual microscopic tumor burden in the surgical field and prevent any potential recurrence. Radiation-induced cytotoxicity is via several pathways including a combination of those mechanisms. These mechanisms include mitotic cell death, apoptosis, immunogenic cell death, and senescence via direct molecular bond breakage and/or generation of free radicals. Mitotic cell death is believed to be the primary pathway in radiation-induced cell death. Electromagnetic radiation consists of electron and photon therapy with the latter being the most often used therapy for oral cancers. Other forms of radiation include particle therapy, which consists of either protons, neutrons, and heavily charged ions such as helium. Different radiation techniques can be administered postoperatively for the oral cancer patient. Some of these treatment techniques include brachytherapy, intraoperative radiation therapy, and intensity-modulated radiation therapy. Intensity-modulated radiation therapy (IMRT) using is the most commonly used radiation modality used in the adjunctive treatment of oral cancer. Different fractionation schedules or the amount of radiation delivered to the tumor site exist; the standard fractionation schedule for oral cancer used in the United States consists of 1.8–2 Gy per fraction given once a day, 5 days a week for 7–8 weeks totaling to a total of 35–39 treatments in total. Radiation treatment can be used as a primary or an adjunct to surgery. Early stage tumors that are T1 and some select T2 tumors can be treated with radiation alone with comparable success rates to surgery with a control rate that ranges from 85% to 90%. Tumor cell survival after radiation is multivariable and is

M. Awadallah (✉) · K. J. Patel
Department of Oral and Maxillofacial Surgery, North Memorial Medical Center, Minneapolis, MN, USA
e-mail: Michael.Awadallah@northmemorial.com; Ketan.Patel@northmemorial.com

K. Nisi
Minneapolis Radiation Oncology, Minneapolis, MN, USA
e-mail: Knisi@mropa.com

D. Kademani (ed.), *Improving Outcomes in Oral Cancer*, https://doi.org/10.1007/978-3-030-30094-4_8

contingent upon the type of radiation, frequency of radiation, amount of radiation, inherent radiation sensitivity of the tumor, and oxygen tension. Radiation-induced damage is most pronounced during the M and G2 phase of the mitotic cycle, hence actively dividing tumors are more sensitive to radiation-induced death of the as compared to slowly dividing or senescent ones. An oxygen-rich environment is radiosensitizer and will lead to more radiation-induced cell death as compared to a hypoxic environment.

8.2 Contemporary Radiation Therapy for Oral Cancer

By far the most common radiation delivery mechanism for oral cancer is via intensity-modulated and image-guided radiation therapy (IMRT). This tcchniquc is a form of highly conformational radiation therapy in which high dose volumes are adapted closely to the target area while minimizing collateral damage to the adjacent healthy tissues. The basic principles in achieving IMRT include outlining the target volume and margins using computed tomography and image guidance programs, using multiple beam directions to cross fire on targets, and customization of each of those radiation beams to deliver the conformed dose while modulating intensity. The pivotal step in this process is defining the volume and margins of the target. There are three volumes that are measured between the radiation oncologist and the medical physicist. The gross tumor volume (GTV) is delineated using multiple slices using CT, PET/CT, and/or MRI in multiple planes, and this is where the macroscopic disease is situated. Once the gross tumor volume is outlined, the clinical target volume (CTV)is then estimated. The CTV is the GTV margin in addition to the estimated microscopic disease not visualized on imaging, usually a 0.5–1 cm extension beyond the GTV (see Figs. 8.1, 8.2, and 8.3). The CTV is dependent on aggressiveness of the disease, pattern of local infiltration, pattern of regional spread, and pattern of locoregional failure in the oral cavity. The most applicable situation of this concept in oral cancer is in the neck where occult spread to the lymphatic basins can occur up to 30% of the time. The planning target volume (PTV) is the area to be irradiated to confirm treatment of the CTV. This is usually achieved by enlarging the CTV by a 0.5–1 cm margin. The CTV and PTV are considered to be comparable to surgical margins in the radiation oncology realm (see Fig. 8.4).

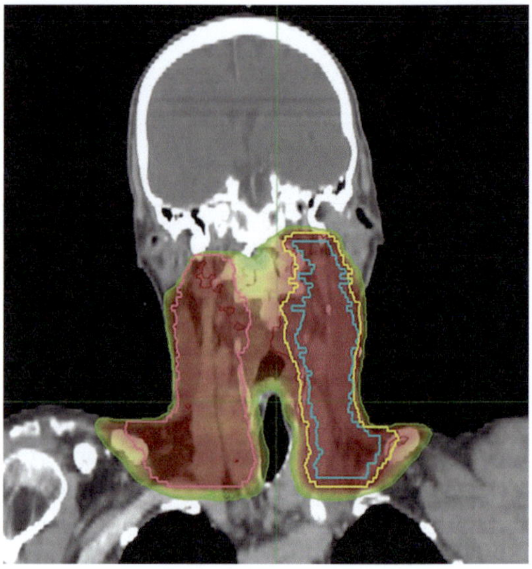

Fig. 8.1 IMRT treatment volumes of an anterior FOM with pathologically proven bilateral neck nodes in sagittal view

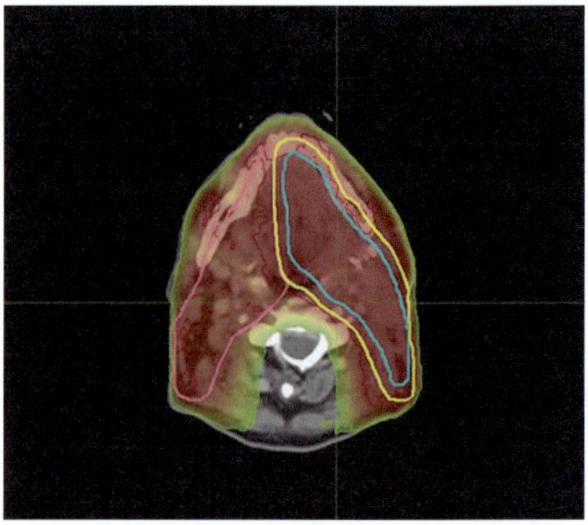

Fig. 8.2 IMRT treatment volumes of an anterior FOM with pathologically proven bilateral neck nodes in axial view

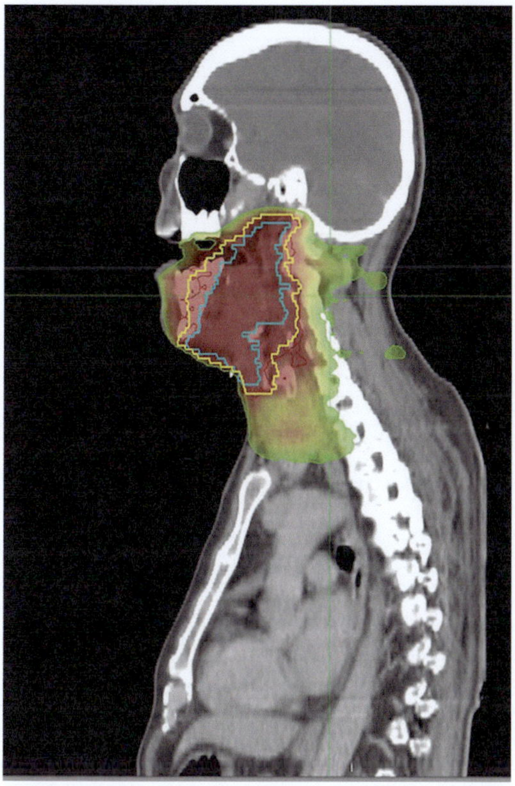

Fig. 8.3 IMRT treatment volumes of an anterior FOM with pathologically proven bilateral neck nodes in coronal view

There are several different fractionation protocols used for management of residual or primary disease for oral cancer according to the National Comprehensive Cancer Network (NCCN) guidelines (see Fig. 8.5). Standard fractionation treatment is modulated based on treatment modality and high- vs. intermediate- vs. low-risk tumors. For definitive treatment with radiation alone, 66–70 Gy is delivered Monday through Friday over 6–7 weeks for high-risk tumors, 54–63 Gy for intermediate-risk tumors, and 44–50 Gy for low-risk tumors. The standard postoperative radiation fractionation schedule is Monday through Friday at 2.0 Gy fractions per day for a total dose of 60–66.6Gy of overall treatment over 6 weeks for high-risk tumors, 54–63 Gy for intermediate-risk tumors, and 44–50 Gy for low-risk tumors. This treatment is usually performed within 6 weeks after surgery to allow for complete wound healing and prevention of wound breakdown. The overall goal of postoperative irradiation is to control locoregional persistence or recurrence at the primary and regional sites. Altered fractionation schedules are used to address the problem of accelerated re-population; which is the concept of a

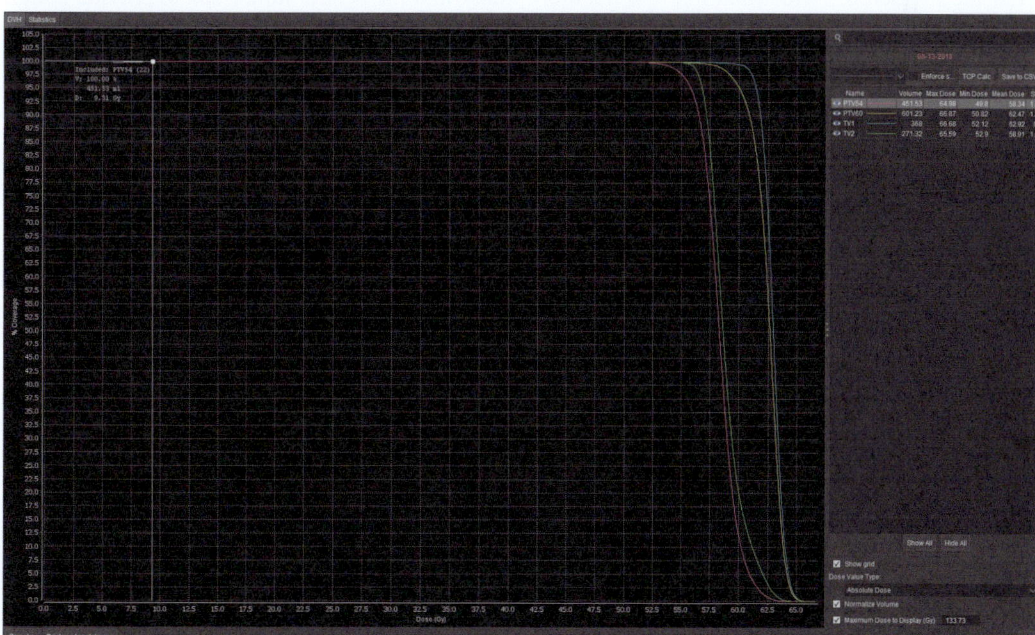

Fig. 8.4 Different dosage curves based on planned their respective IMRT treatment volumes

	Total dose	Gy/fractionation	Days/ week	fractionations/day	Time of treatment
Definitive RT high risk	66-70	2	5	1	6-7 weeks
Definitive RT hyperfractionation	81.6	1.2	5	2	7 weeks
Definitive RT Intermediate risk	54-63	1.6-1.8	5	1	5-6 weeks
Definitive RT low risk	44-50	2	5	1	4-5 weeks
Adjunctive RT high risk	60-66 Gy	2	5	1	6-6.5 weeks
Adjunctive RT intermediate risk	54-63	2	5	1	5-6 weeks
Adjunctive RT low risk	44-50	2	5	1	4-5 weeks

Fig. 8.5 IMRT schedules for primary therapy and post-operative therapy as per NCCN guidelines

tumor cell regenerative response to chemotherapy, radiation, and surgery leading to increased cell division by residual tumor cells ultimately leading to locoregional failure. This response is more accentuated in mucosal tissues that normally have a higher turnover rate at base line as compared to other bodily tissues. Patients with treatment delays either from increased time from surgery to radiation treatment or from prolonged radiation treatment are good candidates for the altered fractionation schedule. Hyperfractionation is the delivery of multiple small doses in a given day instead of one large dose. Accelerated fractionation delivers two or more doses per day to allow for faster completion of the total radiation dose. Both hyper and accelerated fractionation will lead to a greater total radiation dose delivery over the course of treatment as compared to conventional fractionation. Overall, the concept is to decrease the time interval between radiation dosing to control for accelerated re-population. Hyperfractionation is usually used for oral cavity cancers as a definitive therapy for high-risk tumors. The total fractionation dose is 81.6 Gy over 7 weeks with 1.2 Gy given twice a day according to the National Comprehensive Cancer Network (NCCN) guidelines.

Multiple retrospective studies have shown a statistically and a clinically survival benefit of postoperative radiation treatment for non-locally advanced tumors with lymph node metastasis and locally advanced tumors with lymph node metastasis. According to these studies, there was an 11% and 10% increase in 5-year overall survival in the nonlocally advanced and locally advanced groups, respectively [1–3].

Other radiation treatment modalities include brachytherapy, proton beam therapy, neutron beam therapy, and stereotactic radiation therapy. Brachytherapy involves the placement of a radioactive isotope via a carrier and placing it interstitially into the central tumor bed to provide a high but localized dose of radiation. It can be used alone or in conjuction with external beam radiation. It works via calculated radioactive decay of that specific isotope thereby emitting radiation to the tumor bed. Different isotopes can be used and include but are not limited to Iodine-125, Iridium 192, Palladium-103, Cesium 131, Gold 108, and Ruthenium 106. The technique of the procedure itself involves the temporary placement of hollow plastic catheters or tubes into the tumor bed, and the radioactive isotope is placed into the catheters. Fractionation schedule when using brachytherapy is 0.4–0.5 Gy per hour for several hours given 5 days a week to a total dose of 60–70 Gy if given for definitive treatment. However, because of more advanced techniques in using conformational radiation therapy, brachytherapy has fallen out of favor by most if not all radiation oncologists.

Proton beam therapy (PBT) is a promising relatively new technique in particle radiation in which highly charged protons are delivered to the tumor bed. The inherent physical characteristics allow for constant dose delivery without attenuation of energy then a rapid and steep decrease in energy beyond their target; allowing for less collateral damage to healthy tissue and hence has an improved toxicity profile as compared to IMRT. However; this does not translate to better efficacy in repect to locoregional control at the primary or regional sites. The fractionation schedule for PBT is the same as that for IMRT. In respect to oral cancer, there is no major advantage in using PBT over IMRT. The primary benefits of PBT are in the reduction or even the elimination of catastrophic radiation sequela to nearby critical structures like the brain, brain stem, and the orbital/periorbital tissues during the treatment of sinonasal malignancies or other malignancies that extend cephalad. The total fractionation dose of PBT in the head and neck ranges from 66 to 83 Cobalt-gray equivalent (CGE) depending on tumor site.

Stereotactic body radiation therapy (SBRT) is a type of external beam radiation that delivers greater doses of radiation to the tumor bed. Some of the advantages of SBRT are a sharp dose fall off, good local control rates, shorter overall treatment time as compared to other radiation treatment modalities, and acceptable toxicities. The fractionation regimine can be either single dose SBRT or fractionated SBRT. In the single dose SBRT, a 13–18 Gy fraction is given at one time. While in the fractionated SBRT, a total of 36–48 is given over five to eight fractions. At this time, the use of SBRT in the head and neck is limited to select patients that cannot undergo surgery due to poor functional status or in recurrent tumors of the head and neck.

Neutron and heavy ion therapy are a form of high linear energy transfer. Heavy ion dose distribution is similar to that in proton therapy because they deposit little energy until they reach the end of their range. Most heavy particle therapy use either carbon, helium, or neon as their charged particles. However, neutron particles are uncharged, and their dose distribution is similar to that of traditional photon therapy but with at least a 20-fold increase of energy deposition at the target site. The implementation of these techniques are currently under investigation globally, but it will be sometime before light is shed on their efficacy.

8.3 Indications

Approximately 60–70% of oral cancer patients present with late-stage disease, stage 3 or 4, all of which will have at least one of the following characteristics: frank bone invasion, extensive tumor infiltration into the surround soft and hard tissues, nodal metastasis, and extracapsular extension of which all are indications for adjunct radiation therapy. Other indications for adjunct radiation therapy include microscopic positive margins, lympho-vascular invasion, and perineural invasion. Primary radiation treatment is usually reserved for those patients that cannot undergo surgery secondary to severe comorbidities and/or a poor functional status. For tumors including oropharynx, hypopharynx, nasopharynx, and larynx, radiation is usually used for primary management with addition of chemotherapy.

8.4 Prognostic Factors in Radiation Therapy

Tumor biological factors, surgical treatment adequacy, patient-specific factors, and type of radiation treatment all play a role in affecting the response to radiation treatment and the survival of the oral cancer patient. Tumor-specific factors include the oxygen tension in the microenvironment, radiosensitivity, tumor burden, epidermal growth factor expression, nodal involvement, extranodal extension, and molecular composition of the tumor [4]. Surgical treatment factors mainly revolve around the presence of positive margins after resection. Patient-specific variable include functional status and concurrent use of tobacco during radiation. Radiation factors include type of fractionation and timing to fractionation [5].

8.5 Oxygenation

As stated previously, the primary mechanism of radiation tumor cell lysis is by direct killing via the formation of free radicals. This mechanism is further enhanced by the amount of oxygenation in the tumor environment; more oxygen leads to more free radicals and hence tumor cell death. Hence, oxygen is a potent modulator of radiosensitivity. Multiple methods have been developed to quantify oxygenation in a tumor bed environment with the initial being polyarographic electrodes. More contemporary techniques use exogenous and endogenous and exogenous hypoxia markers by immunohistochemistry. These techniques do not require any further intervention other than the initial incisional biopsy. Immunohistochemistry is used to detect the upregulation of certain genes that are modulated by hypoxia. These genes are responsible for glucose transport, pH regulation, and angiogenesis. The presence and degree of hypoxia in oral cancer are associated with poorer outcomes after radiation treatment [6].

8.6 Tumor Volume

Tumor volume can be quantitively measured indirectly by integrated F-fluorodeoxy glucose (FDG) uptake with positron emission tomography (PET) and computed tomography in combination with computer-aided software like RT image. This software will translate the amount of FDG uptake to a semiquantitative standard uptake value (SUV) [7]. Tumors with increased SUV is a prognostic indicator and inversely associated with survival and poorer treatment response [8]. Multiple mechanisms have been put worth as to explain this phenomenon and include degree of hypoxia in a dense tumor, degree of proliferative potential, degree of metabolic activity, tumor cell density, low apoptosis rate, or a combination of these elements. All of these elements are adverse factors in locoregional control with radiation treatment [9].

8.7 Molecular Markers

Molecular markers independently correlate with radiotherapy locoregional control and survival [10]. Immunohistochemical staining is the method of choice to test the expression and the degree of expression of these markers; the markers are then profiled upon degree of expression using a cluster analysis. Biological factors involved in modulating tumor response are those that affect proliferation, progression, cell cycle deregulation, apoptosis, and angiogenesis [10, 11]. The p53 tumor suppressor molecule regulates the cell cycle and programmed cell death. In normal cells, the p53 tumor suppressor gene is not expressed but following an insult to the cell the gene is translated to halt cell cycle division and promotes DNA repair mechanisms [12]. About 50% of head and neck SCC have mutations on the p53 gene leading to the expression of a mutant protein that is nonfunctional/dysfunctional or it can lead to the absence of the protein [13]. The presence of p53 derangements leads to the obtunded ability of the cell to initiate or complete apoptosis and to arrest the cell cycle. These characteristics then lead to less susceptibility to radiation treatment and propels a self-propagating cycle of cellular mutations and transformation leading to further deregulation of the cell division cycle. This leads to tumor polyclonality and further radio-resistance [4]. P53 mutations have a strong correlation with locoregional failure and primary radiation but not surgery [12]. The mutant type of p53 or the lack of p53 can lead to a overexpression of Bcl2 [14]. This molecule plays an important role in promoting cellular immortality by inhibiting apoptosis. This overexpression has been associated with increased radio-resistance [15]. Detecting the molecule ki-67 is an indirect immunohistochemical method measuring tumor growth rate. Ki-67 antibody is used to detect a certain cell nucleus antigen that becomes abundant during the G2 and M phase [16]. Several investigations have shown a correlation between an increased ki-67 index and survival, time to relapse, radio-resistance, and regional spread to lymph nodes [17, 18].

Epidermal growth factor receptor is a transmembrane glycoprotein of the tyrosine kinase family. Activation of which leads to multiple downstream signaling pathways that modulate growth, differentiation, and apoptosis. The majority if not all of oral squamous cell carcinomas have elevated expression of the EGFR glycoprotein. This is detected by immunohistochemistry. It has been demonstrated that radiation induces auto-stimulation of the EGFR leading to downstream epidermal growth factor which in turn leads to an increase in proliferation, colony formation, and ultimately re-population leading to radio-resistance [4]. This characteristic of the EGFR has been associated with locoregional relapse in vitro and in vivo. However, it has not been associated with distant metastasis [19].

8.8 Timing of Radiation Therapy and Fractionation Schedule

Tumor cells that survive prior to the initiation of radiation therapy or during gaps in between fractionation therapy can repopulate the tumor colony given their potential to divide. Multiple head and neck cancer studies have shown worse local control rate if timing to initiation of radiation therapy is prolonged [20–22]. A recent retrospective study looking at 15,064 patients showed worse outcomes for those patients with prolonged radiation treatment and prolonged postoperative interval between surgery and initiation of radiation therapy. In respect to postoperative interval time and time in radiation therapy, mortality increased after 5.7 and 7.9 weeks respectively [21]. Hence prolongation of the overall radiation treatment time which includes time to initiation of postoperative radiotherapy in addition to the time needed for completion of radiation therapy can have a negative impact on local control rate and survival of the patient [23–25]. For those patients who have prolonged overall radiation treatment time, then they might be candidates for accelerated fractionation [26].

The optimal type of fractionation has been the topic of controversy for oral cancer and other head and neck cancers. The question is whether or not the conventional fractionation schedule is less effective in local control than the alternate fractionation schedules which includes accelerated or hyperfractionation. Naturally, the next question is which of the two types of the alternate fractionation schedule is optimal for the oral cancer patient. The MARCH meta-anaylsis trial that included 34 trails with 11,969 patients found that alternative fractionation therapy was associated with an 3.1% improvement of overall survival at 5 years as compared to conventional fractionation. This difference is even more pronounced with the use of hyperfractionation where the absolute difference in overall survival at 5 years is 8.1% [27]. The Radiation Therapy Oncology Group (RTOG) phase 3 randomized study 9003 comparing hyperfractionation and accelerated fraction to conventional fractionation in head and neck squamous cell carcinomas showed improved locoregional control rate with the alternate schedule but no improvement in overall survival [20]. A Cochrane review concluded that alternate fractionation schedule has more efficacy in control of tumor burden at the primary site which translated to better overall survival [28].

8.9 Smoking and Malnutrition

It is well established that tobacco use is a significant risk factor for developing oral squamous cell carcinoma. One systematic review study estimated that the population attributable risk for developing oral squamous cell carcinoma from smoking alone was 25%; being dose-dependent with a life time cumulative use that is positively correlated with developing oral cancer [29]. However, does this also translate to worse outcomes in the efficacy of irradiation treatment? A study performed by Brown et al. on patients with locally advanced stage III and stage IV head and neck cancer showed patients that continued to smoke throughout their course of postoperative radiation therapy had a lower response and overall survival rate than those who abstained from smoking during therapy [30]. A retrospective chart review of a 101 patients with a mean follow-up time of 49 months performed by Chen et al. showed patients that active smokers throughout radiation therapy had poorer disease-free survival (42% vs. 65%), 5-year overall survival (23% vs. 55%), and locoregional control (58% vs. 69%) as compared to smokers that stopped smoking prior to the initiation of radiation therapy [31]. Multiple theories of why smoking during radiation therapy predisposes to a worse prognosis and these include the continued potentiation and propagation of p53 mutations, continued hypoxia in the tumor environment and less free radical production by radiation therapy due to decreased oxygenation, potential upregulation of EGFR, and the repercussions of the overall field cancerization effect that can lead metachronous or synchronous primaries.

Malnutrition and wasting are significant and prevalent problems for the oral cancer patient secondary to not only the disease sequela but also due to comorbidities and social factors like tobacco and/or alcohol abuse. This is compounded by the dysphagia, odynophagia, and mucositis brought on during and after radiation therapy which at the very least negatively impacts the patient's quality of life (QOL). In addition, all patients will have some degree of decreased solid and liquid oral intake after surgical ablation alone. Hence, patients planned for surgical and adjunctive radiation treatment may benefit from alternative routes of supplemental nutrition that include a nasogastric or a gastric feeding tube. According to the NCCN guidelines, intervention with feed tube placement should be implemented in patients with severe weight loss prior to treatment, patients with 5% weight loss or greater over one month, and patients woth 10% weight loss or greater over 6 months. Multiple studies have shown that malnutrition not affects QOL but is associated with poorer treatment outcomes. An analysis study of the RTOG phase III prospective trial 90–93 done by Rabinovitch et al. was performed to evaluate nutritional support with cancer outcomes in patients with locally advanced head and neck cancer treated with definitive radiation therapy. In their study, patients that were malnourished to the point where pretreatment nutritional support was needed, had a worse 5 year locoregional control rate as compared to patient who did not require any nutritional support (29% vs. 57%, respectively) [32]. A retrospective study by Pai et al. also showed similar results when using radiation therapy for curative intent on 1,562 patients by using their pretreatment body mass index (BMI) as an indirect measure of their nutritional status. Their study showed patients with lower preradiotherapy BMI (<25 kg/m^2) had statistically significant decrease in cancer-specific survival and overall survival as compared to those patients with higher pretreatment BMI (>25 kg/m^2) [33]. Multiple theories on why malnutrition is correlated with worse outcomes after radiation therapy have been proposed and include association with increased tumor burden at the locoregional site with higher T and N classifications, increased incidence of anemia, and worse functional status outcomes.

8.10 Pathologic Factors

In general, the same indications used to treat oral cancer with postoperative radiation therapy are the ones that negatively affect the prognosis after radiation therapy. These same factors contribute to the advanced staging of oral cancers. Even with improved survival rates due to earlier detection and more robust treatment like IMRT, immunotherapy, altered fractionation, and other treatment modalities, the overall 5-year survival rates for OSCC ranges from 34% to 42% and locoregional recurrence of 16–35% [34–36]. Cervical lymph node metastasis, extracapsular extension, and positive or close surgical margins are the most critical prognostic factors in 5-year overall survival rate, disease-specific survival, locoregional recurrence, and death follow postoperative radiation therapy for patients. The predominant site of failure is local recurrence at the primary site followed by regional spread/recurrence in the neck [37]. The majority of locoregional failure will occur in the first 2 years.

Local control rate is dependent on primary site, and clinical T stage. The 5-year local control rate of the oral tongue, the retromolar trigone, the floor of the mouth, and other sites ranged from 77% to 84%, 74–76%, 81–85%, 70–81%, respectively [38, 39]. Local control rate based on T stage at 5 years for T1–T2 and T3–T4 tumors were 88–90% and 70–79%, respectively [38, 39].

Locoregional control rates were influenced by margin status, American Joint commission on Cancer clinical stage, and Extranodal Extension (ENE). The 5-year locoregional control rate for negative margins and positive margins ranged from 77% to 79% and 47–52%, respectively [38, 39]. In respect to the AJCC clinical stage on presentation, the locoregional control rate ranged from 87% to 100% for stage I, 74–88% for stage II, 68% for stage III, and 62–72% for stage IV. The 5-year locoregional control incrementally decreases with each additional indication for postoperative radiation, and this is more pronounced after three or more indications [38, 39]. ENE leads to a drastic decrease in locoregional control and overall survival in patients with oral squamous cell carcinoma treated with postoperative radiation. The 5-year locoregional control is 61% as compared to 73% in patients without ENE. The 5-year overall survival in patients with ENE was 21% as compared to 58% in patients without ENE. The 5-year cause-specific survival was in patients with ENE was 38% as compared to 81% in patients without ENE [39].

8.11 Additional Adjunctive Treatment with Chemotherapy

The RTOG 9501 and European Organization for Research and Treatment of Cancer (EORTC) 22,301 randomized trials showed improvement in locoregional control and disease-free survival with concurrent administration of the chemotherapeutic agent cisplatin, especially for high-risk squamous cell carcinoma of the head and neck. A randomized trial by Bernier et al. placed 334 patients with stage 3 and 4 head and neck cancer in two groups of a 167 patient each; one group received postoperative radiation therapy and the other group received postoperative concurrent chemoradiation with Cisplastin. Progression-free survival was 47% for the concurrent chemoradiation group as compared to 36% for the radiation alone group. The overall survival was 53% in the combined therapy group compared to the 40% in the radiation alone group [40]. The overall incidence of relapse was also decreased for the combined therapy group as compared to the radiation alone group; 31% and 18%, respectively. Target therapy with epidermal growth factor inhibitor like Cetuximab also showed improved locoregional control, disease progression-free survival, and overall survival for head and neck cancer patients as compared to radiation therapy alone [41].

8.12 Conclusion

For locally advanced oral cancers surgery in combination with postoperative radiation therapy achieves optimal results in respect to locoregional control, 5-year overall survival, and disease-free specific survival. IMRT with 3-D conformation has shown to provide an optimality in delivering the correct amount of radiation to the tumor bed and the surrounding environment, while minimizing unwanted damage and toxicity to the healthy surrounding tissue, especially sparing the major and minor salivary glands. The goals of postoperative radiation therapy are primarily two-fold at the primary and regional sites; to eradicate residual microscopic and macroscopic disease and to prevent recurrence. Ongoing trials with escalation therapy and different fractionation doses and frequency will have future therapy implications especially in patients with high-risk features like nodal load and ENE.

References

1. Lavaf A, et al. Adjuvant radiotherapy improves overall survival for patients with lymph node-positive head and neck squamous cell carcinoma. Cancer. 2008;112(3):535–43.
2. Kao J, et al. Adjuvant radiotherapy and survival for patients with node-positive head and neck cancer: an analysis by primary site and nodal stage. Int J Radiat Oncol Biol Phys. 2008;71(2):362–70.
3. Sanguineti G, Forastiere AA. Determining the survival benefit of adjuvant radiotherapy in patients with node-positive head and neck cancer. Nat Clin Pract Oncol. 2008;5:694.
4. Perri F, et al. Radioresistance in head and neck squamous cell carcinoma: biological bases and therapeutic implications. Head Neck. 2015;37(5):763–70.
5. Silva P, et al. Clinical and biological factors affecting response to radiotherapy in patients with head and neck cancer: a review. Clin Otolaryngol. 2007;32(5):337–45.

6. Nordsmark M, Overgaard J. A confirmatory prognostic study on oxygenation status and loco-regional control in advanced head and neck squamous cell carcinoma treated by radiation therapy. Radiother Oncol. 2000;57(1):39–43.
7. Allal AS, et al. Standardized uptake value of 2-[18F] fluoro-2-deoxy-D-glucose in predicting outcome in head and neck carcinomas treated by radiotherapy with or without chemotherapy. J Clin Oncol. 2002;20(5):1398–404.
8. La TH, et al. Metabolic tumor volume predicts for recurrence and death in head-and-neck cancer. Int J Radiat Oncol Biol Phys. 2009;74(5):1335–41.
9. Jeong J, et al. Estimate of the impact of FDG-avidity on the dose required for head and neck radiotherapy local control. Radiother Oncol. 2014;111(3):340–7.
10. Buffa FM, et al. Molecular marker profiles predict locoregional control of head and neck squamous cell carcinoma in a randomized trial of continuous hyperfractionated accelerated radiotherapy. Clin Cancer Res. 2004;10(11):3745–54.
11. Begg AC. Predicting recurrence after radiotherapy in head and neck cancer. Semin Radiat Oncol. 2012;22(2):108–18.
12. Alsner J, Sorensen SB, Overgaard J. TP53 mutation is related to poor prognosis after radiotherapy, but not surgery, in squamous cell carcinoma of the head and neck. Radiother Oncol. 2001;59(2):179–85.
13. Somers KD, et al. Frequent p53 mutations in head and neck cancer. Cancer Res. 1992;52(21):5997–6000.
14. Csuka O, et al. Predictive value of p53, Bcl2 and bax in the radiotherapy of head and neck cancer. Pathol Oncol Res. 1997;3(3):204–10.
15. Haffty BG, Glazer PM. Molecular markers in clinical radiation oncology. Oncogene. 2003;22(37):5915–25.
16. Sittel C, et al. Prognostic significance of Ki-67 (MIB1), PCNA and p53 in cancer of the oropharynx and oral cavity. Oral Oncol. 1999;35(6):583–9.
17. Jacob R, et al. Heterogeneity of squamous cell carcinomas of the head and neck-analysis of tumor biologic factors and proliferation rates. Laryngoscope. 1996;106(9):1170–5.
18. Raybaud H, et al. Nuclear DNA content, an adjunct to p53 and Ki-67 as a marker of resistance to radiation therapy in oral cavity and pharyngeal squamous cell carcinoma. Int J Oral Maxillofac Surg. 2000;29(1):36–41.
19. Ang KK, et al. Impact of epidermal growth factor receptor expression on survival and pattern of relapse in patients with advanced head and neck carcinoma. Cancer Res. 2002;62(24):7350–6.
20. Fu KK, et al. A Radiation Therapy Oncology Group (RTOG) phase III randomized study to compare hyperfractionation and two variants of accelerated fractionation to standard fractionation radiotherapy for head and neck squamous cell carcinomas: first report of RTOG 9003. Int J Radiat Oncol Biol Phys. 2000;48(1):7–16.
21. Ho AS, et al. Quantitative survival impact of composite treatment delays in head and neck cancer. Cancer. 2018;124(15):3154–62.
22. Overgaard J, et al. Five compared with six fractions per week of conventional radiotherapy of squamous-cell carcinoma of head and neck: DAHANCA 6 and 7 randomised controlled trial. Lancet. 2003;362(9388):933–40.
23. González Ferreira JA, et al. Effect of radiotherapy delay in overall treatment time on local control and survival in head and neck cancer: review of the literature. Rep Pract Oncol Radiother. 2015;20(5):328–39.
24. Harris JP, et al. Association of survival with shorter time to radiation therapy after surgery for US patients with head and neck cancer. JAMA Otolaryngol Head Neck Surg. 2018;144(4):349–59.
25. Graboyes EM, et al. Effect of time to initiation of postoperative radiation therapy on survival in surgically managed head and neck cancer. Cancer. 2017;123(24):4841–50.
26. Sanguineti G, et al. Accelerated versus conventional fractionated postoperative radiotherapy for advanced head and neck cancer: results of a multicenter phase III study. Int J Radiat Oncol Biol Phys. 2005;61(3):762–71.
27. Lacas B, et al. Role of radiotherapy fractionation in head and neck cancers (MARCH): an updated meta-analysis. Lancet Oncol. 2017;18(9):1221–37.
28. Baujat B, et al. Hyperfractionated or accelerated radiotherapy for head and neck cancer. Cochrane Database Syst Rev. 2010;12:Cd002026.
29. Radoi L, Luce D. A review of risk factors for oral cavity cancer: the importance of a standardized case definition. Community Dent Oral Epidemiol. 2013;41(2):97–109, e78–91.
30. Browman GP, et al. Influence of cigarette smoking on the efficacy of radiation therapy in head and neck cancer. N Engl J Med. 1993;328(3):159–63.
31. Chen AM, et al. Tobacco smoking during radiation therapy for head-and-neck cancer is associated with unfavorable outcome. Int J Radiat Oncol Biol Phys. 2011;79(2):414–9.
32. Rabinovitch R, et al. Impact of nutrition support on treatment outcome in patients with locally advanced head and neck squamous cell cancer treated with definitive radiotherapy: a secondary analysis of RTOG trial 90-03. Head Neck. 2006;28(4):287–96.
33. Pai PC, et al. Impact of pretreatment body mass index on patients with head-and-neck cancer treated with radiation. Int J Radiat Oncol Biol Phys. 2012;83(1):e93–e100.
34. Amit M, et al. Improvement in survival of patients with oral cavity squamous cell carcinoma: an international collaborative study. Cancer. 2013;119(24):4242–8.
35. Zhang H, et al. Survival outcomes of patients with advanced oral cavity squamous cell carcinoma treated with multimodal therapy: a multi-institutional analysis. J Otolaryngol Head Neck Surg. 2013;42:30.

36. Iyer NG, et al. Randomized trial comparing surgery and adjuvant radiotherapy versus concurrent chemoradiotherapy in patients with advanced, nonmetastatic squamous cell carcinoma of the head and neck: 10-year update and subset analysis. Cancer. 2015;121(10):1599–607.
37. Daly ME, et al. Intensity-modulated radiotherapy for oral cavity squamous cell carcinoma: patterns of failure and predictors of local control. Int J Rad Oncol Biol Phys. 2011;80(5):1412–22.
38. Parsons JT, et al. An analysis of factors influencing the outcome of postoperative irradiation for squamous cell carcinoma of the oral cavity. Int J Radiat Oncol Biol Phys. 1997;39(1):137–48.
39. Hinerman RW, et al. Postoperative irradiation for squamous cell carcinoma of the oral cavity: 35-year experience. Head Neck. 2004;26(11):984–94.
40. Bernier J, et al. Postoperative irradiation with or without concomitant chemotherapy for locally advanced head and neck cancer. N Engl J Med. 2004;350(19):1945–52.
41. Ooishi M, et al. Patterns of failure after postoperative intensity-modulated radiotherapy for locally advanced and recurrent head and neck cancer. Jpn J Clin Oncol. 2016;46(10):919–27.

Novel and Emerging Chemotherapeutic Agents in Head and Neck Cancer

9

Arielle Elkrief, Nicholas Makhoul, and Nathaniel Bouganim

9.1 Introduction

Head and neck cancers are a heterogeneous group of malignancies, and their management requires a multidisciplinary approach including input from medical oncologists, radiation oncologists, surgeons, dentists, specialized nursing care, speech and language pathologists, physiotherapists, nutritionists, as well as psychologists [1]. Overall survival (OS) is improved when patients are treated at high-volume centers [2].

Patients with early stage disease (stage I or II) are treated with surgical resection or definitive radiation therapy (RT) to the primary site. Locoregionally advanced disease (stage III or IV) is treated with a combined modality approach such as surgery and RT with or without chemotherapy given the increased risk of local recurrence and distant metastasis in this patient population. Patients with metastatic disease require systemic therapy as well as best supportive care. Patient prognosis is often poor with median survival between 6 and 12 months. Therapeutic options for head and neck cancer patients with metastatic disease include cytotoxic chemotherapeutic agents or molecularly targeted agents.

This chapter will describe the novel and emerging chemotherapeutic agents in head and neck cancer. The role for immunotherapy will be outlined in a later chapter.

A. Elkrief · N. Bouganim (✉)
Department of Oncology, McGil University, Montreal, QC, Canada
e-mail: arielle.elkrief@mail.mcgill.ca; nathaniel.bouganim@mcgill.ca

N. Makhoul
Department of Oral and Maxillofacial Surgery, McGil University, Montreal, QC, Canada
e-mail: nicholas.makhoul@mcgill.ca

9.2 Systemic Therapy for Locoregionally Advanced Disease

Locoregionally advanced squamous head and neck cancer is associated with high rates of local recurrence of up to 50% [3–5] and rates of distant metastases between 4% and 26% [6–8]. Chemotherapy has therefore been integrated into the multimodality treatment plans in an effort to improve the rates of both locoregional and distant recurrence, as well as to reduce patient morbidity related to surgery and radiation using a functional organ preservation approach. These approaches can be classified into induction chemotherapy (neoadjuvant chemotherapy), concurrent chemoradiotherapy, and sequential chemoradiotherapy (combined induction chemotherapy followed by concurrent chemoradiotherapy). Prior to initiation of a multimodality treatment regimen, individual patient characteristics such as age, comorbidities, performance status, and support system should be assessed.

D. Kademani (ed.), *Improving Outcomes in Oral Cancer*,
https://doi.org/10.1007/978-3-030-30094-4_9

Various prospective studies have validated the role for chemotherapy in this patient population. Although there was no survival benefit for single-agent induction chemotherapy in comparison to surgery or RT alone, it was found that there was an OS benefit in patients receiving cisplatin plus fluorouracil [9]. Concurrent chemotherapy significantly improved OS in comparison to surgery or RT alone [9]. In contrast, the benefit for sequential chemoradiotherapy is still unclear [10–13] with suggested benefit for high-risk patients with bulky N2b, N3 nodal status, or those with T3 or T4 disease [12].

9.3 Chemotherapy Regimens for Locoregionally Advanced Disease

For induction chemotherapy, a three-drug combination of cisplatin, fluorouracil, plus a taxane is most commonly used and is the approach of choice [3, 14, 15]. Important toxicities include myelosuppression, febrile neutropenia, stomatitis, dysphagia, nausea, and anorexia [16].

For concurrent therapy in patients with good performance status, high-dose bolus cisplatin (100 mg/m^2 on days 1, 22, 43) can be administrated concurrently with RT [17]. Given the frequent onset of both acute and late-onset adverse events, other dosing regimens are sometimes used. The most commonly associated toxicities included hematological toxicities, stomatitis, dysphagia, as well as nausea and vomiting, neurotoxicity, and nephrotoxicity [18]. Although not as effective as cisplatin in the treatment of locally advanced squamous head and neck cancer [19], weekly carboplatin (AUC of 1.5–2) is an appropriate choice for patients with renal disease or poor performance status [20]. Myelosuppression is an important limitation; however, there is less neurotoxicity associated with this treatment. Carboplatin in combination with fluorouracil given concurrently with RT is another approach [21].

9.4 Treatment Regimens for Recurrent Metastatic Disease in Previously Untreated Patients

The median survival in patients with metastatic head and neck cancer is poor and approaches 6–12 months depending on disease and individual patient factors, such as performance status, presence of comorbidities, and disease-related factors. Systemic treatment options are chosen based on whether the patient has already received systemic treatment as part of organ preservation strategy or if they have already received a first-line agent for presence of systemic or recurrent disease. The role of traditional cytotoxic agents, targeted molecular agents, and checkpoint inhibitor therapy in the treatment of metastatic or recurrent head and neck cancer will be discussed in detail herein. A small subgroup of patients with good performance status who recur may be candidates for "salvage" therapy with curative intent, but most patients require a palliative approach using the regimens discussed in this chapter. It is important to note that best supportive care is also an important component to the management plan in all of these patients.

In otherwise healthy patients with a good performance status and those with advanced disease who are not appropriate candidates for curative therapy, combinations of platinum-based chemotherapy with fluorouracil or a taxane is the preferred approach [22–25]. The data supporting this recommendation are discussed in detail below.

Cisplatin (100 mg/m^2 intravenous on day 1) and fluorouracil (1000 mg/m^2/day continuous infusion over 4 days), and in comparison to single-agent cisplatin or methotrexate, this doublet regimen was associated with higher response rates across all studies, albeit no survival benefit was shown. For example, the EORTC Head and Neck Cancer Cooperative Group conducted a randomized controlled trial three arms (1) cisplatin, methotrexate, bleomycin, and vincristine (CABO), (2) combination cisplatin and fluorouracil (CF), and (3) cisplatin alone in previously untreated head and neck metastatic squamous cell cancer. Both CABO and CF were superior in terms of overall response rates with no difference in progression-free survival or overall survival. The Southwest Oncology Group (SWOG) performed a randomized controlled trial of (1) CF, (2) carboplatin plus fluorouracil, and (3) single-agent methotrexate. Once again, both the combination regimens (CF and carboplatin plus fluorouracil) were associated with improved response rates in comparison to methotrexate alone with similar median survival times across all three groups. There was however increased incidence of adverse events in the combination treatment groups. Further adding to the data supporting a doublet treatment regimen approach, a study by Jacobs et al. randomized patients to receive either cisplatin alone, fluorouracil alone, or their combination and once again found improved overall response rates with no significant difference in survival outcomes. Toxicities were more important in the combination treatment arm, with alopecia and myelosuppression being the most important. One study by Gibson et al. failed to show any statistically significant difference in response rate or survival between the single-agent and combination arms, and toxicities were similar in both groups.

We have seen above the data for combination therapy for fluorouracil and cisplatin or carboplatin; however, both cisplatin and carboplatin have been combined with a taxane regimen, either paclitaxel or docetaxel. No statistically significant benefit in response rate or overall survival exists with this regimen; however, common gastrointestinal adverse events and lack of need for prolonged infusion time make the taxane regimen more convenient.

Cisplatin is sometimes replaced for carboplatin in the taxane combination for more frail individuals as the side effect profile is more favorable with less ototoxicity, kidney failure, vomiting, and neuropathy; however, this has not been validated in phase III trials.

Single-agent therapy is reserved for patients with poor performance status and options include single-agent taxane, cisplatin, carboplatin, or methotrexate. Cetuximab (discussed later in this chapter) can be added to these regimens, and as seen in the EXTREME trial, when added to platin-fluorouracil, confers an OS and PFS improvement when compared to cisplatin-fluorouracil alone [26]. Best supportive care is also an important component to the management plan.

The role of immune checkpoint inhibition with pembrolizumab in the first-line setting is discussed in the final section of this chapter.

9.5 Epidermal Growth Factor Receptor (EGFR)-Targeted Therapy

EGFR is a member of the ErbB/Her group of ligand-activated receptor tyrosine kinases (RTKs) [27]. Through ligand-binding and activation of various downstream pathways, these receptors promote cancer cell proliferation, migration, angiogenesis, and tumor resistance to chemotherapy [28–32]. EGFR expression occurs in over 90% of squamous head and neck cancers, and overexpression is associated with decreased survival, resistance to radiotherapy, locoregional recurrence, and increased rate of distant metastases [27, 33].

9.5.1 Monoclonal Antibodies (mAb) Against EGFR

Monoclonal antibodies targeting EFGR and used in the treatment of locoregionally advanced squamous head and neck cancer include cetuximab, panitumumab, zalatumumab, and nimotuzumab. Their mechanism of action is through direct inhibition of ligand-receptor binding [27].

9.5.1.1 Cetuximab

Cetuximab is a highly specific, human-murine chimeric immunoglobulin G (IgG) mAb targeting EGFR [27]. As demonstrated in this landmark randomized controlled trial by Bonner et al., when administered at a dose of 400 mg/m^2 1 week prior to RT followed by 250 mg/m^2 weekly during high-dose RT in patients with locally advanced squamous head and neck cancer, cetuximab was associated with improved OS (49.0 months compared to 29.3 months HR0.74; $p = 0.03$) and locoregional control (24.4 months compared to 14.9 months (HE 0.68; $p = 0.05$) [34]), in comparison to high-dose radiation therapy alone. Progression-free survival was also improved in the combination treatment arm. This improvement in outcome was particularly important in patients 65 years of age or less with good performance status, albeit the study was not powered to detect differences in subgroups. In this study, there were no statistically significant difference in the incidence of grade 3 or higher adverse events; however, patients treated with cetuximab may have higher incidence of serious radiation dermatitis and another rare, but important side effect is the occurrence of cetuximab-induced infusion reaction, particularly in the first cycle. Interstitial lung disease was also an important side effect [35]. Current available data did not show any benefit to the use of concurrent cetuximab plus cisplatin with RT and is therefore not currently indicated in the treatment of locally advanced squamous head and neck cancer [36]. In the metastatic setting, a randomized, phase III clinical trial in patients with recurrent or metastatic squamous head and neck cancer the addition of cetuximab was compared with cisplatin/carboplatin plus fluorouracil. Chemotherapy plus cetuximab was associated with prolonged OS, PFS, and response rates. The main toxicities associated with the addition of cetuximab in this trial were severe hypomagnesemia, rash, and sepsis [26].

9.5.1.2 Panitumumab

Panitumumab is a fully humanized IgG anti-EGFR mAb, and like cetuximab, it inhibits EGFR ligand-dependant activation. Multiple prospective and randomized studies have failed to show an overall survival benefit in adding panitumumab to concurrent regimens in head and neck cancer, and its use is also associated with increased toxicity such as grade 3 rash or mucosal inflammation [37–40]. There was however a survival benefit p16-negative patients in the metastatic setting [41].

9.5.1.3 Zalutumumab

Zalutumumab, another fully humanized IgG anti-EGFR, works in a similar fashion as cetuximab and zalutumumab. Similar to panitumumab, zalutumumab has failed to show any benefit in the treatment of patients with squamous cell head and neck cancer in multiple phase III randomized controlled trials [42–44].

9.5.1.4 Nimotuzumab

Nimotuzumab, another fully humanized IgG anti-EGFR is now being compared to the administration of cisplatin in phase III trials in the management of locally and regionally advanced nasopharyngeal carcinoma when administered during radiotherapy following preoperative chemotherapy.

9.5.2 Tyrosine Kinase Inhibitors (TKI) Against EGFR

The intracellular domain of EGFR has important tyrosine kinase activity. TKIs serve to inhibit the activation and subsequent phosphorylation of EGFR [27]. In contrast to EGFR mAb, the small nature of these molecules allow for good GI absorption and therefore are prescribed orally in a daily fashion [27]. At the time of writing of this text book, TKIs are under review in several randomized, controlled trials, and none of the TKIs have been approved in the treatment for squamous head and neck cancer.

9.5.2.1 Gefitinib

In a randomized phase III trial, the addition of gefitinib to docetaxel did not improve survival for patients with recurrent or metastatic head and neck cancer [45] despite a phase II trial showing an overall response rate of 10.6% [46].

9.5.2.2 Erlotinib

Erlotinib, the second most common TKI was combined with cisplatin and compared to cisplatin alone in a phase II trial in which the cisplatin was given concurrently with definitive RT. In this study, there was no improvement in the response rate or survival [47].

9.5.2.3 Lapatinib

Lapatinib, a dual TKI, selectively inhibits the activation of EGFR as well as HER-2 [27]. A phase II trial compared the addition of lapatinib to standard chemoradiotherapy and showed promising results for the complete response rate in patients with locally advanced squamous head and neck cancer [48]. At this time, no benefit was shown in survival. In the metastatic setting, no objective response rate was observed in a phase II trial [49].

9.5.2.4 Afatinib

Afatinib is an irreversible TKI and, similarly to lapatinib, binds to the Erb2 receptor to inhibit EGFR [27]. Preliminary results from a phase II trial in the metastatic setting showed that there is significant disease activity for afatinib, and that it may be comparable to cetuximab [50]. It is currently being studied in the locally advanced setting.

9.5.2.5 Dacomitinib

Dacomitinib is an irreversible tyrosine kinase inhibitor for both EGFR and HER2. Two phase II clinical trials in recurrent or metastatic head and neck cancer demonstrated important clinical activity with the most common grade 3 adverse event being diarrhea [51, 52]. Exploratory analyses suggest that certain subgroups of patients with specific biomarkers may have improved responses to dacomitinib, but these findings need to be validated in phase III randomized control trials before their implementation into clinical practice.

9.6 Vascular Endothelial Growth Factor Receptor (VEGFR)-Directed Therapies

Vascular endothelial growth factor is an important cytokine for tumor angiogenesis, which is essential for tumor growth and metastatic dissemination [27]. Overexpression of VEGFR in patients with squamous head and neck cancer is associated with worse OS [53], making the VEGFR pathway an appealing therapeutic target. The VEGFR-directed therapies currently being studied in clinical models in squamous head and neck cancer include bevacizumab, sorafenib, sunitinib, and vandetanib. Other VEGF inhibitors that are currently under investigation for head and neck cancers include pazopanib, axitinib, nilotinib, and linifanib [54–57].

9.6.1 Monoclonal Antibodies (mAb) Against the VEGFR

9.6.1.1 Bevacizumab

Bevacizumab is an antiangiogenic mAb against VEGFR. A phase II study in patients with locally advanced squamous head and neck cancer compared the addition of bevacizumab to concurrent radiation therapy with cetuximab and pemetrexed. The addition of bevacizumab increased toxicity without improvement in efficacy or clinical outcomes [58]. Another phase II trial in squamous head and neck patients with locally advanced disease studying the addition of bevacizumab to concurrent intensity-modulated RT with cetuximab and cisplatin was associated with favorable clinical outcomes with the most common grade 3 adverse events being lymphopenia, mucositis, and dysphagia [59]. In the metastatic setting, a phase II trial showed an overall response rate of 30% with the addition of bevacizumab to pemetrexed with frequent (15%) bleeding adverse events [60].

9.6.2 Tyrosine Kinase Inhibitors (TKIs) Against VEGFR

9.6.2.1 Sorafenib

Sorafenib is a multiple kinase inhibitor targeting VEGFR, RAF, and platelet-derived growth factor receptor (PDGFR) [27]. To date, evidence has been conflicting with two phase II trials in the recurrent or metastatic setting showing little clinical activity [61, 62] and a more recent phase II trial showing an overall response rate of 55% with the combination of sorafenib with paclitaxel and carboplatin [63].

9.6.2.2 Sunitinib

Sunitinib, a second multiple kinase inhibitor targeting VEGFR, PDGFR, RET, and c-kit was evaluated as palliative monotherapy in patients with metastatic head and neck cancer [27]. Outcomes were poor with a significant amount of grade 3–5 hemorrhage [64]. A second study was closed after interim analysis due to only one out of the 19 patients in the study showing partial response [65].

9.6.2.3 Vandetanib

Vandetanib has activity against EGFR, VEGFR, and RET [27]. Currently its use has only been shown to be feasible in the phase I setting [66] with preclinical data showing it may overcome resistance to EGFR as well as RT [67].

9.7 P13K/AKT/mTOR Pathway Inhibitors

An important therapeutic hurdle to the use of EGFR and VEGFR inhibition is resistance to these molecules, either primarily or by prolonged use [68]. Prolonged treatment with EGFR can induce initiation of feedback loops thereby activating the P13/AKT pathway which promotes protein synthesis, cell survival, and tumor growth [27]. The mTOR pathway is another important pathway promoting tumor growth through regulation of cell proliferation, cell motility, and protein synthesis and has shown to be stimulated in 57–81% of patients with squamous head and neck cancer [27]. Temsirolimus is an mTOR inhibitor that was studied in a phase II trial in patients with cetuximab-resistant metastatic squamous head and neck cancer. This study showed a nonstatistically significant improvement in response rate. Two other studies evaluating the combination of temsirolimus with erlotinib and everolimus (a second mTOR inhibitor) with cetuximab and cisplatin were terminated early due to toxicity [69–71].

9.8 Palbociclib

Palbociclib, a selective cyclin-dependant kinase (CDK) 4/6 inhibitor was evaluated in a phase II trial of patients with platinum-resistant recurrent or metastatic head and neck squamous cell carcinoma. This study showed encouraging response rates of 35% with improved PFS and OS in comparison with similar patient cohorts [72].

9.9 Immune Checkpoint Inhibitors

The advent of immune checkpoint inhibitors has revolutionized the therapeutic landscape in many solid tumors and is now emerging as an important therapeutic option in the treatment of metastatic head and neck cancer.

At the time of writing of this text, the data on the use of immune checkpoint inhibitors in the first-line setting have been presented in abstract form only and therefore should be interpreted with caution until regulatory authorities approve these agents in this setting. Nevertheless, the preliminary results are promising and merit discussion.

In an open-label, phase III, randomized controlled study (NCT02358031), patients were randomly assigned to single-agent pembrolizumab, a PD-L1 inhibitor, versus pembrolizumab plus flourouracil/platinum combination, versus cetuximab and a fluorouracil/platinum combination. Patients were stratified based on PD-L1 score which was evaluated using the combined positive score (CPS). Single-agent pembrolizumab improved OS in comparison to the cetuximab and fluorouracil/platinum combination in patients with a high CPS score (above 20). Overall survival in the pembrolizumab arm was 14.9 months compared to 10.7 months. Strangely, this OS benefit did not translate in an improvement in PFS or response rate. As expected, toxicity was less in the single-agent pembrolizumab arm. A similar benefit in OS was seen in the pembrolizumab and fluorouracil/cisplatin arm (13.0 months compared to 10.7 months), and once again no significant differences were seen in response rates or PFS.

In the second-line setting, pembrolizumab was recently approved in the second-line setting for patients with metastatic head and neck squamous carcinoma. The KEYNOTE-040 randomized controlled, phase III trial of patients who had failed standard platinum-based chemotherapy was randomized to either pembrolizumab or standard of care with either methotrexate, docetaxel, or cetuximab [73]. Crossover was allowed at progression. There was a small but non-negligible improvement in overall survival in the pembrolizumab group of 8.4 months versus 6.9 months, and this benefit was most important in those with PDL-1 expression greater than 50%. There were less grade 3 or higher adverse events in the chemotherapy arm, but as expected a higher incidence of grade 1–2 immune-related adverse events, hypothyroidism being the most common. As a result of these studies and two other studies showing favorable response rate, pembrolizumab was approved by the FDA for the treatment of recurrent or metastatic head and neck squamous cell carcinoma at a dose of 200 mg intravenous every 3 weeks.

In a phase III randomized controlled study in the second- and later-line settings in patients with recurrent or metastatic head and neck squamous cell carcinoma, nivolumab, a PD-1 inhibitor demonstrated an overall survival benefit (7.7 months versus 5.1 months), and this was most important for patients with PDL-1 status more than 1% [74]. It is important to note that crossover was not allowed in this study. Based on the results of this study, the FDA approved nivolumab in this setting, at a dose of 240 mg intravenous every 2 weeks.

Darvalumab, another PD-1 inhibitor, has shown clinical activity in a phase II study of patients with recurrent or metastatic and previously treated squamous cell head and neck cancer [75]. The role for ipilimumab, a CTLA-4 inhibitor, is currently undergoing investigation (NCT02369874).

9.10 Oligometastatic Disease

In carefully selected patients with oligometastatic disease (limited metastatic disease) good performance status and who are good candidates for aggressive management, it may be reasonable to consider metastasectomy. As seen above, one of the most common sites of metastasis for head and neck squamous cell carcinoma is the lung. Around 30% of patients with metastatic head and neck squamous cell carcinoma who undergo pulmonary metastatecomy experience long-term survival. Poor prognostic factors in this approach include male sex, oral cavity lesions, lymph node involvement, and incomplete resection [76–78].

9.11 Drug Resistance

Despite significant improvements in the survival rates and organ preservation seen in the treatment of head and neck cancer care, significant challenges still exist as many patients experience drug resistance. Sensitivity to chemotherapeutic agents is associated with tumor heterogeneity, which is a result of patient factors (ethnic differences, age, weight, gender), and genetic differences in clonal tumor cells [79]. Mechanisms of resistance will be discussed in this section of this chapter.

Firstly, decreased concentration of antineoplastic agent within the tumor cells is an important mechanism of resistance and is thought to occur through a ATB-Binding Cassette (ABC)-mediated mechanism [80]. The ABC plays an important role in the transportation of antineoplastic treatments outside of the cell and also transports nutrients within the tumor cells thus allowing for drug resistance.

Secondly, head and neck squamous carcinoma cells are able to perform DNA repair, mediated by base-excision repair (BER). For example, polymorphisms in genes encoding BERs have been described, such as ERCC1 (C8092A), which plays a role in mRNA stability and DNA reparation capability, and ERCC1 expression may be associated with improved chemoradiation sensitivity perhaps clinical outcome as well [81].

Thirdly, there is an increased capability of tumor dissemination through a variety of mechanisms. For example, tumors that show an overexpression of p53 are resistant to both chemo and radiation therapy, and this has been associated with increased tumor progression and decreased survival rates [82]. There may also be increased chemoresistance through matrix metalloproteinase (MMP) through a Fas/FasL-mediated fashion, as some studies have indicated that polymorphisms in MMPs are independently associated with increased chemotherapy resistance [83].

Lastly, inactivation of antineoplastic drugs within the tumor cells can occur, also contributing to resistance. This may be particularly important for EGFR-mediated resistance, as EGF expression may be critical for maintaining tumor cell proliferation, and thus perhaps resistance to cetuximab [84]. However, it is still not been determined which of the EGFR ligands predict response to anti-EGFR treatment in patients with squamous cell carcinoma head and neck cancer. Resistance may also be due to autocrine growth factor production [85]. More data are required in order to fully elucidate the mechanisms of resistance to single-agent cetuximab, but this may be related to the capability of EGF to inhibit epithelial differentiation, and this may be in a cancer stem cell-related fashion [86, 87].

These findings prompt the need for continued search for biomarkers for resistance, with the goal of a personalized approach when prescribing therapy for head and neck squamous cell carcinoma patients.

9.12 Conclusions and Future Directions

The treatment of head and neck cancer continues to be challenging due to its heterogeneous nature as well as its increased incidence of resistance to conventional chemoradiation as well as targeted therapy. The distinct responses of HPV-positive and HPV-negative patients require further study. Advancements in elucidation of cancer cell biology have allowed for the development of several targeted therapies; however, more phase III trials need to be undertaken in order to implement these targeted therapies in daily practice.

References

1. Wheless SA, McKinney KA, Zanation AM. A prospective study of the clinical impact of a multidisciplinary head and neck tumor board. Otolaryngol Head Neck Surg. 2010;143(5):650–4.
2. Wuthrick EJ, Zhang Q, Machtay M, Rosenthal DI, Nguyen-Tan PF, Fortin A, et al. Institutional clinical trial accrual volume and survival of patients with head and neck cancer. J Clin Oncol. 2015;33(2):156–64.
3. Posner MR, Hershock DM, Blajman CR, Mickiewicz E, Winquist E, Gorbounova V, et al. Cisplatin and fluorouracil alone or with docetaxel in head and neck cancer. N Engl J Med. 2007;357(17):1705–15.
4. Brockstein B, Haraf DJ, Rademaker AW, Kies MS, Stenson KM, Rosen F, et al. Patterns of failure, prognostic factors and survival in locoregionally advanced head and neck cancer treated with concomitant chemoradiotherapy: a 9-year, 337-patient, multi-institutional experience. Ann Oncol. 2004;15(8):1179–86.
5. Bourhis J, Le Maitre A, Baujat B, Audry H, Pignon JP. Meta-analysis of chemotherapy in head NCCG, et al. Individual patients' data meta-analyses in head and neck cancer. Curr Opin Oncol. 2007;19(3):188–94.
6. Alvi A, Johnson JT. Development of distant metastasis after treatment of advanced-stage head and neck cancer. Head Neck. 1997;19(6):500–5.
7. Bhatia R, Bahadur S. Distant metastasis in malignancies of the head and neck. J Laryngol Otol. 1987;101(9):925–8.
8. Garavello W, Ciardo A, Spreafico R, Gaini RM. Risk factors for distant metastases in head and neck squamous cell carcinoma. Arch Otolaryngol Head Neck Surg. 2006;132(7):762–6.
9. Pignon JP, le Maitre A, Maillard E, Bourhis J, Group M-NC. Meta-analysis of chemotherapy in head and neck cancer (MACH-NC): an update on 93 randomised trials and 17,346 patients. Radiother Oncol. 2009;92(1):4–14.
10. Haddad R, O'Neill A, Rabinowits G, Tishler R, Khuri F, Adkins D, et al. Induction chemotherapy followed by concurrent chemoradiotherapy (sequential chemoradiotherapy) versus concurrent chemoradiotherapy alone in locally advanced head and neck cancer (PARADIGM): a randomised phase 3 trial. Lancet Oncol. 2013;14(3):257–64.
11. Hitt R, Grau JJ, Lopez-Pousa A, Berrocal A, Garcia-Giron C, Irigoyen A, et al. A randomized phase III trial comparing induction chemotherapy followed by chemoradiotherapy versus chemoradiotherapy alone as treatment of unresectable head and neck cancer. Ann Oncol. 2014;25(1):216–25.
12. Cohen EE, Karrison TG, Kocherginsky M, Mueller J, Egan R, Huang CH, et al. Phase III randomized trial of induction chemotherapy in patients with N2 or N3 locally advanced head and neck cancer. J Clin Oncol. 2014;32(25):2735–43.
13. Ghi MG, Paccagnella A, Ferrari D, Foa P, Alterio D, Codeca C, et al. Induction TPF followed by concomitant treatment versus concomitant treatment alone in locally advanced head and neck cancer. A phase II-III trial. Ann Oncol. 2017;28(9):2206–12.
14. Lorch JH, Goloubeva O, Haddad RI, Cullen K, Sarlis N, Tishler R, et al. Induction chemotherapy with cisplatin and fluorouracil alone or in combination with docetaxel in locally advanced squamous-cell cancer of the head and neck: long-term results of the

TAX 324 randomised phase 3 trial. Lancet Oncol. 2011;12(2):153–9.
15. Vermorken JB, Remenar E, van Herpen C, Gorlia T, Mesia R, Degardin M, et al. Cisplatin, fluorouracil, and docetaxel in unresectable head and neck cancer. N Engl J Med. 2007;357(17):1695–704.
16. Blanchard P, Bourhis J, Lacas B, Posner MR, Vermorken JB, Cruz Hernandez JJ, et al. Taxane-cisplatin-fluorouracil as induction chemotherapy in locally advanced head and neck cancers: an individual patient data meta-analysis of the meta-analysis of chemotherapy in head and neck cancer group. J Clin Oncol. 2013;31(23):2854–60.
17. Adelstein DJ, Li Y, Adams GL, Wagner H Jr, Kish JA, Ensley JF, et al. An intergroup phase III comparison of standard radiation therapy and two schedules of concurrent chemoradiotherapy in patients with unresectable squamous cell head and neck cancer. J Clin Oncol. 2003;21(1):92–8.
18. Forastiere AA, Goepfert H, Maor M, Pajak TF, Weber R, Morrison W, et al. Concurrent chemotherapy and radiotherapy for organ preservation in advanced laryngeal cancer. N Engl J Med. 2003;349(22):2091–8.
19. Fountzilas G, Ciuleanu E, Dafni U, Plataniotis G, Kalogera-Fountzila A, Samantas E, et al. Concomitant radiochemotherapy vs radiotherapy alone in patients with head and neck cancer: a Hellenic Cooperative Oncology Group Phase III Study. Med Oncol. 2004;21(2):95–107.
20. Posner MR, Norris CM, Wirth LJ, Shin DM, Cullen KJ, Winquist EW, et al. Sequential therapy for the locally advanced larynx and hypopharynx cancer subgroup in TAX 324: survival, surgery, and organ preservation. Ann Oncol. 2009;20(5):921–7.
21. Bourhis J, Sire C, Graff P, Gregoire V, Maingon P, Calais G, et al. Concomitant chemoradiotherapy versus acceleration of radiotherapy with or without concomitant chemotherapy in locally advanced head and neck carcinoma (GORTEC 99-02): an open-label phase 3 randomised trial. Lancet Oncol. 2012;13(2):145–53.
22. Clavel M, Vermorken JB, Cognetti F, Cappelaere P, de Mulder PH, Schornagel JH, et al. Randomized comparison of cisplatin, methotrexate, bleomycin and vincristine (CABO) versus cisplatin and 5-fluorouracil (CF) versus cisplatin (C) in recurrent or metastatic squamous cell carcinoma of the head and neck. A phase III study of the EORTC Head and Neck Cancer Cooperative Group. Ann Oncol. 1994;5(6):521–6.
23. Forastiere AA, Metch B, Schuller DE, Ensley JF, Hutchins LF, Triozzi P, et al. Randomized comparison of cisplatin plus fluorouracil and carboplatin plus fluorouracil versus methotrexate in advanced squamous-cell carcinoma of the head and neck: a Southwest Oncology Group study. J Clin Oncol. 1992;10(8):1245–51.
24. Jacobs C, Lyman G, Velez-Garcia E, Sridhar KS, Knight W, Hochster H, et al. A phase III randomized study comparing cisplatin and fluorouracil as single agents and in combination for advanced squamous cell carcinoma of the head and neck. J Clin Oncol. 1992;10(2):257–63.
25. Gibson MK, Li Y, Murphy B, Hussain MH, DeConti RC, Ensley J, et al. Randomized phase III evaluation of cisplatin plus fluorouracil versus cisplatin plus paclitaxel in advanced head and neck cancer (E1395): an intergroup trial of the Eastern Cooperative Oncology Group. J Clin Oncol. 2005;23(15):3562–7.
26. Rivera F, Garcia-Castano A, Vega N, Vega-Villegas ME, Gutierrez-Sanz L. Cetuximab in metastatic or recurrent head and neck cancer: the EXTREME trial. Expert Rev Anticancer Ther. 2009;9(10):1421–8.
27. Dorsey K, Agulnik M. Promising new molecular targeted therapies in head and neck cancer. Drugs. 2013;73(4):315–25.
28. Hynes NE, Horsch K, Olayioye MA, Badache A. The ErbB receptor tyrosine family as signal integrators. Endocr Relat Cancer. 2001;8(3):151–9.
29. Kruger JS, Reddy KB. Distinct mechanisms mediate the initial and sustained phases of cell migration in epidermal growth factor receptor-overexpressing cells. Mol Cancer Res. 2003;1(11):801–9.
30. Masuda M, Toh S, Koike K, Kuratomi Y, Suzui M, Deguchi A, et al. The roles of JNK1 and Stat3 in the response of head and neck cancer cell lines to combined treatment with all-trans-retinoic acid and 5-fluorouracil. Jpn J Cancer Res. 2002;93(3):329–39.
31. Vivanco I, Sawyers CL. The phosphatidylinositol 3-Kinase AKT pathway in human cancer. Nat Rev Cancer. 2002;2(7):489–501.
32. Ellerbroek SM, Halbleib JM, Benavidez M, Warmka JK, Wattenberg EV, Stack MS, et al. Phosphatidylinositol 3-kinase activity in epidermal growth factor-stimulated matrix metalloproteinase-9 production and cell surface association. Cancer Res. 2001;61(5):1855–61.
33. Agulnik M. New approaches to EGFR inhibition for locally advanced or metastatic squamous cell carcinoma of the head and neck (SCCHN). Med Oncol. 2012;29(4):2481–91.
34. Bonner JA, Harari PM, Giralt J, Azarnia N, Shin DM, Cohen RB, et al. Radiotherapy plus cetuximab for squamous-cell carcinoma of the head and neck. N Engl J Med. 2006;354(6):567–78.
35. Bonner JA, Harari PM, Giralt J, Cohen RB, Jones CU, Sur RK, et al. Radiotherapy plus cetuximab for locoregionally advanced head and neck cancer: 5-year survival data from a phase 3 randomised trial, and relation between cetuximab-induced rash and survival. Lancet Oncol. 2010;11(1):21–8.
36. Ang KK, Zhang Q, Rosenthal DI, Nguyen-Tan PF, Sherman EJ, Weber RS, et al. Randomized phase III trial of concurrent accelerated radiation plus cisplatin with or without cetuximab for stage III to IV head and neck carcinoma: RTOG 0522. J Clin Oncol. 2014;32(27):2940–50.
37. Saloura V, Vokes EE. EGFR-based bioradiotherapy in SCCHN. Lancet Oncol. 2015;16(2):129–30.
38. Mesia R, Henke M, Fortin A, Minn H, Yunes Ancona AC, Cmelak A, et al. Chemoradiotherapy with or with-

out panitumumab in patients with unresected, locally advanced squamous-cell carcinoma of the head and neck (CONCERT-1): a randomised, controlled, open-label phase 2 trial. Lancet Oncol. 2015;16(2):208–20.

39. Siu LL, Waldron JN, Chen BE, Winquist E, Wright JR, Nabid A, et al. Effect of standard radiotherapy with cisplatin vs accelerated radiotherapy with panitumumab in locoregionally advanced squamous cell head and neck carcinoma: a randomized clinical trial. JAMA Oncol. 2017;3(2):220–6.
40. Giralt J, Trigo J, Nuyts S, Ozsahin M, Skladowski K, Hatoum G, et al. Panitumumab plus radiotherapy versus chemoradiotherapy in patients with unresected, locally advanced squamous-cell carcinoma of the head and neck (CONCERT-2): a randomised, controlled, open-label phase 2 trial. Lancet Oncol. 2015;16(2):221–32.
41. Vermorken JB, Stohlmacher-Williams J, Davidenko I, Licitra L, Winquist E, Villanueva C, et al. Cisplatin and fluorouracil with or without panitumumab in patients with recurrent or metastatic squamous-cell carcinoma of the head and neck (SPECTRUM): an open-label phase 3 randomised trial. Lancet Oncol. 2013;14(8):697–710.
42. Bastholt L, Specht L, Jensen K, Brun E, Loft A, Petersen J, et al. Phase I/II clinical and pharmacokinetic study evaluating a fully human monoclonal antibody against EGFr (HuMax-EGFr) in patients with advanced squamous cell carcinoma of the head and neck. Radiother Oncol. 2007;85(1):24–8.
43. Machiels JP, Subramanian S, Ruzsa A, Repassy G, Lifirenko I, Flygare A, et al. Zalutumumab plus best supportive care versus best supportive care alone in patients with recurrent or metastatic squamous-cell carcinoma of the head and neck after failure of platinum-based chemotherapy: an open-label, randomised phase 3 trial. Lancet Oncol. 2011;12(4):333–43.
44. Schick U, Gujral DM, Richards TM, Harrington KJ, Nutting CM. Zalutumumab in head and neck cancer. Expert Opin Biol Ther. 2012;12(1):119–25.
45. Argiris A, Ghebremichael M, Gilbert J, Lee JW, Sachidanandam K, Kolesar JM, et al. Phase III randomized, placebo-controlled trial of docetaxel with or without gefitinib in recurrent or metastatic head and neck cancer: an eastern cooperative oncology group trial. J Clin Oncol. 2013;31(11):1405–14.
46. Cohen EE, Rosen F, Stadler WM, Recant W, Stenson K, Huo D, et al. Phase II trial of ZD1839 in recurrent or metastatic squamous cell carcinoma of the head and neck. J Clin Oncol. 2003;21(10):1980–7.
47. Martins RG, Parvathaneni U, Bauman JE, Sharma AK, Raez LE, Papagikos MA, et al. Cisplatin and radiotherapy with or without erlotinib in locally advanced squamous cell carcinoma of the head and neck: a randomized phase II trial. J Clin Oncol. 2013;31(11):1415–21.
48. Harrington KJ, Berrier A, Robinson M, Remenar E, Housset M, Mendoza FH, et al. Phase II study of oral lapatinib, a dual-tyrosine kinase inhibitor, combined with chemoradiotherapy (CRT) in patients (pts) with locally advanced, unresected squamous cell carcinoma of the head and neck (SCCHN). J Clin Oncol. 2010;28(15 Suppl):5505.
49. Abidoye OO, Cohen EE, Wong SJ, Kozloff MF, Nattam SR, Stenson KM, et al. A phase II study of lapatinib (GW572016) in recurrent/metastatic (R/M) squamous cell carcinoma of the head and neck (SCCHN). J Clin Oncol. 2006;24(18 Suppl):5568.
50. Seiwert TY, Fayette J, Cupissol D, del Campo JM, Clement PM, Hitt R, et al. A randomized, phase II study of afatinib versus cetuximab in metastatic or recurrent squamous cell carcinoma of the head and neck†. Ann Oncol. 2014;25(9):1813–20.
51. Abdul Razak AR, Soulières D, Laurie SA, Hotte SJ, Singh S, Winquist E, et al. A phase II trial of dacomitinib, an oral pan-human EGF receptor (HER) inhibitor, as first-line treatment in recurrent and/or metastatic squamous-cell carcinoma of the head and neck†. Ann Oncol. 2013;24(3):761–9.
52. Kim HS, Kwon HJ, Jung I, Yun MR, Ahn M-J, Kang BW, et al. Phase II clinical and exploratory biomarker study of dacomitinib in patients with recurrent and/or metastatic squamous cell carcinoma of head and neck. Clin Cancer Res. 2015;21(3):544–52.
53. Kyzas PA, Stefanou D, Batistatou A, Agnantis NJ. Prognostic significance of VEGF immunohistochemical expression and tumor angiogenesis in head and neck squamous cell carcinoma. J Cancer Res Clin Oncol. 2005;131(9):624–30.
54. Brands RC, Knierim LM, De Donno F, Steinacker V, Hartmann S, Seher A, et al. Targeting VEGFR and FGFR in head and neck squamous cell carcinoma in vitro. Oncol Rep. 2017;38(3):1877–85.
55. Swiecicki PL, Zhao L, Belile E, Sacco AG, Chepeha DB, Dobrosotskaya I, et al. A phase II study evaluating axitinib in patients with unresectable, recurrent or metastatic head and neck cancer. Investig New Drugs. 2015;33(6):1248–56.
56. Hsu HW, de Necochea-Campion R, Williams V, Duerksen-Hughes PJ, Simental AA Jr, Ferris RL, et al. Linifanib (ABT-869), enhances cytotoxicity with poly (ADP-ribose) polymerase inhibitor, veliparib (ABT-888), in head and neck carcinoma cells. Oral Oncol. 2014;50(7):662–9.
57. Kramer B, Hock C, Birk R, Sauter A, Stuck BA, Hormann K, et al. Targeted therapies in HPV-positive and -negative HNSCC – alteration of EGFR and VEGFR-2 expression in vitro. Anticancer Res. 2016;36(6):2799–807.
58. Argiris A, Bauman JE, Ohr J, Gooding WE, Heron DE, Duvvuri U, et al. Phase II randomized trial of radiation therapy, cetuximab, and pemetrexed with or without bevacizumab in patients with locally advanced head and neck cancer. Ann Oncol. 2016;27(8):1594–600.
59. Fury MG, Xiao H, Sherman EJ, Baxi S, Smith-Marrone S, Schupak K, et al. Phase II trial of bevacizumab + cetuximab + cisplatin with concurrent

intensity-modulated radiation therapy for patients with stage III/IVB head and neck squamous cell carcinoma. Head Neck. 2016;38(Suppl 1):E566–70.
60. Argiris A, Karamouzis MV, Gooding WE, Branstetter BF, Zhong S, Raez LE, et al. Phase II trial of pemetrexed and bevacizumab in patients with recurrent or metastatic head and neck cancer. J Clin Oncol. 2011;29(9):1140–5.
61. Williamson SK, Moon J, Huang CH, Guaglianone PP, LeBlanc M, Wolf GT, et al. Phase II evaluation of sorafenib in advanced and metastatic squamous cell carcinoma of the head and neck: Southwest Oncology Group Study S0420. J Clin Oncol. 2010;28(20):3330–5.
62. Elser C, Siu LL, Winquist E, Agulnik M, Pond GR, Chin SF, et al. Phase II trial of sorafenib in patients with recurrent or metastatic squamous cell carcinoma of the head and neck or nasopharyngeal carcinoma. J Clin Oncol. 2007;25(24):3766–73.
63. Blumenschein GR, Glisson BS, Lu C, Sabichi AL, Ginsberg LE, Bartos CI, et al. Final results of a phase II study of sorafenib in combination with carboplatin and paclitaxel in patients with metastatic or recurrent squamous cell cancer of the head and neck (SCCHN). J Clin Oncol. 2012;30(15 Suppl):5592.
64. Machiels JP, Henry S, Zanetta S, Kaminsky MC, Michoux N, Rommel D, et al. Phase II study of sunitinib in recurrent or metastatic squamous cell carcinoma of the head and neck: GORTEC 2006-01. J Clin Oncol. 2010;28(1):21–8.
65. Choong NW, Kozloff M, Taber D, Hu HS, Wade J 3rd, Ivy P, et al. Phase II study of sunitinib malate in head and neck squamous cell carcinoma. Investig New Drugs. 2010;28(5):677–83.
66. Papadimitrakopoulou VA, Frank SJ, Cohen EW, Hirsch FR, Myers JN, Heymach JV, et al. Phase I study of vandetanib with radiation therapy with or without cisplatin in locally advanced head and neck squamous cell carcinoma. Head Neck. 2016;38(3):439–47.
67. Sano D, Matsumoto F, Valdecanas DR, Zhao M, Molkentine DP, Takahashi Y, et al. Vandetanib restores head and neck squamous cell carcinoma cells' sensitivity to cisplatin and radiation in vivo and in vitro. Clin Cancer Res. 2011;17(7):1815–27.
68. Zibelman M, Mehra R. Overview of current treatment options and investigational targeted therapies for locally advanced squamous cell carcinoma of the head and neck. Am J Clin Oncol. 2016;39(4):396–406.
69. Chawla A, Adkins D, Worden FP, Rao KA, Hu HS, Price KAR, et al. Effect of the addition of temsirolimus to cetuximab in cetuximab-resistant head and neck cancers: results of the randomized PII MAESTRO study. J Clin Oncol. 2014;32(15 Suppl):6089.
70. Bauman JE, Arias-Pulido H, Lee SJ, Fekrazad MH, Ozawa H, Fertig E, et al. A phase II study of temsirolimus and erlotinib in patients with recurrent and/or metastatic, platinum-refractory head and neck squamous cell carcinoma. Oral Oncol. 2013;49(5):461–7.
71. Chung CH, Wang H, Tsottles N, Gourin CG, Agrawal N, Molinolo A, et al. A phase I study of everolimus in combination with cetuximab and cisplatin as first-line therapy in recurrent and metastatic (R/M) head and neck squamous cell carcinoma (HNSCC). J Clin Oncol. 2012;30(15 Suppl):e16061.
72. Adkins D, Oppelt PJ, Ley JC, Trinkaus K, Neupane PC, Sacco AG. Multicenter phase II trial of palbociclib, a selective cyclin dependent kinase (CDK) 4/6 inhibitor, and cetuximab in platinum-resistant HPV unrelated (−) recurrent/metastatic head and neck squamous cell carcinoma (RM HNSCC). J Clin Oncol. 2018;36:6008.
73. Cohen EEW, Soulieres D, Le Tourneau C, Dinis J, Licitra L, Ahn MJ, et al. Pembrolizumab versus methotrexate, docetaxel, or cetuximab for recurrent or metastatic head-and-neck squamous cell carcinoma (KEYNOTE-040): a randomised, open-label, phase 3 study. Lancet. 2019;393(10167):156–67.
74. Ferris RL, Blumenschein G Jr, Fayette J, Guigay J, Colevas AD, Licitra L, et al. Nivolumab for recurrent squamous-cell carcinoma of the head and neck. N Engl J Med. 2016;375(19):1856–67.
75. Zandberg DP, Algazi AP, Jimeno A, Good JS, Fayette J, Bouganim N, et al. Durvalumab for recurrent or metastatic head and neck squamous cell carcinoma: Results from a single-arm, phase II study in patients with >/=25% tumour cell PD-L1 expression who have progressed on platinum-based chemotherapy. Eur J Cancer. 2019;107:142–52.
76. Shiono S, Kawamura M, Sato T, Okumura S, Nakajima J, Yoshino I, et al. Pulmonary metastasectomy for pulmonary metastases of head and neck squamous cell carcinomas. Ann Thorac Surg. 2009;88(3):856–60.
77. Liu D, Labow DM, Dang N, Martini N, Bains M, Burt M, et al. Pulmonary metastasectomy for head and neck cancers. Ann Surg Oncol. 1999;6(6):572–8.
78. Mochizuki T, Okumura S, Ishii G, Ishikawa Y, Hayashi R, Kawabata K, et al. Surgical resection for oral tongue cancer pulmonary metastases. Interact Cardiovasc Thorac Surg. 2010;11(1):56–9.
79. Lopez-Verdin S, Lavalle-Carrasco J, Carreon-Burciaga RG, Serafin-Higuera N, Molina-Frechero N, Gonzalez-Gonzalez R, et al. Molecular markers of anticancer drug resistance in head and neck squamous cell carcinoma: a literature review. Cancers. 2018;10(10):pii: E376.
80. Becker M, Levy D. Modeling the transfer of drug resistance in solid tumors. Bull Math Biol. 2017;79(10):2394–412.
81. Quintela-Fandino M, Hitt R, Medina PP, Gamarra S, Manso L, Cortes-Funes H, et al. DNA-repair gene polymorphisms predict favorable clinical outcome among patients with advanced squamous cell carcinoma of the head and neck treated with cisplatin-based induction chemotherapy. J Clin Oncol. 2006;24(26):4333–9.
82. Cutilli T, Leocata P, Dolo V, Altobelli E. Evaluation of p53 protein as a prognostic factor for oral cancer surgery. Br J Oral Maxillofac Surg. 2013;51(8):922–7.

83. Blons H, Gad S, Zinzindohoue F, Maniere I, Beauregard J, Tregouet D, et al. Matrix metalloproteinase 3 polymorphism: a predictive factor of response to neoadjuvant chemotherapy in head and neck squamous cell carcinoma. Clin Cancer Res. 2004;10(8):2594–9.
84. Ansell A, Jedlinski A, Johansson AC, Roberg K. Epidermal growth factor is a potential biomarker for poor cetuximab response in tongue cancer cells. J Oral Pathol Med. 2016;45(1):9–16.
85. Roepstorff K, Grandal MV, Henriksen L, Knudsen SL, Lerdrup M, Grovdal L, et al. Differential effects of EGFR ligands on endocytic sorting of the receptor. Traffic. 2009;10(8):1115–27.
86. Setubal Destro Rodrigues MF, Gammon L, Rahman MM, Biddle A, Nunes FD, Mackenzie IC. Effects of cetuximab and erlotinib on the behaviour of cancer stem cells in head and neck squamous cell carcinoma. Oncotarget. 2018;9(17):13488–500.
87. Gemenetzidis E, Gammon L, Biddle A, Emich H, Mackenzie IC. Invasive oral cancer stem cells display resistance to ionising radiation. Oncotarget. 2015;6(41):43964–77.

Immunotherapy in Oral Cancer: A Fourth Dimension of Cancer Treatment

10

Marcus A. Couey, Rom S. Leidner, Simon W. Young, and R. Bryan Bell

10.1 The Immune System in Head and Neck Cancer

Although many components of the immune system are involved in the antitumor immune response, the most critical immune cell is the T cell. The Cancer Immunity Cycle, as described by Chen and Mellman, explains the steps required for the adaptive immune system to target tumors, including uptake and presentation of antigens by dendritic cells (DC), priming and activation of T cells in the lymph nodes, homing of T cells to the site of the tumor, and T cell recognition and destruction of tumor cells [1] (Fig. 10.1). Cancer cell death then exposes more potential antigens to immune recognition, which can perpetuate the cycle. Each step in this sequence has biochemical stimulators and inhibitors, and appreciation of these steps is critical in developing strategies to overcome immune evasion by tumors.

M. A. Couey · R. S. Leidner · R. B. Bell (✉)
Earle A. Chiles Research Institute in the Robert W. Franz Cancer Center, Providence Cancer Institute, Portland, OR, USA
e-mail: Marcus.Couey@providence.org; Rom.Leidner@providence.org; Richard.Bell@providence.org

S. W. Young
Department of Oral and Maxillofacial Surgery, University of Texas Health Science Center at Houston, Houston, TX, USA
e-mail: Simon.Young@uth.tmc.edu

D. Kademani (ed.), *Improving Outcomes in Oral Cancer*,
https://doi.org/10.1007/978-3-030-30094-4_10

The central role of the immune system in both the prevention and evolution of cancer has been described by Schreiber et al. in the concept of immunoediting [2]. Immunoediting starts with the surveillance of the body for abnormal cells by the immune system. In some cases, the immune system is successful in targeting and eliminating a tumor and preventing the occurrence of clinically detectable cancer. However, sometimes the immune system cannot eliminate a subset of the tumor cells, as those cells have acquired phenotypes that subvert immune targeting. After a period of equilibrium, where these resistant tumor cells exist in quiescence, they may begin to proliferate and spread. This is called immune escape and is now recognized as one of the hallmarks of cancer [3].

Advances in whole-exome sequencing have provided great insights into the molecular landscape of head and neck cancer. Remarkable efforts by several groups, including The Cancer Genome Atlas (TCGA), have identified the most commonly altered molecular pathways involved in head and neck squamous cell carcinoma (HNSCC). These data have shown that HNSCCs have a moderate-to-high mutational burden and are heterogeneous tumors. The most common involved pathways are tumor-suppressor genes such as p53, which are either inactivated or mutated. Successful restoration of functional tumor-suppressor pathways in HNSCC through targeted therapy has so far remained elusive.

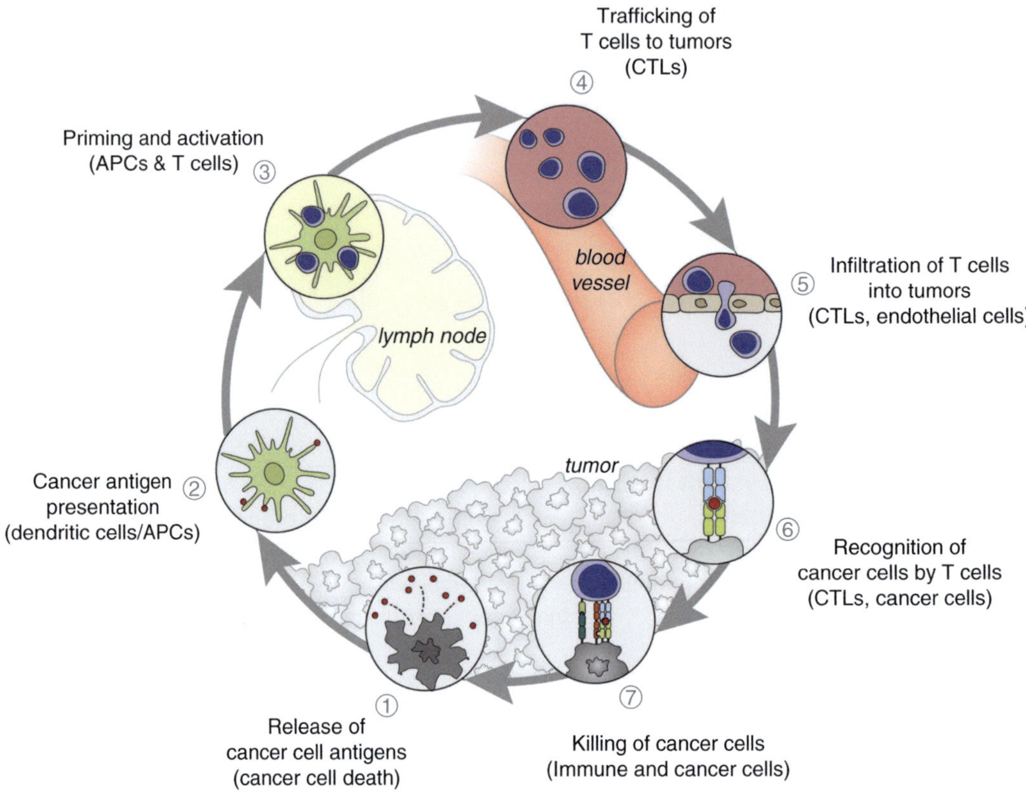

Fig. 10.1 Therapies that might affect the cancer immunity cycle. (From: Chen DS., Mellman I. "Oncology meets immunology: the cancer immunity cycle." *Immunity* 39.1 (2013): 1–10)

Oncogenic pathways which have been identified in a significant percentage of tumors, such as PI3K, are theoretically more targetable than tumor suppressors. However, results of therapies such as PI3K and mTOR inhibitors have been mostly disappointing [4]. The heterogeneity of cells within a tumor, even those tumors that test positive for targetable mutations, may play an important role in the difficulties encountered with targeted therapies [5].

While the relatively high mutational rate of HNSCC creates difficulty in applying targeted therapies, it may be advantageous for the application of immunotherapy through the presence of more mutations that may be recognized as nonself by the immune system. However, there are numerous escape mechanisms that tumors employ to suppress the natural antitumor capabilities of immune cells. Impaired antitumor responses in HNSCC may be caused by alterations in the generation, processing, and/or presentation of T cell epitopes derived from tumor-associated antigens (TAA) by human leukocyte antigen (HLA) class I and/or class II molecule [6]. Other mechanisms for evading immune targeting by tumors include upregulation of immune-suppressive "checkpoint" ligands (e.g., PD-L1) [7], release of inhibitory cytokines by suppressive immune cells including regulatory T cells (Treg), myeloid-derived suppressor cells (MDSC) and tumor-associated macrophages (TAM) in the tumor microenvironment [8–10], or the secretion of immune-suppressive mediators (e.g., TGF-beta) [11]. Knowledge of the specific

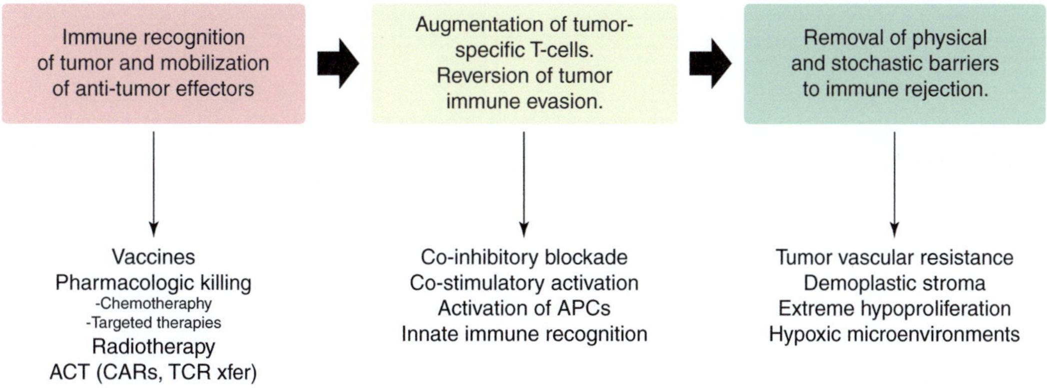

Fig. 10.2 Strategies for immune checkpoint combinations: different classes of therapeutic approaches that have synergistic potential for future combination immunotherapies are depicted. (Modified from: Ai, M, Curran MA. "Immune checkpoint combinations from mouse to man." *Cancer Immunology, Immunotherapy* 64.7 (2015): 885–892)

mechanisms of immune suppression in HNSCC has led to numerous approaches to overcome immune suppression in the tumor microenvironment (Fig. 10.2).

Treatment and prognosis of HNSCC vary depending on anatomical location. For oropharyngeal SCC, carcinogenesis is often driven by infection with high-risk strains of HPV, usually HPV-16. It has been shown that the molecular pathways and immunobiology of HPV-positive tumors are distinct from HPV-negative disease [12]. In addition, HPV-positive HNSCCs respond better to standard therapies and most immunotherapies [13]. The significance of HPV in oral cancer specifically remains uncertain, and there is currently no standard method for identifying HPV as the etiologic agent in oral cavity SCC that is both accepted and available universally [14]. This chapter is meant to focus on cancers arising in the oral cavity and therefore will limit the discussion to HPV-negative HNSCC.

Current therapies and those in development are focused on strategic targeting of the various steps in the Cancer Immunity Cycle. The great promise of immunotherapy lies with the potential for lasting, or durable, responses. This is referred to as the "tail at the end of the survival curve" (Fig. 10.5) and is perhaps the most exciting prospect of immunotherapy.

10.2 A New Standard of Care in Recurrent or Metastatic Head and Neck Cancer

10.2.1 PD-1 Inhibitors

One of the ways that tumors can halt the immune response is through signaling molecules called checkpoints. These inhibitory cell receptors block T cell activity and lead to T cell apoptosis. This is normally a safeguard against autoimmunity. However tumors can upregulate these inhibitory receptors, which promote evasion of immune targeting. Monoclonal antibodies that block the interaction between these receptors and their ligands, known as checkpoint inhibitors (CPI), have shown great promise for many types of solid tumors in recent years (Fig. 10.3).

The most well-studied checkpoint inhibitors in HNSCC are the antiprogrammed cell death protein 1 (anti-PD-1) antibodies nivolumab and pembrolizumab. Through interaction with its ligands programmed death ligand 1 (PD-L1) and 2 (PD-L2), PD-1 acts as an immune rheostat that modulates the immune response within the tumor [1]. The blockade of PD-1 has been shown to prevent the inhibition of T cell activity in the tumor microenvironment, thereby permitting cellular cytotoxicity against tumor cells.

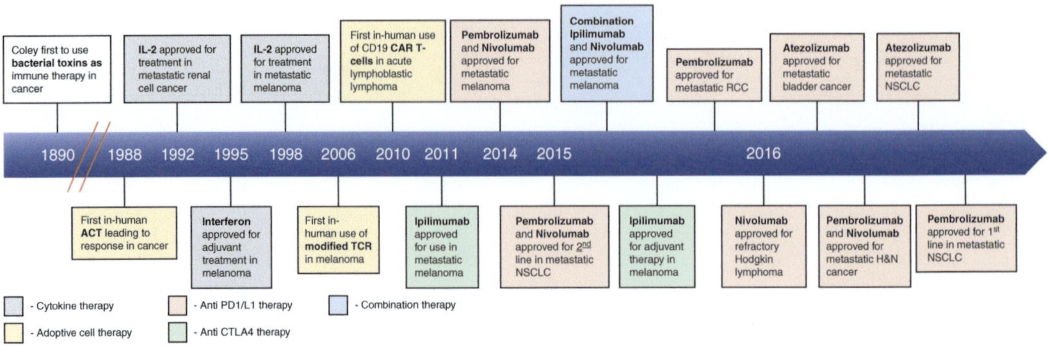

Fig. 10.3 Timeline of breakthroughs in cancer immunotherapy. (From: Wang, Daniel Y., Gosife Donald Okoye, Thomas G. Neilan, Douglas B. Johnson, and Javid J. Moslehi. "Cardiovascular Toxicities Associated with Cancer Immunotherapies." Current Cardiology Reports 19:21. 2017)

In late 2016, the FDA granted approval of nivolumab, following the results from the randomized phase III trial, CheckMate141 [15]. This study evaluated nivolumab versus investigator's choice (IC) chemotherapy in patients with recurrent or metastatic (R/M) HNSCC that had progressed within 6 months of platinum-based chemotherapy. This was the first randomized, controlled data showing a survival benefit in R/M HNSCC since the EXTREME regimen, consisting of the combination of platinum, 5-fluorouracil and cetuximab [16]. The study was ended early after meeting its primary endpoint of overall survival (OS), and patients from the control arm were then allowed to crossover to receive nivolumab. A recent update reported 2-year OS of 16.9% in nivolumab-treated patients, which was more than double the rate for patients that received standard therapy (6.0%) [17]. Significant OS benefit was seen regardless of HPV or PD-L1 status.

In mid-2016, the FDA granted accelerated approval of pembrolizumab for platinum-refractory R/M HNSCC based on results from the phase Ib KEYNOTE-012 trial [18]. This trial studied pembrolizumab in patients with R/M disease whose tumors had progressed within 6 months of platinum-based cytotoxic chemotherapy. The objective response rate (ORR) for pembrolizumab was 18%, with 71% of responses lasting 12 months or more. The KEYNOTE-055 trial studied pembrolizumab in R/M HNSCC who had progressed on platinum and the anti-epidermal growth factor receptor (EGFR) antibody, cetuximab. ORR was 16% with a median duration of response of 8 months [19]. A survival benefit with pembrolizumab in platinum-refractory R/M disease was later confirmed in KEYNOTE-040. In this randomized, controlled phase III trial, patients receiving pembrolizumab had a median OS of 8.4 months, vs 6.9 months for IC chemotherapy. Patients with >50% of tumor cells expressing PD-L1 experienced increased benefit with pembrolizumab (median OS 11.6 months) [20].

Recently, results were announced from the first phase III trial of anti-PD-1 therapy in *first-line* R/M HNSCC. KEYNOTE-048 randomized patients to one of three arms: pembrolizumab monotherapy, pembrolizumab plus platinum and 5-FU, or cetuximab plus platinum and 5-FU (EXTREME regimen). This trial showed that in PD-L1-expressing patients (~85% of patients in this population), pembrolizumab monotherapy was superior to the EXTREME regimen, with 2-year OS of 30.2% vs 18.6%. Further, when looking at the total population (regardless of PD-L1 status), patients who received pembrolizumab with cisplatin and 5-FU had 29% 2-year survival compared with 18.7% with the EXTREME regimen. In June 2019, the FDA approved the use of pembrolizumab with or without cisplatin/5-FU (determined by PD-L1 status) based on data from this trial [21].

Importantly, the anti-PD-1 agents are much better tolerated than cytotoxic chemotherapy, with grade 3–5 drug-related adverse events occurring in 13–14% of patients receiving anti-PD-1 versus 36% with standard of care in phase III, randomized trials. The most common adverse events associated with these agents are fatigue, nausea, rash, decreased appetite, and pruritus. Hypothyroidism occurs in 7.7–13% of patients, vs. about 1% with standard treatment. Pneumonitis is the most severe adverse event associated with anti-PD-1 and can be life-threatening if not recognized early and treated. Numerous physical and social quality of life (QOL) measures were assessed in CheckMate141 which showed advantages of PD-1 inhibitors across the board compared with standard of care chemotherapy. While pembrolizumab and nivolumab have been the most highly studied anti-PD-1 therapies, there are other anti-PD-1 agents currently in development. Spartalizumab (PDR001) and cemiplimab (REGN2810) are being tested alone and in combination with other immunotherapies in multiple solid tumor types including HNSCC.

10.3 Additional Checkpoint Inhibitors

10.3.1 PD-L1

Blockade of checkpoints can be achieved through targeting either the receptor (e.g., PD-1), or the ligand. Of the two ligands for PD-1, PD-L1 is generally thought to play a more prominent role in immunosuppression than PD-L2 [22]. In addition, PD-L1's binding is not exclusive to the PD-1 receptor; it can also block the immune-stimulating ligand B7–1, causing immune suppression by a separate mechanism (Fig. 10.4) [23]. Furthermore, targeting PD-L1 specifically may reduce the risk of pneumonitis compared with anti-PD-1 therapy, as pneumonitis is thought to be at least partially mediated by PD-L2 [24]. Therefore, the blockade of PD-L1 is expected to confer a different treatment response and adverse-effect profile than anti-PD-1 therapy. Several anti-PD-L1 antibodies are currently being stud-

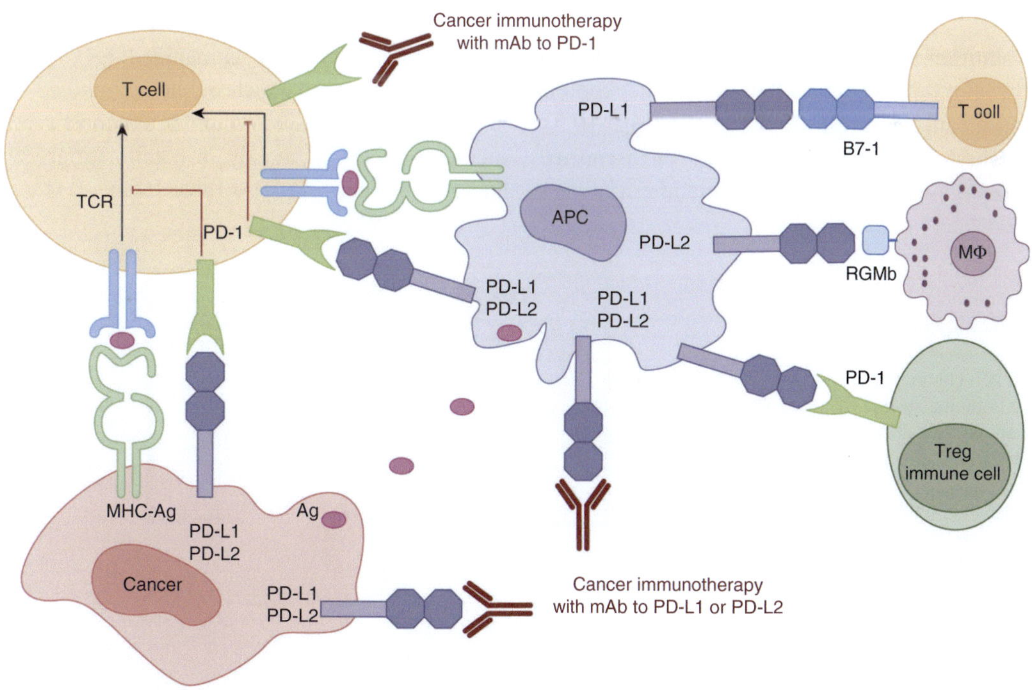

Fig. 10.4 Human cancer immunotherapy with anti-PD-1 and anti-PD-L1/L2 antibodies. (From: Ohaegbulam, KC., et al. "Human cancer immunotherapy with antibodies to the PD-1 and PD-L1 pathway." *Trends in molecular medicine* 21.1 (2015): 24–33)

ied in HNSCC, including durvalumab, avelumab, and atezolizumab.

Recently, the results were announced from the phase II HAWK trial of durvalumab in platinum-refractory R/M HNSCC with high PD-L1 expression, defined as greater than 25% tumor cell expression (NCT02207530). ORR was 16%, and 55% of responses were ongoing at data cutoff. Overall survival at 1 year was 33.6%. There was a striking difference in response rate based on HPV status, with an ORR of 29.4% in HPV-positive disease and 10.8% in HPV-negative disease. The incidence of grade 3 or higher adverse events was relatively low at 8%. One patient discontinued therapy because of a treatment-related adverse event, and there were no treatment-related deaths [25]. There are a large number of clinical trials studying durvalumab in combination with other immune-modulating agents, as well as chemotherapy and radiation, which will be discussed later in the chapter.

10.3.2 CTLA-4

In addition to PD-1/PD-L1, there are numerous other immune receptors that act as checkpoints through inhibition of immune cells (Fig. 10.5). The first immune checkpoint to be identified and targeted for cancer immunotherapy was Cytotoxic T-lymphocyte-Associated Protein 4 (CTLA-4). CTLA-4 is a receptor expressed on the surface of T cells that binds with B7 ligands on antigen-presenting cells (APC), causing T cell anergy and apoptosis. While PD-1 inhibits effector cells within the tumor microenvironment (TME), CTLA-4 inhibits T cell activation within the periphery, largely in the lymph nodes [26]. Blockade of CTLA-4 prevents immune-suppressive signaling, while also freeing the B7 ligands to bind the costimulatory receptor CD28. Additionally, antibodies targeting CTLA-4 cause Treg depletion through antibody-dependent cell-mediated cytotoxicity (ADCC), thereby reducing immunosuppressive influences in the TME [27].

Ipilimumab, a fully humanized IgG1 anti-CTLA-4 antibody, was the first checkpoint inhibitor to demonstrate improved survival in melanoma and subsequently became the first drug in this class to gain FDA approval [28]. Ipilimumab has since shown activity in numerous solid tumor types; however, immune-related adverse events are more common and more severe than with the anti-PD-1 agents. Tremelimumab is fully humanized IgG2 anti-CTLA-4 antibody, which is being studied in many clinical trials across numerous cancer types including HNSCC, mostly in combination with durvalumab (anti-PD-L1) (Table 10.1).

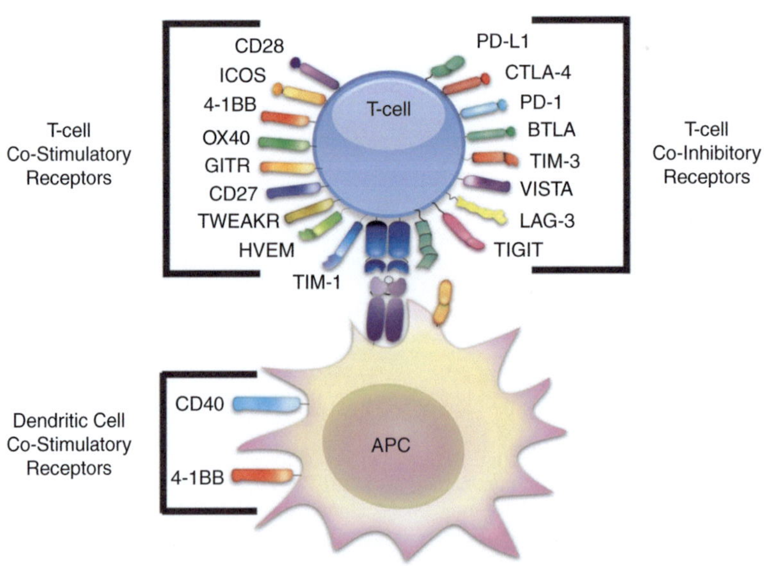

Fig. 10.5 T cell costimulatory and coinhibitory receptors. Shown are the families of T cell costimulatory and immune checkpoint receptors as well as those which affect dendritic cells responsible for T cell activation. (From: Ai, M, Curran MA. "Immune checkpoint combinations from mouse to man." *Cancer Immunology, Immunotherapy* 64.7 (2015): 885–892)

Table 10.1 Clinical trials: other checkpoint inhibitors

	Phase	Tumor type	Combination	Comparison	Trial	Expected completion date
CTLA-4						
Ipilimumab	III	R/M HNSCC	Nivolumab	Ipi placebo	NCT02823574	08/2020
	III	R/M HNSCC	Nrvolumab	Plat/5FU/Cetux	NCT02741570	08/2020
Tremelimumab	II	R/M HNSCC	Durvalumab	Mono vs combo	NCT02319044	09/2018
	III	R/M HNSCC	Durvalumab	SOC chemo	NCT02369874	11/2018
	III	R/M HNSCC	Durvalumab	SOC chemo	NCT02551159	12/2018
TIM-3						
TSR-022	I	Advanced solid tumors		Anti-PDl	NCT02817633	06/2020
LY3321367	I	Advanced		LY3300054	NCT03099109	06/2020
MBG453	I/II	Advanced malignancies		PDR001	NCT02608268	03/2019
LAG-3						
Relatlimab	I	Advanced solid tumors		Nivolumab	NCT02966548	07/2020
	I/IIa	Advanced solid tumors		Nivolumab	NCT01968109	12/2020
TSR-033	I	Advanced solid tumors		Anti-PDl	NCT03250832	05/2021
REGN3767	I	Advanced malignancies		REGN2810	NCT03005782	03/2022
LAG525	I/II	Advanced malignancies		PDR001	NCT02460224	08/2019
TIGIT						
BMS-986207	I/IIa	Advanced solid tumors		Nivolumab	NCT02913313	12/2022
OMP-313M32	I	LA/M solid tumors		Nivolumab	NCT03119428	10/2019
MTIG7192A	I	LA/M tumors		Atezolizumab	NCT02794571	09/2019

LA locally advanced, *R* recurrent, *M* metastatic, *Ipi* ipilimumab, *plat* platinum, *cetux* cetuximab, *mono* monotherapy, *SOC* standard of care

10.3.3 TIM-3

T cell Immunoglobulin and Mucin Domain 3 (TIM-3) is another immune checkpoint expressed on the surface of T cells. High TIM-3 is a marker of T cell exhaustion, similar to PD-1, and has been shown in preclinical and clinical studies to be upregulated in cases of progressive disease after anti-PD-1 therapy [29]. Preclinical models have also shown increased cytokine production and activity of cytotoxic T cells with blockade of TIM-3 and PD-1 pathways in combination compared with PD-1 pathway blockade alone [30]. Therefore, there is sound rationale for studying TIM-3 in combination with therapies targeting the PD-1/PD-L1 pathway. Additionally, blockade of TIM-3 has been shown in preclinical models to promote immune responses and reduce suppressive forces via multiple targets aside from $CD8^+$ T cells, including $CD4^+$ T cells, natural killer (NK) cells, Tregs, MDSCs, and DCs. At least three monoclonal antibodies are currently in phase I-II trials for advanced solid malignancies (Table 10.1).

10.3.4 LAG-3

The immune checkpoint Lymphocyte Activation Gene-3 (LAG-3) has been shown to suppress responses of $CD8^+$ cytotoxic T cells and NK cells and to promote the suppressive influence of Tregs. LAG-3 is co-expressed with PD-1 on dysfunctional or exhausted T cells, and anti-LAG-3 in preclinical studies has demonstrated synergy with anti-PD-1/PD-L1 to improve anti-tumor immune responses [31]. There are at least four monoclonal antibodies being evaluated in phase I–II clinical trials for advanced solid tumors including HNSCC (Table 10.1).

10.3.5 TIGIT

T cell Immunoglobulin and ITIM Doman (TIGIT) is another immune checkpoint that dampens the immune response through interactions with multiple cell types, including effector T and NK cells, DC cells, and suppressive Tregs. The combined blockade of TIGIT and PD-L1 synergistically promotes CD8+ T cell effector function within tumors [32]. There are at least three anti-TIGIT antibodies currently being evaluated in phase I–II clinical trials for advanced solid tumors (Table 10.1).

10.4 Combinations of Checkpoint Inhibitors

There is abundant preclinical evidence supporting a combinatorial approach to cancer immunotherapy. For example, CTLA-4 acts relatively early in the cancer immunity cycle during T cell priming and activation, while PD-1 comes into play later in the cycle by modulating immune effector cell function within tumors. Additionally, blockade of one immune checkpoint can lead to the increased expression of other checkpoints by tumor cells leading to immune escape [29]. Therefore, it has been hypothesized that adding one or more additional CPI to PD-1/PD-L1 therapy may improve response rates, particularly in PD-L1-negative patients, and prevent resistance to single-agent therapy (Fig. 10.6).

Two large studies are currently testing nivolumab (anti-PD-1) alone or in combination with ipilimumab (anti-CTLA-4) in R/M HNSCC. CheckMate714 is a double-blinded, randomized, phase II study in both the platinum-refractory and first-line settings, and CheckMate651 is an open-label, randomized phase III study of the same combination as first-line therapy compared to chemotherapy (NCT02823574, NCT02741570). This combination has been approved for the treatment of patients with advanced melanoma and advanced renal cell carcinoma. Combination nivolumab + ipilimumab has also shown significant promise in the treatment of patients with advanced non-small-cell lung cancer [33]. Data from these trials are not yet mature and will be presented at future meetings.

Tremelimumab (anti-CTLA-4) is now being tested in numerous clinical trials for HNSCC in combination with durvalumab (anti-PD-L1). The CONDOR trial was a phase II, randomized trial of durvalumab and tremelimumab alone and in combination in patients with platinum-refractory R/M HNSCC who had low PD-L1 levels. Median overall survival was 7.6 months in the combination arm, 6.0 months for durvalumab alone, and 5.5 months for tremelimumab alone [34]. EAGLE (NCT02369874) and KESTREL (NCT02551159) are randomized phase III trials studying this combination in platinum-refractory disease and as first-line treatment of R/M HNSCC, respectively.

There is a large body of preclinical evidence for the antitumor activity of other combinations of C. In fact, many of the newer CPI are being developed as combinations from the start, most commonly in combination with PD-1/PD-L1 pathway antagonists. For example, all the current anti-TIM-3, anti-TIGIT, and anti-LAG-3 trials evaluating tolerability and efficacy in advanced solid tumors are testing these agents in combination with

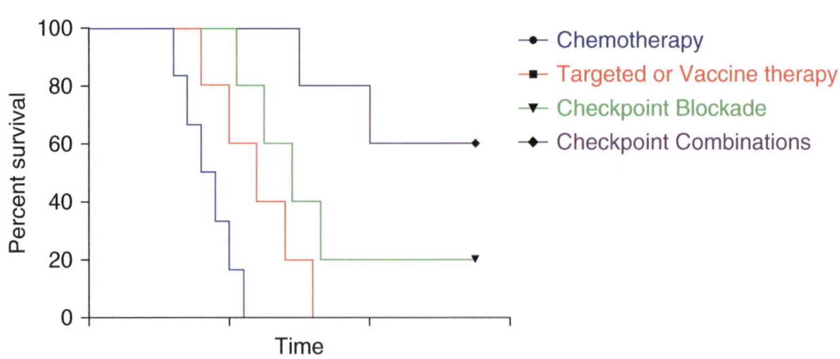

Fig. 10.6 Strategies for immune checkpoint combinations: Shown is the current goal of the field of immunotherapy to increase the percentage of patients experiencing durable, complete responses through combination therapy approaches. (Modified from: Ai, M, Curran MA. "Immune checkpoint combinations from mouse to man." *Cancer Immunology, Immunotherapy* 64.7 (2015): 885–892)

anti-PD-1 or anti-PD-L1 antibodies. While clinical trials for these other combinations are still in early phases for the most part, there are early reports of success such as the phase I/IIa trial of relatlimab (anti-LAG-3) with nivolumab (anti-PD-1) in advanced solid tumors. In an expansion cohort of melanoma patients who were refractory to PD-1 therapy alone, 11.5% had objective responses and 37.7% had stable disease with the combination. Patients with ≥1% LAG-3 expression had an ORR of 18%, and patients who also had prior exposure to CTLA-4 had an ORR of 24% [35]. This trial includes head and neck patients as well, and study completion is expected in late 2019.

10.5 Costimulatory Agonists

In addition to T cell receptor (TCR) recognition of MHC-presented antigens, the activation of T cells requires specific costimulatory signals (Fig. 10.5). TCR ligation without the second costimulation signal leads to T cell anergy and immune tolerance [36]. The development of agonist antibodies that activate costimulatory receptors has added a new dimension to cancer immunotherapy. While the activity of checkpoint inhibitors has been described as "releasing the breaks" on the immune system, costimulatory agonists have been described as "stepping on the gas." Preclinical studies have shown that costimulatory agonists have synergistic activity with CPI, and there are currently many such agents being tested in clinical trials alone and in combination with other immunotherapies.

10.5.1 CD28 Superfamily

Inducible T cell costimulator (ICOS) is a member of the CD28 superfamily that promotes CD4$^+$ T cell growth, differentiation and effector function, as well as survival and memory of both CD4$^+$ and CD8$^+$ T cells [37]. ICOS is only expressed at low levels on naïve T cells but is rapidly upregulated upon TCR ligation [38]. It is also highly expressed on Tregs, and ICOS signaling can therefore contribute to immune suppression, contrary to its action on effector T cells. Preclinical studies have shown effector T cell -mediated antitumor immune responses and Treg depletion with antibodies from subclasses capable of ADCC, as well as synergy with both CTLA-4 and PD-1 blocking agents. There are currently two antibodies in clinical trials in advanced solid tumors (Table 10.2). JTX-2011, a humanized IgG1 monoclonal ICOS agonist antibody, is the furthest along in development. It was found to be well tolerated in phase I trials and is currently undergoing phase II testing in several tumor types including HNSCC [39].

10.5.2 Tumor Necrosis Factor (TNF) Receptor Superfamily

The TNF superfamily of receptors (TNFRs) are involved in immune cell activation, proliferation, and survival. There are several members of this group that are being targeted with agonist pharmaceuticals in cancer immunotherapy clinical trials, including OX40, 4-1BB, CD27, glucocorticoid-induced TNFR-related protein (GITR), and CD40.

OX40 is transiently expressed on CD4$^+$ and CD8$^+$ T cells and Tregs following TCR ligation. OX40 is also expressed on NK cells, NKT cells, and neutrophils, and its ligand OX40L is transiently expressed on APCs and some T cells. OX40 appears to be important for T cell survival and expansion, and for differentiation of T cells, skewing toward an effector phenotype [40]. OX40 has shown synergistic activity with checkpoint blockade in preclinical studies [41]. Furthermore, OX40 is highly expressed in tumor-infiltrating lymphocytes (TILs) in HNSCC, particularly CD4$^+$ T cells, providing strong rationale for testing in clinical trials in this disease [42, 43]. There are six OX40-targeting antibodies in pharmaceutical pipelines that are currently in clinical trials for advanced solid tumors, including HNSCC (Table 10.2). Interestingly, one such agent was recently tested in a phase Ib neoadjuvant trial prior to surgery: MEDI6469 was administered intravenously at various time intervals prior to definitive surgical resection in 17 patients with stage II–IVA HNSCC [44]. Fifty percent of the patients treated experienced an increase in the percentage of tumor-reactive CD8$^+$ T cells in the

Table 10.2 Clinical trials: costimulatory agonists

	Phase	Tumor type	Combination	Trial	Expected completion date
ICOS					
GSK3359609	I	Advanced solid tumors	Pembrolizumab	NCT02723955	05/2020
JTX-2011	I/II	Advanced malignancies	Ipilimumab or nivolumab or pembrolizumab	NCT02904226	12/2022
OX40					
MEDI0562	I	Advanced solid tumors	None	NCT02318394	Completed, pending publication
	I	Advanced solid tumors	Durvalumab or tremelimumab	NCT02705482	12/2019
	Ib	HNSCC or melanoma (neoadjuvant)	None	NCT03336606	12/2024
PF-4518600	I	LA/M cancers	Utomilumab	NCT02315066	01/2021
	Ib/II	Advanced solid tumors	Avelumab +/− utomilumab	NCT02554812	05/2020
MOXR0916	Ib	LA/M solid tumors	Atezolizumab	NCT02410512	08/2018
GSK3174998	I	Advanced solid tumors	Pembrolizumab	NCT02528357	01/2020
BMS-986178	I/IIa	Advanced solid tumors	Nivolumab and/or ipilimumab	NCT02737475	10/2021
INCAGN1949	I	A/M solid tumors	None	NCT02923349	02/2019
4-1BB					
Urelumab	III	A/M solid tumors/ NHL	Nivolumab	NCT02253992	09/2019
	I	Malignant tumors	Nivolumab	NCT02534506	06/2019
	I	Metastases in advanced solid tumors	Nivolumab + SBRT	NCT03431948	02 2020
Utomilumab	I	LA/M cancers	PF-4518600	NCT02315066	01/2021
	Ib/II	Advanced solid tumors	Avelumab +/− PF-4518600	NCT02554812	05 2020
GITR					
TRX518	I	Melanoma and other solid tumors	None	NCT01239134	12/2018
	I	Advanced solid tumors	Pembrolizumab or nivolumab or gemcitabine	NCT02628574	09/2020
GWN323	I	Advanced solid tumors	PDR001	NCT02740270	12/2019
MK-4166	I	Advanced solid tumors	Pembrolizumab	NCT02132754	10/2019
MK-1248	I	Advanced solid tumors	Pembrolizumab	NCT02553499	10/2018
MEDI1873	I	Advanced solid tumors	None	NCT02583165	01/2021
INCAGN01876	I/II	Advanced malignancies	None	NCT02697591	08/2018
BMS-986156	I/IIa	Advanced solid tumors	Nivolumab	NCT02598960	05/2020
CD27					
Varlilumab	I/II	Advanced refractory solid tumors	Nivolumab	NCT02335918	01/2020

Table 10.2 (continued)

	Phase	Tumor type	Combination	Trial	Expected completion date
CD40					
SEA-CD40	I	Advanced malignancies	Pembrolizumab	NCT02376699	09/2022
CDX-1140	I	Advanced solid tumors	None	NCT03329950	12/2020
Selicrelumab	Ib	LA/M solid tumors	Atezolizumab	NCT02304393	10/2019
	Ib	Advanced solid tumors	Emactuzumab	NCT02760797	Completed, pending publication
APX005M	I	Solid tumors	None	NCT02482168	12/2018
ABBV-927	I	Advanced solid tumors	ABBV-181	NCT02988960	11/2019

tumor after anti-OX40 treatment. Early-phase clinical trials are underway with the goal of understanding how best to incorporate OX40 into combination trials with CPI and conventional therapies.

4-1BB is can be found on many cell types, including cells of hematopoietic and neuronal origins. Like OX40, 4-1BB is transiently expressed on $CD4^+$ and $CD8^+$ T cells following activation. Binding to 4-1BB ligand induces cell proliferation and survival, promotes effector functions, and stimulates memory cell differentiation. Preclinical studies have shown potent antitumor responses predominantly mediated by cytotoxic $CD8^+$ T cells. 4-1BB agonists have also demonstrated enhancement of NK-mediated ADCC [45], making these agents attractive for combinations with targeted therapies and immunotherapies capable of tumor killing or Treg depletion through ADCC. Two 4-1BB agonists are currently in clinical trials in solid tumors (Table 10.2).

GITR, similarly to OX40 and 41-BB, is transiently expressed on $CD4^+$ and $CD8^+$ T cells following TCR ligation. Like these other TNFRs, GITR appears to be less important for T cell priming, and more involved with promoting effector cell functions. GITR is also expressed on DCs, monocytes, granulocytes, and NK cells and is constitutively expressed on Tregs. Preclinical studies have shown that GITR ligation can overcome Treg-mediated immunosuppression, and agonists have shown impressive antitumor efficacy in several cancer models [46]. There are currently seven GITR agonist monoclonal antibodies in phase I–II clinical trials for patients with advanced solid tumors (Table 10.2).

CD27 is a costimulatory receptor that is constitutively expressed on lymphoid cells, including T cell s, B-cells, and NK cells and is upregulated on $CD4^+$ and $CD8^+$ after activation. Binding of CD27 with its ligand CD70 on activated APCs promotes clonal expansion of T cells, in addition to effector and memory T cell differentiation and survival. Contrary to the above TNFRs, CD27 also stimulates T cell priming. Preclinical studies of CD27 agonists have shown efficacy in several tumor models [47]. Varlilumab, a humanized IgG1 monoclonal antibody agonist to CD27, is currently being tested in clinical trials for a variety of cancers, including one study with a phase II cohort in combination with nivolumab in HNSCC (Table 10.2).

CD40 is a member of the TNF-receptor superfamily expressed on multiple cell types including dendritic cells, B cells, monocytes, and some tumor types including HNSCC [48]. Rather than directly activating T cells, CD40 agonists have been shown to activate dendritic cells to induce T cell responses. These agents can also activate macrophages to mount a T cell independent antitumor response and can induce ADCC and complement-dependent cytotoxicity (CDC) through interaction with NK cells [49]. Phase I studies have shown favorable toxicity profiles and therapeutic promise in targeting CD40 [50].

There is a strong rationale for combining CD40 agonists with other immunotherapies, including CPI. Currently, there are at least five of these agents in active clinical trials, alone and in combination with other immunotherapies (Table 10.2).

10.6 Cytokines

Cytokine therapy with IFN-α or IL-2 has been utilized in the treatment of cancer for over 30 years. IFN-α use has greatly diminished due to marginal effectiveness and concerns for acute toxicities [51]. High-dose IL-2 (HD-IL2) is also associated with severe, although generally reversible, acute toxicities including hypotension, renal failure, and thrombocytopenia. However, HD-IL2 is capable of producing durable responses in a minority of patients with metastatic melanoma and renal cell carcinoma (RCC). Patients must be selected for good functional status and organ function, and the therapy must be administered in specialized centers with hospitalization required for the duration of treatment [52]. The antitumor activity of intravenous HD-IL2, however, has not been demonstrated in cancers outside of melanoma and RCC.

The well-established immune-stimulating effects of various cytokines have sustained interest in researching clinical applications for cancers outside of melanoma and RCC, including HNSCC. In 2002, results were published from a randomized phase III trial of perioperatively administered perilymphatic IL-2 in Stage II-IVb oral or oropharyngeal SCC. This therapy appeared to be safe and efficacious, significantly improving disease-free survival and OS. The 5-year survival rate in the perilymphatic IL-2 group was 73%, compared with 55% in the control group, and disease-free survival (DFS) rates were 64% and 51%, respectively [53]. Despite the impressive improvement in outcomes from this randomized, phase III study, perilymphatic IL-2 has not received much attention in the field. One possible reason for this includes the intensive dosing regimen used in the study, including daily injections into the neck for 10 days prior to surgery, and injections five times a month for up to a year after surgery.

Building on this work, another group is investigating in HNSCC, a blend of cytokines termed IRX-2, which primarily consists of IL-2, IL-1β, IFN-γ, and TNF-α. The formulation is administered perilymphatically and is combined with systemic low-dose cyclophosphamide for Treg depletion, along with indomethacin and zinc to inhibit immunosuppressive elements within the systemic circulation and TME. In 2011, nonrandomized phase II data were presented from 27 patients with Stage II-IVa HNSCC receiving perilymphatic IRX-2. The regimen was found to be well-tolerated, with no grade 4 or higher toxicities. 3-year OS and DFS rates were 69% and 62%, respectively; median DFS and OS were not reached after follow-up of at least 3 years [54]. A larger, phase II trial in HNSCC is currently underway (NCT02609386) and a phase Ib trial in combination with durvalumab (anti-PD-1L) and tremelimumab (anti-CTLA-4) is planned to commence in October 2018 (NCT03381183).

Another cytokine mixture-dubbed Multikine has been tested in HNSCC. This formulation contains 14 interleukins, interferons (IFN), chemokines, and colony-stimulating factors. In 2005, published data from a phase II clinical trial in T2-3, N0-2, M0 HNSCC showed an ORR of 41% in 17 patients treated with neoadjuvant perilymphatic Multikine injections [55]. A large phase III trial of Multikine in HNSCC completed enrollment in late 2016, and results are pending (NCT01265849).

IL-15 is cytokine of particular interest currently in cancer immunotherapy. IL-15 shares the immunostimulatory characteristics of IL-2; however, IL-15 does not promote Treg expansion or activation-induced cell death (AICD) of effector T cells, which are characteristics of IL-2 [56]. Two variants of IL-15, modified to improve the pharmacokinetic and pharmacodynamic properties when administered intravenously, are currently in clinical development. Recombinant human IL-15 (rhIL-15) was found to be well-tolerated and produced substantial increases in circulating NK and CD8+ T cells [57]. Additional phase I trials are combining CPI with rhIL-15 or hetIL-15, another modified IL-15, for metastatic or refractory cancer (NCT03388632, NCT02452268).

10.7 Targeting the Innate Immune System

Traditionally, the immune system has been divided into "innate" and "adaptive" components. The term "innate" refers to sensors that do not require rearrangement of genes. Receptors present on innate immune cells, such as dendritic cells and macrophages, are highly conserved between individuals and species. "Adaptive" immune components require rearrangement of genes, leading to great diversity in receptors but are therefore specific to individuals. Adaptive immune components include T cell receptors, B-cell receptors, and antibodies.

The innate and adaptive immune systems are not separate systems but are in fact intimately related. Innate immune cells are involved in the activation of the adaptive immune system through cytokine signaling and antigen presentation [58]. Therefore, the innate immune system is capable of targeting threats directly through "innate" pathways and also of "priming" adaptive immune cells including T cells. Appreciation of this relationship has made targeting the innate immune system attractive for cancer immunotherapy, as well as autoimmune diseases.

10.7.1 TLR Agonists

Toll-like receptors (TLR) are components of innate immunity that recognize foreign molecules (pathogen-associated molecular patterns [PAMPs], e.g., lipopolysaccharide [LPS]) or products of damaged tissues (danger-associated molecular patterns [DAMPs], e.g., HMGB1) [59]. After recognition of a foreign or danger-associated molecule, receptor signaling leads to release cytokines and interferons, which initiate an immune response. Each TLR subtype recognizes a specific type of PAMP or DAMP, for example, LPS for TLR 4 or double-stranded viral RNA for TLR3. While the subtypes TLR can be expressed on a variety of cell types, they are all expressed on dendritic cells [60]. Currently, compounds of clinical interest are agonists of TLR3, 7, 8, or 9, which are present on endosomes, and TLR4, which is present on the cell surface.

TLR7 and 8 are closely related structurally and functionally, recognizing single-stranded RNA from viruses or bacteria. Activation of these TLRs induces production of cytokines and type I interferons [61]. Imiquimod, a topical TLR7 agonist, was FDA-approved in 1997 for the treatment of genital warts after clinical trials showed efficacy against this virus-induced pathology. Imiquimod later demonstrated activity against actinic keratosis, a premalignancy, as well as basal cell carcinoma, and now has FDA approval for both of these conditions [51]. Intratumoral injection of TLR7 and TLR7/8 agonists are undergoing early clinical investigation in multiple tumor types including HNSCC (Table 10.3).

The phase II Active8 trial randomized patients with R/M HNSCC to receive SOC platinum/5FU/cetuximab with or without the TLR8 agonist, motolimod. Although motolimod failed to improve PFS or OS in the intent-to-treat population, HPV+ patients and those with injection site reactions experienced significant benefit [62]. These results suggest that motolimod may benefit certain subgroups of HNSCC patients, based on HPV status or other biomarkers. A phase Ib trial of motolimod combined with cetuximab in the neoadjuvant setting showed evidence of immune response in the peripheral blood and resected tumor specimens [63]. The study protocol was amended in 2016 to add nivolumab to the combination of cetuximab and motolimod, and those results are pending [64].

TLR9 is a subset of TLR that recognizes CpG-rich DNA, a PAMP. Activation of TLR9 leads to TNF and type I IFN production, which in turn

Table 10.3 Clinical trials: innate immune activators

Target	Drug	Phase	Tumor type	Combination	Trial	Completion date
TLR7	LHC165	I	Advanced malignancies	PDR001	NCT03301896	08/2019
TLR7/8	MEDI9197	I	Solid tumors	Durvalumab and/or palliative RT	NCT02556463	08/2020
	NKTR-262	I	Advanced or metastatic solid tumors	NKTR-214 (modified IL-2)	NCT03435640	12/2019
TLR8	Motolimod	I	R/M/ persistent progressive solid tumors	Cyclophosphamide	NCT02050635	05/2021
		Ib	Resectable HNSCC (neoadjuvant)	Cetuximab and nivolumab	NCT02124850	Unknown
TLR9	SD-101	I/II	R/M HNSCC	Pembrolizumab	NCT02521870	02/2020
	IMO-2125	I	Solid tumors	None	NCT03052205	04/2020
	MGN1703	I	Advanced solid malignancies	Ipilimumab	NCT02668770	05/2020
STING	ADU-S100	I	Advanced or metastatic solid tumors	Ipilimumab	NCT02675439	12/2020
		I	Advanced or metastatic solid tumors	PDR001	NCT03172936	05/2019
	MK-1454	I	Advanced or metastatic solid tumors	Pembrolizumab	NCT03010176	10/2021

R recurrent, *M* metastatic

can activate T cells. Preliminary data are available from a phase I/II study of the TLR9 agonist, SD-101, with pembrolizumab in R/M HNSCC. Out of 16 PD-1-naïve patients currently enrolled, ORR in 10 evaluable patients is 40% (four PR, one SD, five PD). Final results of the study after data maturation are anticipated, but these early results are promising [65]. Other TLR9 agonists in phase I studies in solid tumors include IMO-2125 and MGN1703 (Table 10.3). IMO-2125 is also in phase III development in combination with CPI in melanoma.

10.7.2 STING Agonists

The STING (stimulator of interferon genes) pathway has recently been recognized as a critical component of the antitumor response. STING is an endoplasmic reticulum protein which binds to cytosolic (tumor) DNA, causing activation dendritic cells. Experimental studies in STING −/− mice show a markedly defective CD8$^+$ T cell priming [66]. Preclinical studies have also shown that activation of the STING pathway can increase effector T cell tumor infiltration [67]. ADU-S100 is a cyclic dinucleotide (CDN) that was discovered to activate all known human STING alleles and is currently undergoing phase I clinical evaluation in advanced solid tumors in combination with ipilimumab or PDR001 (anti-PD-1). Another CDN STING agonist, known as MK-1454, is also in phase I trials in advanced/metastatic solid tumors, alone or in combination with pembrolizumab (Table 10.3).

STING agonists are local therapy—they are injected into the tumor and have no systemic effect. One group is developing a novel intervention using a biomaterial containing CDN ligands that is called *STINGblade*, which is implanted locally into the resection site at the time of surgery and is extremely effective at preventing local recurrence following total or subtotal surgical resection [68]. Using several different models of

Table 10.4 Targeting of tumor-associated antigens

Class	Advantages	Concerns	Examples
Tissue differentiation antigens	• Shared antigens • "Off the shelf" treatments can be developed	• Expression on normal tissues • Potential for on-target, off-tumor toxicity	MART-1 gp100 CEA CD19
Tumor germline ("tumor-testis") antigens	• Shared antigens • "Off the shelf" treatments can be developed • Potentially tumor-specific	• Potential for on-target off-tumor toxicity • May be expressed in a low frequency of cancers	NY-ESO1 MAGE-A3
Normal proteins overexpressed by cancer cells	• Shared antigens • "Off the shelf" treatments can be developed	• On-target, off-tumor toxicity	hTERT EGFR mesothelin
Viral proteins	• Shared antigens • "Off the shelf" treatments can be developed • Tumor-specific, thus minimal risk of on-target off-tumor toxicity	• Low frequency of virus-associated cancers	HPV EBV MCC
Tumor-specific mutated antigens	• Tumor specific, thus minimal risk of on-target off-tumor toxicity • Shared driver hot-spot mutations can potentially be targeted	• Currently requires surgical resection for next-generation sequencing • Most immunogenic mutations identified so far are patient-specific • Extended time to develop personalized treatment targeting mutations	Mum-1 B-catenin CDK4 ERBB2IP

Modified from: Ilyas S, Yang JC. Landscape of Tumor Antigens in T cell Immunotherapy. *Journal of immunology (Baltimore, Md: 1950)*. 2015;195(11):5117–5122. doi:https://doi.org/10.4049/jimmunol.1501657)

HNSCC, they showed that antitumor activity was host-STING and CD8-dependent, indicating that adaptive immune responses are required for control of disease and improved survival. Subsequent work demonstrated that a novel approach to analyzing cytokine response using tumor explants treated ex vivo identified tumors with variable immune responses to STING ligands, which could enable personalization of the immunotherapy-containing biomaterial to induce tumor cure.

10.8 Vaccines

Just as vaccines can train the immune system to recognize and destroy pathogens, thereby preventing infection, vaccination can also initiate antitumor immune responses [69]. To induce an effective immune response and avoid targeting of self-antigens, vaccination would ideally utilize antigens that are expressed only on tumor cells and not on normal cells, i.e., tumor-specific antigens (TSA) including viral proteins and tumor-specific mutated antigens or "neoantigens." Alternative targets include tumor-associated antigens (TAA) including tissue differentiation antigens, antigens that are overexpressed on tumors compared with normal tissue (e.g., EGFR), and cancer germline antigens that are not normally expressed on somatic cells but are aberrantly expressed in tumor cells [70]. Each type of target antigen caries potential advantages and disadvantages for vaccination, outlined in Table 10.4.

Numerous types of cancer vaccines have been tested in preclinical models and in clinical trials. These include peptide vaccines, tumor lysates, DNA or RNA vaccines, and cellular vaccines including dendritic cells that have been exposed to antigen and danger signals. Sipuleucel-T (Provenge), an autogenous cellular vaccine targeting prostatic acid phosphatase, was approved by the FDA for the treatment of metastatic prostate cancer in 2010. While Sipuleucel-T was shown to increase OS in a randomized phase III trial, there was no increase in PFS [71].

Sipuleucel-T remains the only FDA-approved therapeutic vaccine for the treatment of cancer.

The ability to identify neoantigens through next-generation sequencing (NGS) techniques is appealing, in that neoantigens would theoretically avoid self-reactivity seen with tissue differentiation antigens or overexpressed antigens. However, this approach is based on patient-specific antigens and relies on complex mathematical modeling to predict binding to the patient's MHC types. Short-lived peptides are another potential source of tumor-associated antigens that have not been tolerized, due to the usual rapid degradation in autophagosomes. By "freezing" these vesicles in vitro, preventing fusion with lysosomes and subsequent destruction of the antigens, a source of tumor-associated antigens can be obtained which otherwise would have been "thrown away" by normal cell metabolism. This technique has been used to create a vaccine known as DRibbles, which has been shown to contain shared antigens capable of cross-recognition between different tumors and is currently in phase I clinical trials in multiple tumor types, with plans to expand to oral cancer [72].

Therapeutic vaccines have been tested clinically in HNSCC, mostly showing modest efficacy [73–76]. While vaccination can facilitate antigen presentation, it does not address deficiencies in T cell activation or suppressive forces within tumors. Furthermore, targeting specific antigens may lead to immune editing and shedding of that antigen, unless the mutant target is a true "driver" of oncogenesis. Therefore, vaccination as a monotherapy is unlikely to be successful in most settings and should be approached as an additional tool in the immunotherapy arsenal rather than a standalone therapy. Future directions for cancer vaccines will undoubtedly involve other therapies such as costimulatory agonists or checkpoint blockade to capitalize on antigen presentation or reduce immune-suppressive influences that may prevent immune response despite recognition of a tumor [77]. Ongoing trials in HNSCC are listed in Table 10.5.

Table 10.5 Clinical trials: therapeutic vaccines in HNSCC (including HPV-negative)

Category	Target	Product	Phase	Combination	Trial	Estimated completion date
Tissue differentiation antigen	CEA	CEA(6D)/TRICOM	I	None	NCT02999646	Completed, results pending
Tissue differentiation antigen	CEA	GI-6207	I	None	NCT00924092	Completed, results pending
Tissue differentiation antigen	MUC-l	-	I/II	Tadalafil	NCT02544880	04/2021
Cancer germline antigen	MAGE-A3	Biropepimut-S	II	cyc, GM-CSF, poly ICLC	NCT02873819	12/2020
Tumor lysate	Tumor- derived antigens	Allovax	II	None	NCT02624999	12/2018
Tumor lysate (irradiated)	Tumor- derived antigens	MVX-ONCO-1	II	None	NCT02999646	06/2020
Tumor-associated antigens	CEA, MUC-l, Ras, Brachyury	NANT vaccine	I/II	chemo, RT, CPI, cytokines	NCT03109764	01/2019
Neoantigen—vaccine/antibody hybrid	Patient-specific neoantigens	Vaccibody VB10.NEO	I/IIa	None	NCT03548467	03/2023

cyc cyclophosphamide, *CPI* checkpoint inhibitors

Table 10.6 Clinical trials: adoptive cell therapy in HNSCC (including HPV-negative)

Method	Product	Phase	Combination	Trial	Estimated completion date
TIL	LN-145	II	Lymphodepletion/IL-2	NCT03083873	10/2018
TCR-engineered	IMA201	I	Lymphodepletion/IL-2	NCT03247309	12/2019
CAR-T	T4	I	None	NCT01818323	6/2019

10.9 Adoptive Cell Therapy

Adoptive cell therapy (ACT) is an immunotherapeutic approach that involves the extraction of T cells from a patient, expansion of a T cell population ex vivo, and infusion of the T cells back into the patient, usually after chemotherapeutic lymphocyte depletion and followed by administration of cytokines such as IL-2 [78]. Several methods of ACT are in development, including extracting tumor-infiltrating lymphocytes (TIL), which are expected to include some T cells that have specificity for TAA. Alternatively, T cells may be extracted from the peripheral blood and either (1) selected for tumor reactivity ex vivo, (2) exposed to dendritic cells loaded with specific TAA, (3) transduced with specific T cell receptors (TCR) with affinity for known TAAs, or (4) transduced with a chimeric antigen receptor (CAR) that has the antigen-recognizing domain of an antibody and the signaling domain of a TCR [60]. These approaches essentially skip the majority of the cancer immunity cycle, including antigen recognition, T cell activation and proliferation, by directly introducing cancer-fighting T cells into the patient. ACT is therefore termed "passive immunity," as it circumvents reliance on the patient's immune response.

ACT has proven to be a potent strategy in melanoma, capable of inducing complete responses, and investigation of this method has broadened to include cancers of epithelial origin [79]. There are currently three ACT clinical trials that include patients with HPV-negative HNSCC (Table 10.6). Early results from the LN-145 TIL trial showed an ORR of 38% in eight patients evaluable [80, 81]. Additionally, preliminary data from a phase I dose-escalation study of intratumorally injected pan-ErbB CAR T cell s showed a disease control rate (DCR = CR + PR + SD) of 69%, despite rapidly progressing tumors at trial enrollment [82].

10.10 Oncolytic Viruses

It has been shown that certain viruses can preferentially replicate within malignant cells while preserving normal cells. Some viruses naturally possess this capability (myxoma virus, Newcastle disease virus (NDV), reovirus), while other types of viruses (herpes simplex, vaccinia, adenovirus) can be genetically modified to specifically infect malignant cells [83]. In addition to direct tumor cell killing, oncolytic viruses can induce immunogenic cell death (ICD), essentially acting as a cancer vaccine [84]. As with many new cancer therapies in development, oncolytic viruses will likely find the most utility when combined with immunotherapies such as CPI, and this is reflected by the design of many current clinical trials (Table 10.7).

In 2015, the first FDA approval of an oncolytic virus was granted to a genetically engineered, GM-CSF-transduced Herpes Simplex Virus (HSV-1), Talimogene Laherparepvec or T-VEC, for use in locally advanced or nonresectable melanoma. In HNSCC, T-VEC was tested in a small phase I/II study in combination with chemoradiotherapy in advanced HNSCC, showing an OS of 70.5% at median follow-up of 29 months. Patients all received post-therapy neck dissection, which was not standard of care for many of these patients; however, a pathologic CR rate of 94% in neck dissection specimens was a promising finding [85]. T-VEC is being tested in many other types of cancers and is currently in a phase Ib/III study in HNSCC in combination

Table 10.7 Clinical trials: oncolytic viruses in HNSCC and solid tumors

Virus	Product	Phase	Tumor type	Combination	Trial	Estimated completion date
Herpes virus	T-VEC	Ib/III	R/M HNSCC	Pembrolizumab	NCT02626000	08/2020
Measles	MV-NIS	I	R/M HNSCC	None	NCT01846091	12/2018
Vaccinia	Pexa-Vec	I	A/M solid tumors	Ipilimumab	NCT02977156	11/2019
Vaccinia	p53MVA	I	Refractory solid tumors	Pembolizumab	NCT02432963	02/2019
Adenovirus	Enadenotucirev	I	A/M epithelial tumors	Nivolumab	NCT02636036	03/2019

A advanced, *R* recurrent, *M* metastatic

with pembrolizumab [86]. HF10, a spontaneously occurring mutant HSV-1 virus, was shown to be well-tolerated in a phase I trial in HNSCC [87], and in a phase II trial in advanced melanoma, HF10 combined with nivolumab showed an ORR of 41% with a 16% rate of CR [88].

Another example is Cavatak™, a coxsackievirus developed by Viralytics, which seeks out and attaches itself to a protein that is highly expressed on the surface of many cancer cells, intercellular adhesion molecule-1 (ICAM-1). Since ICAM-1 is expressed in HNSCC [89], a phase 1 clinical trial studying Cavatak with pembrolizumab has been designed and is currently in its final stages of preparation before opening for recruitment. GL-ONC1, an attenuated vaccinia virus, was well-tolerated with concurrent chemoradiotherapy in HNSCC [90] and is in phase II development in recurrent ovarian cancer (NCT02759588). Oncorine (H101), an E1B-deleted adenovirus, was approved in China in 2005 for use in HNSCC after a phase III study showed an ORR of 78% when combined with cisplatin and 5-FU [91, 92]. The use of H101 so far remains limited to China.

A trial called REO 018 trial was initially designed as a randomized phase III study of Reolysin, a reovirus, in combination with carboplatin and paclitaxel in platinum-refractory HNSCC. The study was reformatted after interim analysis found differential responses in patients with locoregional disease versus patients with metastatic disease alone. The company claimed a statistically significant increase in PFS and OS in patients with locoregional disease, but stated that there were too few patients to power a statistical analysis for patients with distal metastases alone [93]. From review of the company's webpage, it appears that further development is currently focused on myeloma, breast, and pancreatic cancer [94].

10.11 The Role of Conventional Therapies in Activating the Immune System

While the efficacy of traditional cancer treatments, including chemotherapy, radiation, and targeted therapies, has historically been ascribed to direct cytotoxicity or inhibition of cellular activities, there is increasing appreciation for the immune-stimulating effects of these treatments. As described above, the Cancer Immunity Cycle begins with the release of cancer cell antigens. This is achieved by a process known as Immunogenic Cell Death (ICD), in which the killing of tumor cells can elicit an antitumor immune response. In addition to promoting recognition of tumor antigens through ICD, many chemotherapeutic agents have been shown to modulate immunosuppressive influences, e.g., through depletion of Tregs or MDSCs [95].

Many chemotherapeutics have been assessed for the various components of ICD. While cisplatin has previously been thought to be incapable of inducing bona fide ICD on its own, recent work on HNSCC models indicate that cisplatin

Table 10.8 Immunotherapy with chemotherapy in HNSCC

Chemo agent	Phase	Settiug	Immunotherapy	Timing of immunotherapy	Trial
Docetaxel + cisplatin + 5FU	I	PULA	Durvalumab	Induction (before chemo/rad)	NCT02997332
Evofosfamide	I	LA or M	Ipilimumab	Concurrent (second line)	NCT03098160
Docetaxel	I/II	R/M	Pembrolizumab	Concurrent (second line)	NCT02718820
Platinum + 5FU	III	R/M	Pembrolizumab	Concurrent (first line)	NCT02358031

Table 10.9 Immunotherapy with radiation in HNSCC

Type of radiation	Phase	Setting	Immunotherapy	Timing in relation to RT	Trial
With surgery					
Neoadjuvant SBRT	I/II	Curative	Nivolumab	Neoadjuvant + adjuvant	NCT03247712
IMRT	II	LA	Pembrolizumab	Neoadjuvant + adjuvant	NCT02296684
Without surgery					
IMRT	II	LA	Pembrolizumab	Concurrent	NCT02707588
"High dose"	II	M	Pembrolizumab	Concurrent	NCT03085719
Re-irradiation	II	R	Pembrolizumab	During and after	NCT02289209
Re-irradiation	I/II	R	Nivolumab	Before, during and after	NCT03317327
SBRT	II	M	Nivolumab	During and after	NCT02684253
Proton SBRT	Observational	R/M	Nivolumab	Before, during and after	NCT03539198

can effectively induce ICD [96]. This strengthens the rationale for combining SOC platinum agents with immunotherapy. KEYNOTE-048 was the first randomized phase III trial of anti-PD-1 therapy plus chemotherapy in HNSCC. As mentioned previously in section 10.2, the positive results from this trial led to approval of pembrolizumab alone or in combination with platinum chemotherapy in first line R/M disease. Additional trials of cytotoxic chemotherapy combined with immunotherapy in HNSCC are listed in Table 10.8.

Radiation may also play a synergistic role in combination with immunotherapy. In addition to induction of ICD, radiation therapy has been shown to recruit T cells to the irradiated tumor and increase susceptibility of tumor cells to cytotoxic effector cells [98]. Radiation also upregulates PD-L1 expression on tumor cells, which may limit the immunogenicity of radiation alone, but offers a therapeutic opportunity for combination with PD-1 inhibitors [99]. In HNSCC, immunotherapy appears to increase the antitumor response from radiation, rather than facilitate distant abscopal responses through an autovaccination effect of radiation [100]. Nonetheless, there is abundant evidence for the synergistic effect of radiation and immunotherapy [101]. There are numerous studies combining immunotherapy and radiation in HNSCC (Table 10.9), including a phase I study of neoadjuvant nivolumab combined with hypofractionated stereotactic body radiotherapy (SBRT) prior to surgical resection in the definitive setting (NCT03247712).

Additionally, there are mechanistic rationales for combining targeted therapies with immunotherapy. The antitumor activity of cetuximab in HNSCC is now appreciated to be primarily ADCC, as opposed to direct cytotoxicity. By combining cetuximab with CPI or other immunotherapies, immune-suppressive forces within the TME could potentially be counteracted leading to increased efficacy over either agent alone [102]. An interim safety analysis of a phase II trial of pembrolizumab and cetuximab in R/M HNSCC showed good tolerability with no DLTs [103]. There are several other efficacy studies underway which combine cetuximab with CPI with or without chemotherapy and radiation.

Lenvatinib is a multiple kinase inhibitor approved for differentiated thyroid cancer and advanced renal cell carcinoma. In addition to its effects on tumor angiogenesis and proliferation, lenvatinib has been shown to decrease suppressive TAM populations within tumors and to increase numbers of effector CD8$^+$ cells [104]. Interim analysis of a phase Ib/II clinical trial of lenvatinib with pembrolizumab in metastatic HNSCC showed an ORR of 41%, although the rate of grade 3–4 adverse events was 73% [105]. Interim analysis of a phase I/II trial of pembrolizumab in combination with vorinostat, a histone deacetylase inhibitor, showed an ORR of 36% with DCR of 56%. Another study of Acalabrutinib, a Bruton's tyrosine kinase inhibitor, in combination with pembrolizumab in advanced HNSCC, is underway. Trials of targeted therapies with immunotherapy in HNSCC are listed in Table 10.10.

There are a number of "preoperative window," neoadjuvant immunotherapy studies underway in HNSCC (Table 10.11). In addition to testing immunotherapies in earlier stages of disease with curative intent, studies such as these provide great potential for understanding the effects of immunotherapy in human cancer. Results from a phase II study of neoadjuvant nivolumab in resectable HNSCC showed good tolerability and tumor reductions within 1 month in nearly half of evaluable patients [106]. Many other neoadjuvant immunotherapy trials in HNSCC are underway, with a focus on analysis of immune effects within the surgical specimens. The histological and clinical comparison of tumors before and after immunotherapy may provide much insight into the effects in vivo, including the potential to identify biomarkers for response and further therapeutic targets.

Due to the large number of clinical trials combining chemotherapy, radiation, and/or targeted therapies with immunotherapy in HNSCC in a variety of settings (neoadjuvant, adjuvant, recurrent/metastatic), much will be learned about the safety and efficacy of combinations. Studies not already listed in previous sections are presented in Table 10.12. Moving forward, a major focus of preclinical research and clinical trials moving

Table 10.10 Immunotherapy with targeted therapy in HNSCC

Targeted therapy	Phase	Setting	Immunotherapy	Timing of immunotherapy	Trial
Acalabrutinib	II	LA[a] or R/M	Pembrolizumab	Concurrent	NCT02454179
Vorinostat	I/II	LA[a] or M	Pembrolizumab	Concurrent	NCT02538510
Cetuximab	I/II	R/M	Nivolumab	Concurrent	NCT03370276
	II	R/M	Pembrolizumab	Concurrent	NCT03082534
Lenvatinib	I/II	M	Pembrolizumab	Concurrent	NCT02501096

[a]Not amenable to surgery

Table 10.11 Preoperative "window of opportunity" immunotherapy trials

Imtnuaotherapy	Phase	Endpoint	Trial	Expected completion date
Nivolumab	II	Response; indicators of immune response in tissue/blood	NCT03021993	03/2020
Nivolumab +/− ipilimumab	II	Response, recurrence	NCT02919683	04/2024
Nivolumab +/− ipilimumab or relatlimab or daratumumab	I/II	Response, recurrence	NCT02488759	12/2019
Cemiplimab (RENG2810)	II	Response, recurrence	NCT03565783	01/2020
Durvalumab	II	Indicators of immune response in tissue/blood	NCT02827838	01/2019
Ipilimumab (intratumoral)	I	Indicators of immune response in tissue/blood	NCT02812524	07/2019
MEDI0562 (anti-OX40)	Ib	Indicators of immune response in tissue/blood	NCT03336606	12/2024

Table 10.12 Immunotherapy with chemotherapy/targeted therapy and radiation in HNSCC

Type of chemotherapy	Phase	Setting	Immunotherapy	Timing of immunotherapy	Trial
With surgery					
Carboplatin + nab-paclitaxel	II	LA	Durvalumab	Neoadjuvant and adjuvant	NCT03174275
Cisplatin	II	LA	Pembrolizumab	Neoadjuvant and adjuvant	NCT02641093
Without surgery					
Cisplatin or cetuximab	I	LA[a]	Nivolumab	Before, during, after CRT	NCT02764593
	I	LA[a]	Durvalumab	During radiation	NCT03509012
Cetuximab	III	PULA	Avelumab	Before, during, after CRT	NCT02999087
	Ib	LA[a]	Ipilimumab	During and after CRT	NCT01860430
Cisplatin	III	LA[a]	Pembrolizumab	Before, during, after CRT	NCT03040999

LA locally advanced, *PULA* previously untreated locally advanced, *R* recurrent, *M* metastatic
[a]Not amenable to surgery

will be to determine the optimal doses and timing of standard therapies to promote responses to different types of immunotherapy.

10.12 Conclusions

Immunotherapy is rapidly changing the standard of care in oncology. The appearance of a tail at the end of the survival curve with checkpoint inhibition in advanced cancers provides a graphic representation of the durable responses that can be achieved with this new group of therapies. *This* is the great promise of cancer immunotherapy, that is, the possibility of achieving lasting responses or even cures.

As evidence of the enthusiasm around immunotherapy, the number of new products in development and early-phase clinical trials has skyrocketed in the last decade. In 2017, it was estimated that there were 800–1000 cancer immunotherapy trials in the US involving over 100,000 patients [107, 108]. The same year, a report from the Pharmaceutical Research and Manufacturers of America found that there were 248 immuno-oncology agents in clinical trials, which only included "the most recognized classes of immunotherapy" [109]. In addition to the therapies described in this chapter, there are many other immunotherapies and immune adjuncts in development, including but not limited to agents that target tumor metabolism (e.g., IDO-1 and the adenosine pathway) [110–112], therapies to deplete or inhibit Tregs, MDSC, or TAM (e.g., anti-CCR4, PDE-5 inhibitors, anti-CSF1R) [113–115], and checkpoint inhibitors that target NK cells (e.g., anti-KIR, anti-NKG2A) [116, 117].

Moving forward in this new era of cancer immunotherapy will require continuing integration between the clinic and laboratory. Not only will preclinical science remain critical in developing new approaches in patient care, but laboratory evaluation of pathologic tumor responses, immune cell infiltrates, and circulating immune components will allow full-circle analysis and understanding of the physiologic effects of experimental treatments. The increasing number of neoadjuvant trials will facilitate this route of scientific discovery by providing postimmunotherapy tissue samples for comparison with pretreatment biopsies. Cutting-edge technologies for specimen analysis, such as NGS allowing whole-exome, RNA and T cell receptor sequencing, as well as advanced imaging techniques for multiplex immunohistochemistry, will allow for greater understanding of the in vivo effects of various immunotherapies on tumor biology. This work, along with clinical outcome correlations, will be critical in identifying predictive biomarkers and prognostic indicators and will provide evidence for future directions in cancer research.

References

1. Chen DS, Mellman I. Oncology meets immunology: the cancer-immunity cycle. Immunity. 2013;39:1–10.
2. Schreiber RD, Ikeda H, Dunn GP, Bruce AT, Old LJ. Cancer immunoediting: from immunosurveillance to tumor escape. Nat Immunol. 2002;3:991–8.

3. Hanahan D, Weinberg R. Hallmarks of cancer: the next generation. Cell. 2011;144:646–74.
4. Isaacsson Velho PH, Castro J, Gilberto CCH. Targeting the PI3K pathway in head and neck squamous cell carcinoma. Am Soc Clin Oncol Meet. 2015;2015:123.
5. Cai Y, Dodhia S, Su GH. Dysregulations in the PI3K pathway and targeted therapies for head and neck squamous cell carcinoma. Oncotarget. 2017;8:22203–17.
6. Tran E, Robbins PF, Lu YC, Prickett TD, Gartner JJ, Jia L, Pasetto A, Zheng Z, Ray S, Groh EM, Kriley IR, Rosenberg SA. T-cell transfer therapy targeting mutant KRAS in cancer. N Engl J Med. 2016;375(23):2255–62. https://doi.org/10.1056/NEJMoa1609279. PubMed PMID: 27959684; PMCID: PMC5178827.
7. Tumeh PC, Harview CL, Yearley JH, Shintaku IP, Taylor EJ, Robert L, Chmielowski B, Spasic M, Henry G, Ciobanu V, West AN, Carmona M, Kivork C, Seja E, Cherry G, Gutierrez AJ, Grogan TR, Mateus C, Tomasic G, Glaspy JA, Emerson RO, Robins H, Pierce RH, Elashoff DA, Robert C, Ribas A. PD-1 blockade induces responses by inhibiting adaptive immune resistance. Nature. 2014;515(7528):568–71. https://doi.org/10.1038/nature13954. PubMed PMID: 25428505; PMCID: PMC4246418.
8. Spranger S, Spaapen RM, Zha Y, Williams J, Meng Y, Ha TT, Gajewski TF. Up-regulation of PD-L1, IDO, and T(regs) in the melanoma tumor microenvironment is driven by CD8(+) T cells. Sci Transl Med. 2013;5(200):200ra116. https://doi.org/10.1126/scitranslmed.3006504. PubMed PMID: 23986400; PMCID: PMC4136707.
9. Jie HB, Gildener-Leapman N, Li J, Srivastava RM, Gibson SP, Whiteside TL, Ferris RL. Intratumoral regulatory T cells upregulate immunosuppressive molecules in head and neck cancer patients. Br J Cancer. 2013;109(10):2629–35. https://doi.org/10.1038/bjc.2013.645. PubMed PMID: 24169351; PMCID: PMC3833228.
10. Gordon SR, Maute RL, Dulken BW, Hutter G, George BM, McCracken MN, Gupta R, Tsai JM, Sinha R, Corey D, Ring AM, Connolly AJ, Weissman IL. PD-1 expression by tumour-associated macrophages inhibits phagocytosis and tumour immunity. Nature. 2017;545(7655):495–9. https://doi.org/10.1038/nature22396. PubMed PMID: 28514441; PMCID: PMC5931375.
11. Mehal WZ, Sheikh SZ, Gorelik L, Flavell RA. TGF-beta signaling regulates CD8+ T cell responses to high- and low-affinity TCR interactions. Int Immunol. 2005;17(5):531–8. https://doi.org/10.1093/intimm/dxh233.
12. Puram SV, Rocco JW. Molecular aspects of head and neck cancer therapy. Hematol Oncol Clin North Am. 2015;29:971–92.
13. Fakhry C, Westra WH, Li S, Cmelak A, Ridge JA, Pinto H, Forastiere A, Gillison ML. Improved survival of patients with human papillomavirus–positive head and neck squamous cell carcinoma in a prospective clinical trial. J Natl Cancer Inst. 2008;100(4):261–9. https://doi.org/10.1093/jnci/djn011.
14. Lingen MW. Low etiologic fraction for high-risk human papillomavirus in oral cavity squamous cell carcinomas. Oral Oncol. 2013;49(1):1–8. https://doi.org/10.1016/j.oraloncology.2012.07.002
15. Nivolumab for SCCHN. U.S. Food and Drug Administration. https://www.fda.gov/Drugs/InformationOnDrugs/ApprovedDrugs/ucm528920.htm.
16. Vermorken JB, Mesia R, Rivera F, et al. Platinum-based chemotherapy plus cetuximab in head and neck cancer. N Engl J Med. 2008;359:1116–27.
17. Ferris RL, Blumenschein Jr GR, Fayette J, et al. Nivolumab (Nivo) vs investigator's choice (IC) in recurrent or metastatic (R/M) squamous cell carcinoma of the head and neck (SCCHN): 2-yr outcomes in the overall population and PD-L1 subgroups of CheckMate 141. Oral presentation at: 2018 American Association for Cancer Research annual meeting, 14–18 Apr 2018, Chicago, IL.
18. Pembrolizumab (KEYTRUDA). U.S. Food and Drug Administration. https://www.fda.gov/Drugs/InformationOnDrugs/ApprovedDrugs/ucm515627.htm. Accessed 25 Nov 2017.
19. Bauml J, Seiwert TY, Pfister DG, et al. Pembrolizumab for platinum- and cetuximab-refractory head and neck cancer: results from a single-arm, phase II study. J Clin Oncol. 2017;35:1542–9.
20. Soulieres D, et al. Updated survival results of the KEYNOTE-040 study of pembrolizumab vs standard-of-care chemotherapy for recurrent or metastatic head and neck squamous cell carcinoma. Abstract CT115. Presented at: American Association for Cancer Research Annual Meeting; 14–18 Apr, Chicago; 2018.
21. Burtness B, Harrington KJ, Greil R, Soulières D, Tahara M, De Castro JG, et al. LBA8_PRKEYNOTE-048: Phase III study of first-line pembrolizumab (P) for recurrent/metastatic head and neck squamous cell carcinoma (R/M HNSCC). Ann Oncol. 2018;29(suppl_8):mdy424.045.
22. Alsaab HO, Sau S, Alzhrani R, et al. PD-1 and PD-L1 checkpoint signaling inhibition for cancer immunotherapy: mechanism, combinations, and clinical outcome. Front Pharmacol. 2017;8:561. https://doi.org/10.3389/fphar.2017.00561.
23. Butte MJ, Keir ME, Phamduy TB, Sharpe AH, Freeman GJ. Programmed death-1 ligand 1 interacts specifically with the B7-1 costimulatory molecule to inhibit T cell responses. Immunity. 2007;27:111–22.
24. Xiao Y, Yu S, Zhu B, et al. RGMb is a novel binding partner for PD-L2 and its engagement with PD-L2 promotes respiratory tolerance. J Exp Med. 2014;211:943–59.
25. European Society for Medical Oncology. ESMO 2017: durvalumab shows promising clinical benefit in recurrent/metastatic head and neck squamous cell carcinoma (11 Sep 2017). Accessed 24 Dec 2017. http://www.esmo.org/Conferences/Past-Conferences/ESMO-2017-Congress/News-Articles/.

26. Buchbinder EI, Desai A. CTLA-4 and PD-1 pathways: similarities, differences, and implications of their inhibition. Am J Clin Oncol. 2016;39(1):98–106. https://doi.org/10.1097/COC.0000000000000239.
27. Du X, et al. A reappraisal of CTLA-4 checkpoint blockade in cancer immunotherapy. Cell Res. 2018;28(4):416.
28. Hodi FS, O'Day SJ, McDermott DF, Weber RW, Sosman JA, Haanen JB, Gonzalez R, Robert C, Schadendorf D, Hassel JC, Akerley W, van den Eertwegh AJ, Lutzky J, Lorigan P, Vaubel JM, Linette GP, Hogg D, Ottensmeier CH, Lebbe C, Peschel C, Quirt I, Clark JI, Wolchok JD, Weber JS, Tian J, Yellin MJ, Nichol GM, Hoos A, Urba WJ. Improved survival with ipilimumab in patients with metastatic melanoma. N Engl J Med. 2010;363(8):711–23. https://doi.org/10.1056/NEJMoa1003466. PubMed PMID: 20525992; PMCID: PMC3549297.
29. Koyama S, Akbay EA, Li YY, et al. Adaptive resistance to therapeutic PD-1 blockade is associated with upregulation of alternative immune checkpoints. Nat Commun. 2016;7:10501.
30. Economopoulou P, Kotsantis I, Psyrri A. The promise of immunotherapy in head and neck squamous cell carcinoma: combinatorial immunotherapy approaches. ESMO Open. 2017;1:e000122.
31. Goldberg MV, Drake CG. LAG-3 in cancer immunotherapy. Curr Top Microbiol Immunol. 2011;344:269–78.
32. Pauken KE, Wherry EJ. TIGIT and CD226: tipping the balance between costimulatory and coinhibitory molecules to augment the cancer immunotherapy toolkit. Cancer Cell. 2014;26(6):785–7.
33. Argiris A, Gillison M, Ferris RL, Harrington K, Sanchez TK, Baudelet C, Geese WJ, Shaw J, Haddad R. A randomized, open-label, phase 3 study of nivolumab in combination with ipilimumab vs extreme regimen (cetuximab + cisplatin/carboplatin + fluorouracil) as first-line therapy in patients with recurrent or metastatic squamous cell carcinoma of the head and neck-CheckMate 651. Ann Oncol. 2016;27(Suppl_6):1016TiP. https://doi.org/10.1093/annonc/mdw376.68.
34. Siu L, et al. A randomized, open-label, multicenter, global phase 2 study of durvalumab (D), tremelimumab (T), or D plus T, in patients with PD-L1 low/negative recurrent or metastatic head and neck squamous cell carcinoma: CONDOR. Int J Rad Oncol Biol Phys. 2017;100(5):1307. https://doi.org/10.1016/j.ijrobp.2017.12.021.
35. Ascierto PA, Bono P, Bhatia S, et al. Efficacy of BMS-986016, a monoclonal antibody that targets lymphocyte activation gene-3 (LAG-3), in combination with nivolumab in pts with melanoma. In: Proceedings from the 2017 ESMO congress, 8–12 Sep 2017, Madrid, Spain. Abstract LBA18.
36. Harding FA, McArthur JG, Gross A, Raulet DH, Allison JP. CD28-mediated signaling co-stimulates murine T cells and prevents induction of anergy in T-cell clones. Nature. 1992;356:607–9.
37. Chen L, Flies DB. Molecular mechanisms of T cell co-stimulation and co-inhibition. Nat Rev Immunol. 2013;13:227.
38. Acton QA. Cytokines. In: Acton QA, editor. Intercellular signaling peptides and proteins – advances in research and application. Atlanta, GA: Scholarly Editions; 2013. p. 278.
39. Burris HA, Callahan MK, et al. Phase 1 safety of ICOS agonist antibody JTX-2011 alone and with nivolumab (nivo) in advanced solid tumors; predicted vs observed pharmacokinetics (PK) in ICONIC. J Clin Oncol. 2017;35(Suppl):abstr 3033.
40. Sturgill ER, Redmond WL. TNFR agonists: a review of current biologics targeting OX40, 4-1BB, CD27, and GITR. AJHO. 2017;13(11):4–15.
41. Guo Z, Wang X, Cheng D, Xia Z, Luan M, Zhang S. PD-1 blockade and OX40 triggering synergistically protects against tumor growth in a murine model of ovarian cancer. PLoS One. 2014;9:e89350.
42. Montler R, Bell RB, Thalhofer C, Leidner R, Feng Z, Fox BA, Cheng AC, Bui TG, Tucker C, Hoen H, Weinberg A. OX40, PD-1 and CTLA-4 are selectively expressed on tumor-infiltrating T cells in head and neck cancer. Clin Transl Immunol. 2016;5(4):e70. https://doi.org/10.1038/cti.2016.16. PubMed PMID: 27195113; PMCID: PMC4855266.
43. Bell RB, Leidner RS, Crittenden MR, et al. OX40 signaling in head and neck squamous cell carcinoma: overcoming immunosuppression in the tumor microenvironment. Oral Oncol. 2016;52:1–10.
44. Bell RB, Duhen R, Ballesteros-Merino C, Duhen T, Bifulco C, Piening BD, Bernard B, Pucilowska J, Tamakawa R, Redmond WL, Koguchi Y, Montler R, Morris G, Fisher B, Shuster M, Cheng A, Patel A, Urba WJ, Fox BA, Curti BD, Leidner RS, Weinberg AD. Neoadjvuant anti-OX40 (MEDI6469) prior to surgery in head and neck squamous cell carcinoma. J Clin Oncol. 2018;36(Suppl):abstr 6011.
45. Kohrt HE, Houot R, Weiskopf K, et al. Stimulation of natural killer cells with a CD137-specific antibody enhances trastuzumab efficacy in xenotransplant models of breast cancer. J Clin Invest. 2012;122:1066–75.
46. Knee DA, Hewes B, Brogdon JL. Rationale for anti-GITR cancer immunotherapy. Eur J Cancer. 2016;67:1–10.
47. van de Ven K, Borst J. Targeting the T-cell co-stimulatory CD27/CD70 pathway in cancer immunotherapy: rationale and potential. Immunotherapy. 2015;7:655–67.
48. Cao W, Cavacini L, Tillman K, Posner M. CD40 function in squamous cell cancer of the head and neck. Oral Oncology. 2005;41:462–9.
49. Vonderheide RH, Glennie MJ. Agonistic CD40 antibodies and cancer therapy. Clin Cancer Res. 2013;19(5):1035–43.
50. Vonderheide R, Dutcher J, Gribben J, et al. Phase I study of recombinant human CD40 ligand in cancer patients. J Clin Oncol. 2001;19(13):3280–7.
51. Hauschild A. Adjuvant interferon alfa for melanoma. Curr Oncol. 2010;17(3):6–7.

52. Payne R, Glenn L, Hoen H, et al. Durable responses and reversible toxicity of high-dose interleukin-2 treatment of melanoma and renal cancer in a Community Hospital Biotherapy Program. J Immunother Cancer. 2014;2:13. https://doi.org/10.1186/2051-1426-2-13.
53. De Stefani A, et al. Improved survival with perilymphatic interleukin 2 in patients with resectable squamous cell carcinoma of the oral cavity and oropharynx. Cancer. 2002;95(1):90–7.
54. Wolf GT, Fee WE, Dolan RW, et al. Novel neoadjuvant immunotherapy regimen safety and survival in head and neck squamous cell cancer. Head Neck. 2011;33(12):1666–74. https://doi.org/10.1002/hed.21660.
55. Tímár J, et al. Neoadjuvant immunotherapy of oral squamous cell carcinoma modulates intratumoral CD4/CD8 ratio and tumor microenvironment: a multicenter phase II clinical trial. J Clin Oncol. 2005;23(15):3421–32.
56. Romano E, Margolin K. T cell modulatory cytokines. In: Butterfield LH, Kaufman HL, Marincola FM, editors. Cancer immunotherapy principles and practice. New York, NY: Demos LLC; 2017.
57. Miller J, Morishima C, Conlon K, et al. A first-in-human phase i study of subcutaneous outpatient recombinant human IL15 (rhIL15) in adults with advanced solid tumors. Clin Cancer Res. 2018;24(7):1525–35.
58. O'Neil LAJ. The innate immune system. In: Paul WE, editor. Fundamental immunology. 7th ed. Philadelphia, PA: Lippincott Williams & Wilkins; 2013.
59. Land WG. The role of damage-associated molecular patterns (DAMPs) in human diseases: part II: DAMPs as diagnostics, prognostics and therapeutics in clinical medicine. Sultan Qaboos Univ Med J. 2015;15(2):e157–70.
60. Gajewski TF. Manipulating innate immune pathways as cancer immunotherapy. In: Butterfield LH, Kaufman HL, Marincola FM, editors. Cancer immunotherapy principles and practice. New York, NY: Demos LLC; 2017.
61. Cervantes JL, et al. TLR8: the forgotten relative revindicated. Cell Mol Immunol. 2012;9:434.
62. Ferris RL, Saba NF, Gitlitz BJ, et al. Effect of adding motolimod to standard combination chemotherapy and cetuximab treatment of patients with squamous cell carcinoma of the head and neck: the Active8 Randomized Clinical Trial. JAMA Oncol. 2018;4:1583–8. https://doi.org/10.1001/jamaoncol.2018.1888.
63. Ferris RL, et al. A phase 1b study of neoadjuvant immune biomarker modulation with cetuximab and motolimod in head and neck cancer (HNC). Int J Radiat Oncol Biol Phys. 2016;94(4):867–8.
64. Garlapow M. Motolimod plus cetuximab proves efficacious in head and neck cancer. Target Oncol. 2016; https://www.targetedonc.com/news/motolimod-plus-cetuximab-efficacious-head-and-neck-cancer. Accessed 19 Aug 2018.
65. Cohen E, et al. Abstract CT098: phase Ib/II, open label, multicenter study of intratumoral SD-101 in combination with pembrolizumab in anti-PD-1 treatment naïve patients with recurrent or metastatic head and neck squamous cell carcinoma (HNSCC). Cancer Res. 2018;78(13 Suppl):CT098.
66. Woo S-R, Fuertes MB, Corrales L, et al. STING-dependent cytosolic DNA sensing mediates innate immune recognition of immunogenic tumors. Immunity. 2014;41(5):830–42. https://doi.org/10.1016/j.immuni.2014.10.017.
67. Demaria O, De Gassart A, Coso S, et al. STING activation of tumor endothelial cells initiates spontaneous and therapeutic antitumor immunity. Proc Natl Acad Sci U S A. 2015;112(50):15408–13. https://doi.org/10.1073/pnas.1512832112.
68. Baird JR, Bell RB, Troesch V, Friedman D, Bambina S, Kramer G, Blair T, Medler T, Wu Y, Sun Z, de Gruijl T, van de Ven R, Leidner RS, Crittenden MR, Gough MJ. Evaluation of explant responses to STING ligands: personalized immunosurgical therapy for head and neck squamous cell carcinoma. Cancer Res. 2018;78(21):6308–19.
69. Church SE, et al. Multiple vaccinations: friend or foe. Cancer J. 2011;17(5):379.
70. Ilyas S, Yang JC. Landscape of tumor antigens in T cell immunotherapy. J Immunol. 2015;195(11):5117–22.
71. Kantoff PW, et al. Sipuleucel-T immunotherapy for castration-resistant prostate cancer. N Engl J Med. 2010;363(5):411–22.
72. Page DB, et al. Glimpse into the future: harnessing autophagy to promote anti-tumor immunity with the DRibbles vaccine. J Immunother Cancer. 2016; 4(1):25.
73. Ferris RL, et al. Phase I dendritic cell p53 peptide vaccine for head and neck cancer. Clin Cancer Res. 2014;2014:2617.
74. Voskens CJ, Sewell D, Hertzano R, et al. Induction of MAGE-A3 and HPV-16 immunity by Trojan vaccines in patients with head and neck carcinoma. Head Neck. 2012;34(12):1734–46. https://doi.org/10.1002/hed.22004.
75. Yoshitake Y, et al. Phase II clinical trial of multiple peptide vaccination for advanced head and neck cancer patients revealed induction of immune responses and improved OS. Clin Cancer Res. 2014;2014:0202.
76. Chindavijak S, Har-Noy M, Lausoontornsiri W. Effect of therapeutic vaccine on CTLA4 and tumor debulking response in recurrent and metastatic HNSCC. Clin Cancer Res. 2018;36(5 Suppl):115.
77. Yu G, et al. Combinational immunotherapy with Allo-DRibble vaccines and anti-OX40 co-stimulation leads to generation of cross-reactive effector T cells and tumor regression. Sci Rep. 2016;6:37558.
78. Redeker A, Arens R. Improving adoptive T cell therapy: the particular role of T cell costimulation, cytokines, and post-transfer vaccination. Front Immunol. 2016;7:345.
79. Rosenberg SA, Restifo NP. Adoptive cell transfer as personalized immunotherapy for human cancer. Science. 2015;348(6230):62–8.
80. Iovance biotherapeutics announces preliminary phase 2 data for TIL Treatment in head and neck and cer-

vical cancers. 2018. http://ir.iovance.com/phoenix.zhtml?c=254507&p=irol-newsArticle&ID=2328242.

81. Leidner R, et al. A phase 2, multicenter study to evaluate the efficacy and safety of autologous tumor infiltrating lymphocytes (LN-145) for the treatment of patients with recurrent and/or metastatic squamous cell carcinoma of the head and neck (HNSCC). J Clin Oncol. 2018;36:TPS6096.
82. Papa S, et al. A phase I trial of T4 CAR T-cell immunotherapy in head and neck squamous cancer (HNSCC). J Clin Oncol. 2018;36:3046.
83. Pikor L, Bell JC, Kaufman HL. Oncolytic viruses. In: Butterfield LH, Kaufman HL, Marincola FM, editors. Cancer immunotherapy principles and practice. New York, NY: Demos LLC; 2017.
84. Yaghchi CA, Zhang Z, Alusi G, Lemoine NR, Wang Y. Vaccinia virus, a promising new therapeutic agent for pancreatic cancer. Immunotherapy. 2015;7(12):1249–58. https://doi.org/10.2217/imt.15.90.
85. Harrington KJ, Hingorani M, Tanay MA, Hickey J, Bhide SA, Clarke PM, Renouf LC, et al. Phase I/II study of oncolytic HSVGM-CSF in combination with radiotherapy and cisplatin in untreated stage III/IV squamous cell cancer of the head and neck. Clin Cancer Res. 2010;16(15):4005. https://doi.org/10.1158/1078-0432.CCR-10-0196.
86. Harrington KJ, et al. Safety and preliminary efficacy of talimogene laherparepvec (T-VEC) in combination (combo) with pembrobrolizumab (Pembro) in patients (pts) with recurrent or metastatic squamous cell carcinoma of the head and neck (R/M HNSCC): a multicenter, phase 1b study (MASTERKEY-232). J Clin Oncol. 2018;36(Suppl):abstr 6036.
87. Gildener-Leapman N, et al. A phase I trial of intratumoral administration of HF10 in patients with refractory superficial cancer: immune correlates of virus injection. J Clin Oncol. 2013;31(15 Suppl):3099. https://doi.org/10.1200/jco.2013.31.15_suppl.3099.
88. Andtbacka, Robert HI, et al. Final results of a phase II multicenter trial of HF10, a replication-competent HSV-1 oncolytic virus, and ipilimumab combination treatment in patients with stage IIIB-IV unresectable or metastatic melanoma. Abstract 166420. Presented at: American Society of Clinical Oncology Annual Meeting, 20 May 2017, Chicago, IL.
89. Usami Y, Ishida K, Sato S, Kishino M, Kiryu M, Ogawa Y, Okura M, Fukuda Y, Toyosawa S. Intercellular adhesion molecule-1 (ICAM-1) expression correlates with oral cancer progression and induces macrophage/cancer cell adhesion. Int J Cancer. 2013;133(3):568–78. https://doi.org/10.1002/ijc.28066.
90. Mell LK, et al. Phase I trial of intravenous attenuated vaccinia virus (GL-ONC1) with concurrent chemoradiotherapy (CRT) for locoregionally advanced head and neck carcinoma. J Clin Oncol. 2015;33:–6026.
91. Xia Z-J, et al. Phase III randomized clinical trial of intratumoral injection of E1B gene-deleted adenovirus (H101) combined with cisplatin-based chemotherapy in treating squamous cell cancer of head and neck or esophagus. Chin J Cancer. 2004;23(12):1666–70.
92. Garber K. China approves world's first oncolytic virus therapy for cancer treatment. J Natl Cancer Inst. 2006;98(5):298–300. https://doi.org/10.1093/jnci/djj111.
93. Oncolytics Biotech Inc. Announces additional data from REO 018 randomized study of REOLYSIN in head and neck cancers. Calgary Oncol Biotech. 2014; https://www.oncolyticsbiotech.com/press-releases/detail/308/oncolytics-biotech-inc-announces-additional-data-from. Accessed 19 Aug 2018.
94. Oncolytics Biotech Inc. Website studies current development plan. https://www.oncolyticsbiotech.com/clinical-trials/studies. Accessed 19 Aug 2018.
95. Kroemer G, et al. Immunogenic cell death in cancer therapy. Annu Rev Immunol. 2013;31:51–72. https://doi.org/10.1146/annurev-immunol-032712-100008.
96. Tran L, et al. Cisplatin alters antitumor immunity and synergizes with PD-1/PD-L1 inhibition in head and neck squamous cell carcinoma. Cancer Immunol Res. 2017;5(12):1141–51.
97. The ASCO Post. KEYNOTE-048: pembrolizumab monotherapy in head and neck squamous cell carcinoma. 2018. http://www.ascopost.com/News/59121. Accessed 8 Aug 2018.
98. Van Limbergen EJ, De Ruysscher DK, Olivo Pimentel V, et al. Combining radiotherapy with immunotherapy: the past, the present and the future. Br J Radiol. 2017;90(1076):20170157. https://doi.org/10.1259/bjr.20170157.
99. Illidge T, et al. Radiation therapy induces an adaptive upregulation of PD-L1 on tumor cells which may limit the efficacy of the anti-tumor immune response but can be circumvented by anti-PD-L1. Int J Rad Oncol. 2014;90(1):S776.
100. McBride SM, et al. A phase II randomized trial of nivolumab with stereotactic body radiotherapy (SBRT) versus nivolumab alone in metastatic (M1) head and neck squamous cell carcinoma (HNSCC). J Clin Oncol. 2018;36(Suppl):abstr 6009.
101. Gong J, et al. Radiation therapy and PD-1/PD-L1 blockade: the clinical development of an evolving anticancer combination. J Immunother Cancer. 2018;6(1):46.
102. Ferris RL, et al. Rationale for combination of therapeutic antibodies targeting tumor cells and immune checkpoint receptors: harnessing innate and adaptive immunity through IgG1 isotype immune effector stimulation. Cancer Treat Rev. 2018;63:48–60.
103. Sacco AG et al. An open-label, non-randomized, multi-arm, phase II trial evaluating pembrolizumab combined with cetuximab in patients with recurrent/metastatic (R/M) head and neck squamous cell carcinoma (HNSCC): results of the interim safety analysis. ASCO 2018 meeting abstract. http://abstracts.asco.org/214/AbstView_214_225517.html

104. Kato Y, et al. Abstract A92: effects of lenvatinib on tumor-associated macrophages enhance antitumor activity of PD-1 signal inhibitors. Mol Cancer Ther. 2015;14(12 Suppl 2):A92.
105. Taylor MH, et al. A phase 1b/2 trial of lenvatinib plus pembrolizumab in patients with squamous cell carcinoma of the head and neck. J Clin Oncol. 2018;36:6016.
106. Ferris RL, et al. LBA46. An open-label, multicohort, phase 1/2 study in patients with virus-associated cancers (CheckMate 358): safety and efficacy of neoadjuvant nivolumab in squamous cell carcinoma of the head and neck (SCCHN). Ann Oncol. 28(Suppl_5):mdx440.041. https://doi.org/10.1093/annonc/mdx440.041.
107. Financial Times. Calling time on the immunotherapy gold rush. Financial Times. 2017.
108. Kolata G. A cancer conundrum: too many drug trials, too few patients. The New York Times. https://www.nytimes.com/2017/08/12/health/cancer-drug-trials-encounter-a-problem-too-few-patients.html. Accessed 5 Sep 2017.
109. Medicines in development for immuno-oncology 2017 Report. PhRMA.org. 2017. https://www.phrma.org/medicines-in-development-immuno-oncology. Accessed 20 Aug 2018.
110. Jochems C, et al. The IDO1 selective inhibitor epacadostat enhances dendritic cell immunogenicity and lytic ability of tumor antigen-specific T cells. Oncotarget. 2016;7(25):37762.
111. Ma SR, et al. Blockade of adenosine A2A receptor enhances CD8(+) T cells response and decreases regulatory T cells in head and neck squamous cell carcinoma. Mol Cancer. 2017;16(1):99.
112. Antonioli L, et al. Anti-CD73 in cancer immunotherapy: awakening new opportunities. Trends Cancer. 2016;2(2):95–109.
113. Vela M, et al. Chemokine receptor-specific antibodies in cancer immunotherapy: achievements and challenges. Front Immunol. 2015;6:12.
114. Weed DT, Vella JL, Reis IM, et al. Tadalafil reduces myeloid-derived suppressor cells and regulatory T cells and promotes tumor immunity in patients with head and neck squamous cell carcinoma. Clin Cancer Res. 2015;21(1):39–48. https://doi.org/10.1158/1078-0432.CCR-14-1711.
115. Gomez-Roca CA, Cassier PA, Italiano A, Cannarile M, Ries C, Brillouet A, Mueller C, Jegg AM, Meneses-Lorente G, Baehner M, et al. Phase I study of RG7155, a novel anti-CSF1R antibody, in patients with advanced/metastatic solid tumors. J Clin Oncol. 2015;33:3005.
116. Beldi-Ferchiou A, Caillat-Zucman S. Control of NK cell activation by immune checkpoint molecules. Int J Mol Sci. 2017;18:2129.
117. Cohen RB, Salas S, Even C, Kotecki N, Jimeno A, Soulié AM, Tirouvanziam-Martin A, Zerbib R, André P, Boyer-Chammard A, Fayette J. Abstract 5666: safety of the first-in-class anti-NKG2A monoclonal antibody monalizumab in combination with cetuximab: a phase Ib/II study in recurrent or metastatic squamous cell carcinoma of the head and neck (R/M SCCHN). Cancer Res. 2017;77(13 Suppl):5666. https://doi.org/10.1158/1538-7445.AM2017-5666.

11 Recurrent Oral Cancer and Salvage Options

Joshua E. Lubek and Michael Nagai

11.1 Introduction

Oral cancer is the sixth most common cancer to occur worldwide, with squamous cell cancer accounting for greater than 90% of these cases histologically. Considered to be a global health problem, there will be more than 300,000 new cases of oral squamous cell cancer (OSCC) diagnosed each year and will be responsible for over 140,000 deaths per year. Once thought to be predominantly a disease of older males with known risk factors such as tobacco use, alcohol use, or betel nut habit (high rates of buccal squamous cell carcinoma in certain countries such as India, China, or Taiwan), recent epidemiologic data would suggest that patients without risk factors such as younger patients (<45 years of age, females and nonsmokers) are developing these cancers. Despite good prognosis for early-stage disease, overall survival and disease relapse for late-stage oral cavity disease remains poor, even with aggressive surveillance and new advances in therapy [1–5].

Recurrence rates for oral squamous cell cancer are reported to occur in up to 30% of patients depending on initial disease stage presentation with most recurrences developing either locally or regionally within 3 years of initial therapy. Successful salvage therapy for recurrent disease will depend on numerous factors to include initial tumor staging, location of recurrence, and initial treatment utilized (i.e., surgery, primary radiotherapy, or multimodality therapy as initial treatment strategy) [6–9].

11.2 Recurrent Disease of the Oral Cavity: General Considerations

Recurrent OSCC is devastating for the patient both from an emotional and physical standpoint. Very often a patient has just recovered from the healing phases of primary therapy to now have to deal with the psychological impact of facing yet further treatment. This fear along with the previous resultant physical sequelae such as trismus, decreased salivary function, dysarthria, dysphagia, or disfigurement will pose significant complexities to quality of life considerations that will factor into patient treatment decisions.

Meta-analysis and pooled prospective data for upper aerodigestive squamous cell carcinoma

J. E. Lubek (✉)
Oral-Head and Neck Surgery/Microvascular Reconstructive Surgery, Department of Oral and Maxillofacial Surgery, University of Maryland, Baltimore, MD, USA
e-mail: jlubek@umaryland.edu

M. Nagai
Oral-Head and Neck Surgery/Microvascular Surgery, University of Maryland, Baltimore, MD, USA
e-mail: mnagai@umaryland.edu

D. Kademani (ed.), *Improving Outcomes in Oral Cancer*,
https://doi.org/10.1007/978-3-030-30094-4_11

suggest that for stage I and II recurrences, the 2-year recurrence-free survival is around 70% with 60–85% achieving or exceeding presurgical quality of life (QOL), with a modest complication rate of 6%. For stage III disease, the 2-year recurrence-free survival drops to 30% with the rates of significant complications also reaching the 30th percentile and only 40% of patients achieving or exceeding their baseline QOL. For stage IV disease recurrences, the outcomes were considerably worse with less than 25% of patients living disease-free for greater than 2 years and more than half of patients dying within 9 months [10]. Ultimately final treatment decisions will be based upon long-term prognosis and patient morbidity as the guide to help stratify those patients who will benefit from salvage therapy with a curative intent versus discussions for a palliative approach.

The classic definition of a locally recurrent head and neck cancer is any lesion that is located within a 2 cm distance from the index tumor or that which occurs within 3 years of the index tumor [11]. This certainly is true for most recurrent OSCC; however, recent data would indicate that aggressive active surveillance is required for much longer duration, as late recurrence and second primary cancers both within the oral cavity and other sites within the head and neck can occur even in patients initially treated for very early stage disease. In a series of 112 Stage I oral squamous cell carcinomas, there was a 19.6% incidence of late local failure (>36 months) despite 75% and 86% of patients having negative margins (≥5 mm and ≥3 mm, respectively). The authors also noted a 11.6% rate of second primaries within the head and neck [12].

Time to recurrence is considered an important factor both in the prognosis of disease and in the ability to successfully salvage a patient. Various studies suggest that recurrent disease within a 6-month interval is a significantly poor prognostic marker. Although this statement holds true, one could ask if this is truly recurrent disease versus recidivistic occult disease [13]. In a large series of over 1600 patients with OSCC, Liu et al. reported a local recurrence rate of 31%, and that recurrence within 18 months of initial surgery was increased risk for decreased survival. The authors also found that recurrence after age greater than 60 years was associated with increased survival [14].

Regional failures are those that occur within the previously treated or untreated draining lymphatic cervical system. In general, the first echelon lymphatics for oral squamous cell cancer are considered to be levels I–III of the anterior neck (submental, submandibular, and supraomohyoid jugular chain lymphatics). Drainage patterns can be altered in cases of previous neck treatment (surgical lymphadenectomy or radiotherapy) resulting in failure to unusual locations such as parotid or axillary lymphatics.

Recurrence within the local site or neck will depend on numerous factors to include margin status, perineural invasion, tumor depth of invasion (DOI), tumor size and location within the oral cavity, pre-existing neck nodal disease, and extranodal tumor extension (ENE). Initial treatment strategies employed will also factor into recurrence rates, salvage options, and overall patient outcomes. Most series would demonstrate that single modality therapy, upfront surgery, negative surgical margins, and the pathologically node negative (N0) neck not only do better in terms of initial prognosis but also will have improved overall survival (OS) and disease-free survival (DFS) when undergoing salvage therapy in those cases that do recur [15, 16]. Benefits of the elective neck dissection in terms of improved survival and decreased neck failure were initially suggested by studies such as Kligerman et al. [17], with confirmatory results in a recent large prospective trial by D'Cruz et al. [18] Patients in these studies with OSCC who underwent elective neck dissection in the N0 neck with DOI ≥ 3 mm not only OS and DFS, but recurrence within the dissected neck tended to be smaller burden of disease. Failure in the dissected neck does bring with a worse prognosis, and rates of successful salvage are more controversial.

Margin status following surgical resection has been considered to be a risk factor for recurrence within OSCC. In a meta-analysis by Anderson et al. Recurrence rates were pooled to give a 21% absolute risk reduction in local recurrence with margins clear by more than 5 mm [19]. This has been challenged with possibility of margins greater than 3 mm as adequate. Further controversy exists with the finding of dysplasia at the surgical margin and risk of recurrent OSCC. Most authors would agree that both carcinoma-in-situ and severe dysplasia are increased risk factors for recurrence; however, the presence of mild or moderate dysplasia is of more questionable significance [20, 21]. In a series by Pu et al. of over 500 patients who were surgically treated for OSCC, positive or dysplastic margins were identified in 20% of patients [22]. The authors concluded on multivariate analysis there was no significant difference in recurrence-free survival (RFS) or disease-free survival (DFS) in patients with mild dysplasia and negative margins; however, patients with mild dysplasia who did not undergo re-excision demonstrated significantly worse DFS and RFS. Another series by Gokavarapu et al. analyzed 425 patients with OSCC resected with negative surgical margins and revealed that patients with mild and moderate dysplasia at the margin had lower rates of survival with moderate dysplasia being an independent risk factor for survival [23]. As the data would suggest, dysplasia at the margin likely represents field cancerization change within the oral cavity and would seem logical that there is increased risk of recurrence.

Recurrence that occurs distantly is associated with a poor long-term prognosis. Considerations for treatment should be based upon patient life expectancy, disease burden, and treatment with the specific purpose of addressing quality of life issues. Patients faced with both local recurrence and simultaneous distant metastatic disease should be considered for definitive treatment for local source control to improve quality of life and to minimize systemic palliative therapies and tumor burden. Clinical trials should also be considered in these situations as well [24–26].

Surveillance for recurrent OSCC requires both a thorough clinical exam to include indirect mirror exam and fiberoptic/rigid endoscopy especially in patients with trismus and periodic imaging. Very often new symptoms such as pain or swelling should alert the clinician to a recurrence. One should have a low threshold for rebiopsy of persistent or new oral leukoplakia, erythroplakia, or ulcerations. Surveillance imaging can be very helpful especially in situations of altered anatomy (flap reconstruction), trismus, or radiation. Computerized tomography (CT) imaging and magnetic resonance imaging (MRI) are generally first-line surveillance. Positron emission tomography (PET) is useful for detection of early recurrence prior to any anatomic changes with other imaging modalities but can generate a false-positive finding if performed too early after surgery or radiation due to inflammation [26]. A 2016 meta-analysis of prospective studies involving PET/CT for detection of recurrent head and neck cancers concluded that PET/CT imaging 3 months post treatment was beneficial in the detection of residual or recurrent disease. Sensitivity and specificity of residual and recurrent regional and distant disease were 72.3%, 88.3% and 84.6%, 94.9%, respectively [27]. Lin et al. retrospectively reviewed 111 patients with advanced resected OSCC who developed recurrences following adjuvant therapy and surveillance PET/CT imaging [28]. The authors concluded that scheduled periodic PET/CT surveillance is a valuable tool for early detection of recurrent lesions in asymptomatic OSCC patients as the presence of clinical symptoms and a short time to positive PET/CT findings were adverse prognostic factors for clinical outcome in patients with advanced OSCC.

11.3 Surgical Salvage

Prior to deciding on a surgical option, one must consider the previous treatment rendered, time to recurrence, location of the recurrence, ease of surgical access, ability to achieve the surgical objective (i.e., negative surgical margin), need for reconstruction, and patient comorbidities.

For patients who recur locally within the oral cavity, complete surgical resection should be considered as a first-line therapy. With active surveillance, these patients can be identified early and surgery offers a good chance of cure, especially in low-volume disease. In a recent published series, Ord et al. reported on a series of 112 patients with T1 oral tongue carcinoma patients followed long-term [12]. Of the 19.6% of patients who recurred locally and of those 50% ($n = 11/22$) were salvaged with a second surgery requiring no further treatment. The other 50% continued to develop multiple failures but were able to be successfully salvaged with surgery provided they did not recur regionally. Surveillance for local disease becomes more problematic in situations that make clinical exam more difficult such as in cases of pre-existing flap reconstruction, trismus, adjuvant radiotherapy, or disease occurring within the maxilla.

Regional recurrence within the neck can be divided into two categories to include recurrence within the previously untreated neck and those that have received treatment. This is further complicated as the previously treated neck can be further subdivided into patients who were treated with definitive surgery alone, definitive radiotherapy, or multimodality therapy. Patients who have only undergone previous surgery generally have better rates of successful salvage as the option for combined modality therapy still exists (i.e., surgery +/− chemoradiotherapy) as opposed to those treated initially with radiotherapy.

In a series by Wong et al. patients who underwent salvage surgery were found to have significant improved recurrent survival time when compared to radiotherapy/chemoradiotherapy. Some may argue that these were patients who were more likely to have unresectable recurrent disease thus biasing the statistical analysis [29]. In a 2018 series from Memorial Sloan Kettering, 190 recurrent OSCC patients (all were initially N0) were evaluated [30]. The authors reported a 15% recurrence rate within the neck and that significantly poorer outcomes in DFS as compared to those who did not recur in the neck (32% vs. 74% DFS, respectively). Patients that were able to receive combined surgery and adjuvant radiotherapy +/− chemotherapy had better overall survival as compared to those who received either surgery or radiotherapy alone. A smaller series of 24 OSCC recurrences by Skelenica et al. noted that salvage surgery significantly improved overall survival; however, in the 50% of patients who received adjuvant radiotherapy, there was no overall or DFS benefit following recurrence [31].

Matsuura et al. [16] compared a cohort of 46 patients with recurrent OSCC who underwent salvage versus 199 patients without recurrence following primary therapy. Independent risk factors for poor prognosis included positive lymph node metastases and positive surgical margins. Patients who developed a recurrence and were successfully salvaged had similar overall survival as compared to those who never developed a recurrence (54.7% vs. 70.7%, overall survival $p = 0.158$ respectively). The authors also note that patients who continued to develop recurrences after salvage surgery had similar overall survival for those who received palliative treatment.

It cannot be overstated that the surgical and reconstructive undertaking for these patients can be daunting. They often require many adjunct services during the course of treatment, and adequate supportive care is a must. It is therefore recommended that these complex cases be completed at centers that regularly manage this type of disease and have the available resources as well as experienced surgical and reconstructive teams. It is important to note that advances in reconstructive techniques and standardization among perioperative protocols at many centers has increased the number of candidates available to undergo salvage surgery and decreased the incidence of some complications. In the 1960s and 1970s, Gilbert and Kagan found that only 18.3% of patients with recurrent carcinoma of the oral cavity or oropharynx were considered eligible for salvage surgery due to limitations related to reconstructive methods [32]. With the advancement of microvascular techniques and availability of reliable donor site options this percentage has dramatically increased, and free flaps are now becoming the standard of care in many salvage operations allowing patients options never before seen with functional outcomes that are exceptional. Dense, fibrotic scar tissue from prior surgery, radiation or a combination of both can make conventional local tissue flaps and nonvascularized grafts unreliable for reconstruction of these defects. Bringing nonirradiated tissue with its native vascular supply to the site of recurrence can lessen the burden of tissue healing and reduce local wound complications. Although it may increase surgical time and is associated with some additional morbidity, the risks of aggressive surgery are often outweighed by the improved quality of life, reported by many patients, following salvage surgery. Over the last decade, the utility, reliability, and function of free tissue transfer has had a significant impact on the functional outcomes for those patients undergoing recurrent cancer care [33]. In a recent study by Smirk and Kyzas, 25 of 29 patients underwent salvage surgery with free flap reconstruction. The authors reported that surgical complications were relatively uncommon with only one total flap failure [34]. Both this current study and a series by Kostrzewa et al. found that over 50% of patients were gastrostomy-dependent after salvage surgery, highlighting the high risk of long-term dysphagia despite successful salvage surgery and reconstruction [35]. This impact will only continue to grow as the population ages and the treatment of cancers improve; patients will be living longer with the desire to surgically treat recurrences when feasible.

Surgical salvage can also include palliative options such as tumor debulking, ablation without reconstruction, and the creation of an elective surgical airway for prolonged comfort in an attempt to improve quality of life. Noncurative surgery, which reduces the primary tumor bulk can reduce pain and bleeding, improve swallowing and nutrition while enhancing airway patency. Surgical resection with application of a simple reconstruction bar or coverage with a pedicled flap such as a pectoralis or supraclavicular may reduce operating time, blood loss and provide sufficient reconstruction of certain defects. In select settings, using newer endovascular techniques, embolization and vessel stenting may offer symptom control for bleeding related to major vascular erosion [24, 25]. Following recurrences, surgical salvage should be explored as the first-line option for treatment, especially if the goal is cure. Despite increased morbidity and lower success rates compared with surgery in the setting of primary disease, surgery among those patients with early T stage tumors, longer disease-free intervals, and favorable comorbidity profile will have a high likelihood of success.

11.4 Radiation Therapy for Salvage

Adjuvant radiotherapy should be utilized in a standard fashion per guidelines for those patients considered radiation-naïve who recur locoregionally during standard surveillance. Patients who meet criteria include advanced T stage disease, perineural/lymphovascular invasion, close margins, and nodal disease/ENE. Recurrent disease within the neck should be treated initially with surgery if possible, irrespective of previous neck dissection or suspicion of extranodal disease, taking into consideration patient morbidity. This approach will help reduce tumor burden and increase the effectiveness of adjuvant radiotherapy. Local recurrence that has been resected to a negative surgical margin without adverse features should continue with close surveillance only [36].

Patients who present with early recurrence or even recidivistic OSCC before planned postoperative radiotherapy (PORT) present with a difficult challenge. The question as to why these patients have developed disease so early within the primary treatment window is paused for concern. Perhaps surgical wounds have not fully healed, or patients are recovering in rehabilitation facilities and are too weak to start adjuvant therapy, or maybe the patient is delaying therapy for personal reasons. Regardless this early recurrence whether within the local site, neck or as dermal or distant metastases should alert the clinician as to the aggressiveness of the tumor. A recent series by Hosni et al. analyzed a cohort of OSCC patients of which 88 patients (15% of patients in the series) developed early recurrence while awaiting the start of PORT. The authors divided the patients into two cohorts; 70 patients in the salvage group (locoregional disease only) and 18 patients in the palliative group (had developed locoregional and distant disease) [37]. Radiation dosages were adjusted accordingly to the specific groups. The authors concluded that significant risk factors for early recurrence included the oral tongue subsite and microscopic positive margin. The 3-year OS salvage and palliative rates were 71% and 41%, respectively. Disease-free survival following salvage PORT was 36% with extranodal disease and volume of gross disease being associated with poor DFS following salvage PORT. This study certainly highlights the importance of "total treatment package time" (85–100 days) with longer surgery-PORT interval times greater than 6 weeks increasing the odds risk for local failure [38].

For patients who may be candidates for surgery but have recurrent tumors that are not amenable to salvage due to anatomic considerations, or for patients who are medically unfit for surgery, then reirradiation with or without concurrent chemotherapy may offer a survival benefit or a palliative alternative [39]. Patient selection is critical, and when choosing reirradiation as a modality, then the risk of acute and late toxicity must be appreciated. Also important is the assessment of tumor characteristics, prognosis, and how willing the patient is to undergo a potentially toxic regime as treatment-related fatalities from bleeding, tissue necrosis, and infection can be substantial. Historically, radiation was thought to be a single use treatment, but with the advancements in modern conformational radiotherapy techniques such as IMRT and volumetric-modulated arch therapy, the therapeutic ratio of reirradiation has changed such that a select group of people may benefit from a second round of treatment, and it is considered safe to do so [40]. Those that may be candidates for reirradiation include patients who have undergone surgical salvage with their tumors showing high-risk features on final pathology, patients who have surgically unresectable disease, or patients whose performance status limits their operative choices. It is generally considered that tumors which have recurred at the site of previous radiation to a full treatment dose (>50 Gy) within 6 months of therapy have radioresistant disease and would be unlikely to benefit from additional dosing. In these patients, the potential risks of radiation-induced adverse events outweigh its therapeutic use and alternative treatments should be sought. Ionizing radiation can have a significant impact on the native tissues of the head and neck, and the risks of serious complications such as carotid stenosis or rupture, neurosensory loss, speech deficits, dysphagia, and osteoradionecrosis must be carefully assessed against any potential benefits, especially in terms of overall survival. In a large multicenter review of reirradiation for recurrent head and neck cancers, Caudell et al. showed a 22.1% risk of grade ≥3 complications, and that late toxicities continue to increase up to 5 years following reirradiation, plateauing at 48–66% [41]. Although there is no general consensus regarding the total dose, fractionation scheme, or mode of delivery, most centers will reirradiate qualifying patients to doses >50 Gy and will often limit the field to the site of recurrence [42, 43]. Another consideration is potential retreatment with proton beam therapy. The unique physical properties of this type of radiation allow for higher doses to be delivered to tumors, while minimizing the dose to previously irradiated normal tissues. While the initial evaluations have been promising [44, 45], further prospective trials with longer follow-up times are needed to assess the efficacy, tolerability, and cost effectiveness of this treatment modality.

Another potential use of reirradiation is in the palliative setting. Although data are limited, palliative radiation could afford patients not candidates for aggressive reirradiation; in specific situations, treatment options geared toward improving symptoms. An effective palliative approach that minimizes the burden of longer protracted courses of treatment is considered in this approach [26]. Often, lower doses of radiation with increased fractions are delivered in an attempt to reduce acute toxicity with the hope that late complications with increased fraction size will be irrelevant [46, 47]. Alleviating pain, dysphagia, bleeding, and impending airway compromise should be the goals of treatment and can have a dramatic impact on a patient's outlook, ability to function, and live in a comfortable setting.

Patients who have undergone treatment of head and neck cancer pose a difficult therapeutic challenge. Surgical clearance of the recurrent or second primary disease will remain the preferred treatment modality of choice, but when disease and patient specific factors are critically evaluated, then the addition of reirradiation can become an important aspect of achieving the greatest survival outcomes. Patients undergoing salvage surgery with curative intent should be considered for repeat radiotherapy when high-risk pathologic features are encountered. These include positive margins, perineural invasion, lymphovascular invasion, and extranodal extension. Radiation alone or the addition of radiation to supplement treatment has well-recognized benefits. This, however, must be balanced against the risks associated with the radiation, and each treatment plan will need to be tailored to each individual patient and their overall therapeutic objectives. Eckardt et al. compared the survival of patients treated with surgery with that of patients treated with multimodality treatment over a 20-year period and found a 31.0% rate of salvage with surgery as compared with a 15.4% rate with surgery and radiotherapy, with a salvage rate of 0% for patients treated with radiotherapy or supportive therapy alone [7].

11.5 Systemic Therapy and Immunotherapy

Systemic therapy to treat head and neck cancer has been well established and has recently seen promising advancements with the development of targeted immunotherapy which has begun to play a significant role in the management of those affected by advanced-stage recurrent disease. Salvage therapy options for patients with unresectable, previously irradiated cancers of the head and neck are limited, and ultimately most patients who recur will require some form of palliative systemic therapy. At present, chemotherapy is the treatment most often used in this population; however, the optimal regimen for these patients has not been clearly defined in randomized clinical trials. Unfortunately, median survival with chemotherapy alone has approximated 6 months, and alternative strategies are needed [48]. Treatment options include single-agent therapy and combination regimens using either conventional cytotoxic chemotherapy and/or molecularly targeted agents combined with best supportive care. Checkpoint inhibitor immunotherapy is an option for patients with progressive disease after they have failed initial platinum-based chemotherapy. Currently, concurrent chemoradiotherapy over chemotherapy or radiation alone is favorable and has demonstrated survival benefits in multi-institutional group settings [49]. There are a multitude of therapeutic drug classes available and include conventional cytotoxic platinum containing compounds (cisplatin and carboplatin), taxanes (docetaxel, paclitaxel, and nabpaclitaxel), methotrexate, fluorouracil, and the monoclonal EGFR receptor inhibitor cetuximab. Varying combinations of these medications have been used with and without reirradiation, and with the exception of combining cetuximab with a platinum-based compound as shown in the EXTREME trial [50], no specific treatment algorithm has shown any significant survival benefit over another [51]. When choosing a systemic therapy, prognostic indicators, such as ECOG performance status, histologic differentiation of the tumor, and prior response to any therapeutic agents, along with patient-specific co-morbidities need to be taken into consideration to help guide prescribing decisions and avoid excessive toxicities.

Immunotherapy has been one of the most discussed and potentially exciting treatments for recurrent advanced stage OSCC in recent years, and the antitumor defense of these medications is widely recognized. Although it is still considered a second-line therapy, the mechanisms through which these agents work are believed to be the key toward recognizing improved host recognition and destruction of cancer, ultimately resulting in effective and sustainable long-term survival outcomes. There has been a paradigm shift in the way cancer is viewed, from a biologic and host interaction standpoint to the way treatment strategies are being implemented. In 2016, based on the results of the phase III CHECKMATE 141 trial and the phase I KEYNOTE 012 trial, the FDA approved the PD-1 checkpoint inhibitors nivolumab (Opdivo, Bristol-Myers Squibb) and pembrolizumab (Keytruda, Merck), respectively, for the treatments of patients with recurrent or metastatic head and neck squamous cell carcinoma that had progressed after treatment with chemotherapy [52, 53]. Ferris et al. reported long-term follow-up data of nivolumab versus chemotherapy and noted an overall 2-year survival of 16.9% in the immunotherapy PD-L1 group versus a 6% overall survival in the chemotherapy cohort. The nivolumab group also reported over 50% less side effects and significant toxicities as compared to the chemotherapy arm. These immune checkpoint inhibitors may represent a ground-breaking advance for treatment of solid tumors including head and neck cancers that exhibit poor responses to chemo- and radiotherapy [54]. Currently, numerous ongoing clinical trials are investigating various immunotherapy agents—alone and in combination—for management of patients with head and neck cancer. Encouraging and pertinent clinical results have been achieved in head and neck cancers, but many challenges remain for the clinical impact of immunotherapy to be improved: predictive biomarkers are needed for patient selection, and associations of several immunotherapies or with conventional drugs need to be tested [35]. At this time, only 10–20% of patients will be responders to immune therapy, and this must be weighed against the high financial costs of these drugs on the healthcare system. As further insight into the tumor-host microenvironment is gained and more specific targeted therapies are developed, there hopes to be a substantial improvement in long-term survival while at the same time reducing adverse events.

11.6 Summary

For patients with recurrent oral cancer, the prognosis remains poor. It is clear that a better understanding of the molecular and biological interactions between the host and various tumor types is needed and will facilitate the development of more precisely targeted agents. As further biomarkers are discovered and results of trials become available, the stratification of particular tumors and or patients into specific treatment groups will hopefully result in a survival benefit and loss of morbidity. While surgical salvage will continue to be the foundation upon which additional treatment choices can be applied, promising novel therapies are on the horizon and undergoing evaluation in large-scale prospective clinical trials, which may alter the scope of the current day approach to cancers of the oral cavity. The oncologic team now has multiple tools at their disposal to help patients throughout the course of their treatment and all options should be explored when delivering care. Treatment plans need to be developed in a multidisciplinary setting and reflect more than just survival outcomes. Patient input and preferences should be a large component of the decision to apply any therapy in the recurrent setting. Quality of life needs to be at the core of the decision-making process, and aggressive tumor surveillance with close patient recall needs to be performed to identify those patients that can be identified with local recurrence and potentially be successfully salvaged.

References

1. National Cancer Institute. Surveillance, epidemiology and end results program. cancer stat facts: oral cavity and pharynx cancer. https://seer.cancer.gov/statfacts/html/oralcav.html.
2. Patel SC, Carpenter WR, Tyree S, Couch ME, Weissler M, Hackman T, et al. Increasing incidence of oral tongue squamous cell carcinoma in young white women, age 18 to 44 years. J Clin Oncol. 2011;29:1488–94.
3. Farquhar DR, Tanner AM, Masood MM, et al. Oral tongue carcinoma among young patients an analysis of risk factors and survival. Oral Oncol. 2018;84:7–11.
4. Hussein AA, Helder MN, de Visscher JG, et al. Global incidence of oral and oropharynx cancer in patients younger than 45 years versus older patients: a systematic review. Eur J Cancer. 2017;82:115–27.
5. Haas I, Hauser U, Ganzer U. The dilemma of follow-up in head and neck cancer patients. Eur Arch Otorhinolaryngol. 2001;58:177–83.
6. Ho AS, Kraus DH, Ganly I, et al. Decision making in the management of recurrent head and neck cancer. Head Neck. 2014;36:144–51.

7. Eckardt A, Barith EL, Kokemueller H, et al. Recurrent carcinoma of the head and neck: treatment strategies and survival analysis in a 20-year period. Oral Oncol. 2004;40:427–32.
8. Liao CT, Chang JT, Wang HM, et al. Salvage therapy in relapsed squamous cell carcinoma of the oral cavity: how and when? Cancer. 2008;112:94.
9. Ord RA, Kolokythas A, Reynolds MA. Surgical salvage for local and regional recurrence in oral cancer. J Oral Maxillofac Surg. 2006;64:1409–14.
10. Goodwin WJ Jr. Salvage surgery for patients with recurrent squamous cell carcinoma of the upper aerodigestive tract: when do the ends justify the means? Laryngoscope. 2000;110:1–18.
11. Warren S, Gates DC. Multiple malignant primary tumors: a survey of the literature. Am J Cancer. 1932;16:1358–414.
12. Ord RA, Isaiah A, Dyalram D, Lubek JE. Is long term follow up mandatory for stage I oral tongue cancer? J Oral Maxillofac Surg. 2018;76:2676–83. https://doi.org/10.1016/j.joms.2018.06.169.
13. Schwartz GJ, Mehta RH, Wenig BL, et al. Salvage treatment for recurrent squamous cell carcinoma of the oral cavity. Head Neck. 2000;22:34–41.
14. Liu SA, Wong YK, Lin JC, et al. Impact of recurrence interval on survival of oral cavity squamous cell carcinoma patients after local relapse. Otolaryngol Head Neck Surg. 2007;136:112–8.
15. Brandwein-Gensler M, Teixeira MS, Lewis CM, et al. Oral squamous cell carcinoma: histologic risk assessment, but not margin status, is strongly predictive of local disease-free and overall survival. Am J Surg Pathol. 2005;29:167.
16. Matsuura D, Valim TD, Kulcsar MAV, et al. Risk factors for salvage surgery failure in oral cavity squamous cell carcinoma. Laryngoscope. 2018;128:1113–9.
17. Kligerman J, Lima RA, Soares JR, et al. Supraomohyoid neck dissection in the treatment of T1/T2 squamous cell carcinoma of the oral cavity. Am J Surg. 1994;168:391.
18. D'Cruz AK, Vaish R, Kapre N, et al. Elective versus therapeutic neck dissection in node negative oral cancer. N Engl J Med. 2015;373:521.
19. Anderson CR, Sisson K, Moncrieff M. A meta-analysis of margin size and local recurrence in oral squamous cell carcinoma. Oral Oncol. 2015;51:464–9.
20. Shah A. Postoperative pathologic assessment of surgical margins in oral cancer a contemporary review. J Oral Maxillofac Pathol. 2018;22:78–85.
21. Sopka DM, Li T, Lang MN, et al. Dysplasia at the margin? Investigating the case for subsequent therapy in 'low-risk' squamous cell carcinoma of the oral tongue. Oral Oncol. 2013;49(11):1083–7.
22. Pu Y, Wang Y, Huang X, et al. The influence of mild dysplasia at the surgical margin on the prognosis of oral squamous cell carcinoma. Int J Oral Maxillofac Surg. 2016;45:1372–7.
23. Gokavarapu S, Parvataneni N, Pavagada S, et al. Mild to moderate dysplasia at surgical margin is significant indicator of survival in patients with oral cancer. Oral Surg Oral Med Oral Pathol Oral Radiol. 2017;123:330–7.
24. Cocks H, Ah-See K, Capel M, et al. Palliative and supportive care in head and neck cancer: United Kingdom national multidisciplinary guidelines. J Laryngol Otol. 2016;130:198–207.
25. Kim J, Kim S, Albergotti W, et al. Selection of ideal candidates for surgical salvage of head and neck squamous cell carcinoma: effects of the Charlson age comorbidity index and oncologic characteristics on a 1-year survival and hospital course. JAMA Otolaryngol Head Neck Surg. 2015;141:1059–65.
26. Lok BH, Jiang G, Gutiontov S, et al. Palliative head and neck radiotherapy with the RTOG 8502 regimen for incurable primary or metastatic cancers. Oral Oncol. 2015;51:957–62.
27. Cheung PK, Chin RY, Eslick GD. Detecting residual/recurrent head neck squamous cell carcinomas using PET or PET/CT systematic review and meta analysis. Otolaryngol Head Neck Surg. 2016;154:421–32.
28. Lin HC, Kang CJ, Huang SF, et al. Clinical impact of PET/CT imaging after adjuvant therapy in patients with oral cavity squamous cell carcinoma. Eur J Nucl Med Mol Imaging. 2017;44:1702–11.
29. Wong LY, Wei WI, Lam LK, Yuen AP. Salvage of recurrent head and neck squamous cell carcinoma after primary curative surgery. Head Neck. 2003;25:953–9.
30. Mizrachi A, Migliacci JC, Montero PE, et al. Neck recurrence in clinically node negative oral cancer: 27 year experience at a single institution. Oral Oncol. 2018;78:94–101.
31. Skelenica S, Gardiner S, Dierks EJ, et al. Survival analysis and risk factors for recurrence in oral squamous cell carcinoma does surgical salvage affect outcome. J Oral Maxillofac Surg. 2010;68:1270–5.
32. Gilbert H, Kagan AR. Recurrence patterns in squamous cell carcinoma of the oral cavity, pharynx and larynx. J Surg Oncol. 1974;6:357–80.
33. Knoetgen J, Choudry U, Finical SJ, et al. Head and neck reconstruction with a second free flap following resection of a recurrent malignance. Ann Plast Surg. 2005;55:378–83.
34. Smirk R, Kyzas P. Outcome of salvage procedures for recurrent oral and oropharyngeal cancer. Br J Oral Maxillofac Surg. 2018;56:847–53.
35. Kostrzewa JP, Lancaster WP, Iseli TA, et al. Outcomes of salvage surgery with free flap reconstruction for recurrent oral and oropharyngeal cancer. Laryngoscope. 2010;120:267–72.
36. Rosenthal DI, Mohamed ASR, Garden AS, et al. Final report of a prospective randomized trial to evaluate the dose response relationship for postoperative radiation therapy and pathologic risk groups in patients with head and neck cancer. Int J Radiat Oncol Biol Phys. 2017;98:1002–11.
37. Hosni A, Huang SH, Chiu K, Xu W, Su J, Bayley A, Bratman SV, Cho J, Giuliani M, Kim J, O'Sullivan B, Ringash J, Waldron J, Spreafico A, Yu E, de Almeida JR, Monteiro E, Chepeha DB, Irish JC, Goldstein DP, Hope A. Predictors of early recurrence prior to planned

post-operative radiation therapy for oral cavity squamous cell carcinoma and outcomes following salvage intensified radiation therapy. Int J Radiat Oncol Biol Phys. 2019, 103:363–73. https://doi.org/10.1016/j.ijrobp.2018.09.013.
38. Rosenthal DI, Liu L, Lee JH, et al. Importance of the treatment package time in surgery and postoperative radiation therapy for squamous carcinoma of the head and neck. Head Neck. 2002;24:115–26.
39. McDonald MW, Lawson J, Garg MK, et al. ACR appropriateness criteria retreatment of recurrent head and neck cancer after prior definitive radiation expert panel on radiation oncology head and neck cancer. Int J Radiat Oncol Biol Phys. 2011;80:1292.
40. Sulman EP, Schwartz DL, Le TT, et al. IMRT reirradiation of head and neck cancer – disease control and morbidity outcomes. Int J Radiat Oncol. 2009;73:399–409.
41. Caudell JJ, Ward MC, Riaz N, et al. Volume, dose and fractionation considerations for IMRT based reirradiation in head and neck cancer: a multi-institution analysis. Int J Radiat Oncol Biol Phys. 2018;100:606–17.
42. Merlotti A, Mazzola R, Alterio D, et al. What is the role of post operative re-irradiation in recurrent and second primary squamous cell cancer of the head and neck? A literature review according to PICO criteria. Crit Rev Oncol Hematol. 2017;111:20.
43. Popovtzer A, Gluck I, Chepeha DB, et al. The pattern of failure after reirradiation of recurrent squamous cell head and neck cancer: implications for defining the targets. Int J Radiat Oncol Biol Phys. 2009;74:1342–7.
44. Phan J, Sio TT, Nguyen TP, et al. Reirradiation of head and neck cancers with proton therapy: outcomes and analysis. Int J Radiat Oncol bio Phys. 2016;96:30–41.
45. Romesser PB, Cahlon O, Scher ED, et al. Proton beam reirradiation for recurrent head and neck cancer: multi-institutional report on feasibility and early outcomes. Int J Radiat Oncol Bio Phys. 2016;95:386–95.
46. Chen AM, Vaughn A, Narayan S, et al. Palliative radiation therapy for head and neck cancer: toward an optimal fractionation scheme. Head Neck. 2008;30:1586–91.
47. Corry J, Peters LJ, Costa ID, et al. The 'QUAD SHOT'—a phase II study of palliative radiotherapy for incurable head and neck cancer. Radiother Oncol. 2005;77:137–42.
48. Jacob C, Layman G, Velez-Garcia E, et al. A phase III randomized study comparing cisplatin and fluorouracil as single agents and in combination for advanced squamous cell carcinoma of the head and neck. J Clin Oncol. 1992;10:257–63.
49. Spencer SA, Harris J, Wheeler RH, et al. Final report of RTOG 9610, a multi-institutional trial of reirradiation and chemotherapy for unresectable recurrent squamous cell carcinoma of the head and neck. Head Neck. 2008;30:281–8.
50. Vermorkin JB, Mesia R, Rivera F, et al. Platinum-based chemotherapy plus cetuximab in head and neck cancer. N Engl J Med. 2008;359:1116–27.
51. Forastiere AA, Metch B, Schuller DE, et al. Randomized comparison of cisplatin plus fluorouracil and carboplatin plus fluorouracil versus methotrexate in advanced squamous cell carcinoma of the head and neck: a southwest oncology group study. J Clin Oncol. 1992;10:1245.
52. Ferris RL, Blumenschein G, Fayette J, et al. Nivolumab vs investigators choice in recurrent metastatic squamous cell carcinoma of the head and neck: 2 year long term survival update of CheckMate 141 with analyses by PD-L1 expression. Oral Oncol. 2018;81:45–51.
53. Hsu C, Lee S-H, Ejadi S, et al. Antitumor activity and safety of pembrolizumab in patients with PD-L1 positive nasopharyngeal carcinoma: interim results from a phase 1b study. Ann Oncol. 2015;26:93–102.
54. Outh-Gauer S, Alt M, Le Tourneau C, et al. Immunotherapy in head and neck cancers: a new challenge for immunologists, pathologists and clinicians. Cancer Treat Rev. 2018;65:54–64.

Oral Reconstruction

12

J. Collin, B. Turner, and R. Fernandes

12.1 General Considerations

The general concept behind reconstructive surgery is to assess what is missing and what is available to replace it, bearing in mind that where possible "like should replace like." For any given defect, the reconstruction options range from simple to complex, along a spectrum frequently referred to as the reconstructive ladder [1]. The reconstructive matrix is an elaboration of this linear concept that considers technical requirements and the potential risks to the patient on additional axes [2].

At the bottom of the reconstructive ladder, some very small defects, especially of the tongue, can be left to heal by secondary intention. This is rarely appropriate for malignant lesions, as even the theoretical lesion of zero volume would still require enough margin to preclude this approach. The second rung is primary closure. This approach is appropriate for small defects that can be closed without significant functional deficit. It should be borne in mind that some small defects, particularly of the tongue, will have better functional results with primary closure than with a flap of excessive bulk for the defect. Similarly, a small lip defect can be closed primarily in a highly esthetic manner. The third rung is occupied by grafts, commonly split or full thickness skin, but also mucosal grafts. The fourth rung includes local advancement or rotation flaps supplied by a random vascular pattern. The fifth includes regional pedicled flaps. These flaps provide a greater area of soft tissue coverage than is possible with local flaps in the mouth, without requiring the facilities and expertise for microvascular reconstruction. They are frequently thought of as less susceptible to failure than microvascular flaps, but it should be pointed out that this is not necessarily the case. For example, pectoralis major myocutaneous flaps are associated with a partial necrosis rate of up to 29% [3, 4]. Furthermore, while pedicled flaps are versatile, they are sometimes esthetically inferior to free flaps. The final rung is free tissue transfer. Free flaps excel the previously mentioned options with respect to versatility, size, and sometimes cosmetic and functional outcomes. Free flaps are available to close any size of defect in the oral cavity, and their freedom from a regional pedicle allows them to be placed in any location. Their disadvantages include the need for costly resources and expertise, increased operative time, donor site morbidity, and a low, but nonzero rate of flap loss.

12.2 Reconstruction of the Lips

The goals of lip reconstruction should be both functional and esthetic. Oral competence is important during mastication and the oral stage

J. Collin · B. Turner · R. Fernandes (✉)
University of Florida College of Medicine
Jacksonville, Jacksonville, FL, USA
e-mail: John.Collin@jax.ufl.edu; Benjamin.Turner@jax.ufl.edu; Rui.Fernandes@jax.ufl.edu

D. Kademani (ed.), *Improving Outcomes in Oral Cancer*,
https://doi.org/10.1007/978-3-030-30094-4_12

of deglutition, particularly with fluids, but also when at rest to prevent drooling. Continuity of the orbicularis oris muscle and adequate perioral sensation are required to fulfill this function. The size of the oral stoma also has a bearing on function. All of these factors contribute to the esthetics of the lower face. Careful reconstruction of the anatomic landmarks of the lip, such as the white roll, vermilion border, and Cupid's bow will facilitate cosmetic reconstruction.

The unique structure and appearance of the lips, involving transition from skin, keratinized dry, and nonkeratinized wet mucosa, means that using existing lip tissue for reconstruction gives better results than when distant tissue is employed. Preservation of contiguous, innervated orbicularis oris muscle, and hence function is also more likely. Local flaps including rotational, advancement, and cross-lip flaps have become mainstays of reconstruction for larger deformities not amenable to direct or sliding lip closure.

12.2.1 A Timeline of Lip Reconstruction Techniques

1000 BC	Shushruta	First mention of lip repair
1597 AD	Tagliacozzi	Upper and lower lip repair using forearm flap
1768	Louie	Wedge excision described
1838	Sabattini	Full thickness switch from lower to upper
1845	Dieffenbach	Cheek advancement for upper lip repair
1857	Von Bruns	Cheek advancement for lower lip repair
1872	Estlander	Upper to lower switch at commissure
1898	Abbe	Lip switch for bilateral cleft lip
1909	Lexer	Tongue flaps for lip repair
1954	Schuchardt	Sliding inferiorly based cheek flaps
!969	Bakamjian	Deltopectoral flap to lower lip defect
1974	Karapandzic	Advancement along nasolabial fold for lower lip defects

12.3 Reconstruction of the Vermillion

Distortion of the vermillion and the white roll is readily apparent; therefore careful reconstruction is important for cosmesis. Small defects that do not involve the underlying orbicularis muscle may heal satisfactorily by secondary intention. However, the process is slow (25 days on average) and can result in contracture [5, 6].

Alternatively, primary closure following small vertically oriented fusiform excisions will give excellent results. Where redundant 'dog-ear' tissue is likely to occur, a V-Y island of mucosa can be advanced from the labial mucosa into the vermillion or laterally from adjacent vermillion [7].

Larger superficial defects of the upper or lower vermillion are best managed by resection of the entire vermillion (lip shave) and advancement of a flap of labial mucosa. This affords a close cosmetic match, and sensation is usually regained; however, atrophy and contracture can be apparent. The vermillion of the opposing lip can also be transferred on a single or double pedicle and can include underlying muscle pedicled on the labial vessels [8]. This technique requires a second procedure for division and inset, arguably for little benefit compared with mucosal advancement. Vermillion reconstruction with tongue [9], buccal mucosal, or myomucosal flaps can give acceptable results. Grafting anal verge mucosa has also been described [10].

12.4 Lower Lip Reconstruction

12.4.1 Defects Less Than 50%

Depending on the laxity of the lower lip (mainly a function of age), most defects of less than one third to half the width of the lower lip can be closed primarily with good cosmetic and functional outcomes. The excision is extended inferiorly to complete a "v" or shield shape. The point of the 'v can be curved laterally to follow the labiomental groove. In wider resections, this groove can be followed on one or both sides of the base of the resection to aid in tissue mobilization. Some surgeons utilize a 'w'-shaped incision, but this gives a less cosmetic outcome.

12.4.2 Defects Greater Than 50%

Lower lip defects of this proportion are unlikely to be able to be closed primarily without causing unacceptable microstomia.

12.4.2.1 Karapandzic Flap

Unilateral or bilateral transdermal curvilinear incisions following the nasolabial crease(s) allow mobilization and approximation of the remaining lower lip [11]. The incision extends through dermis only, leaving the neurovascular supply to the lower lip elements intact. This improves upon Gillie's fan flap and other advancement techniques that employ full thickness incisions that disrupt the neurovasculature. Reconstruction of defects up to 80% of the lower lip have been described [12], with good preservation of function and cosmesis. A degree of micostomia and blunting of the commissures is associated, however.

12.4.2.2 Lip Switch Flaps

A reverse Abbe flap can be employed whereby a segment of upper lip with the same vertical dimension, but around 50% of the width of the lower lip defect is pedicled on the labial artery. Cosmetically, harvest should only be from lateral to the philtrum. In theory bilateral flaps can be harvested, but the two resultant pedicles make oral intake challenging until the flaps are inset.

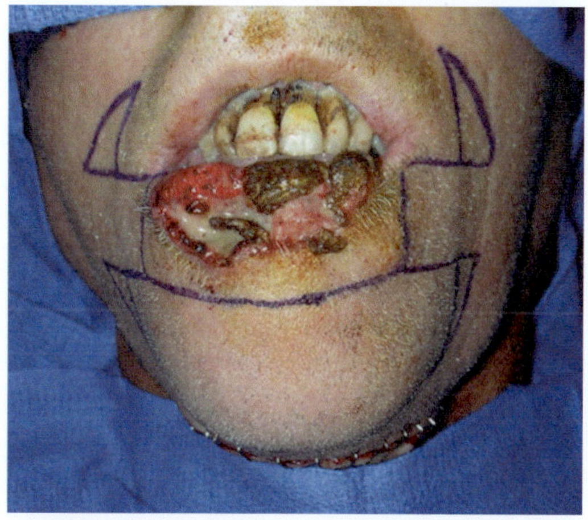

Fig. 12.1 Webster–Bernard Burrow flap markings prior to lower lip resection

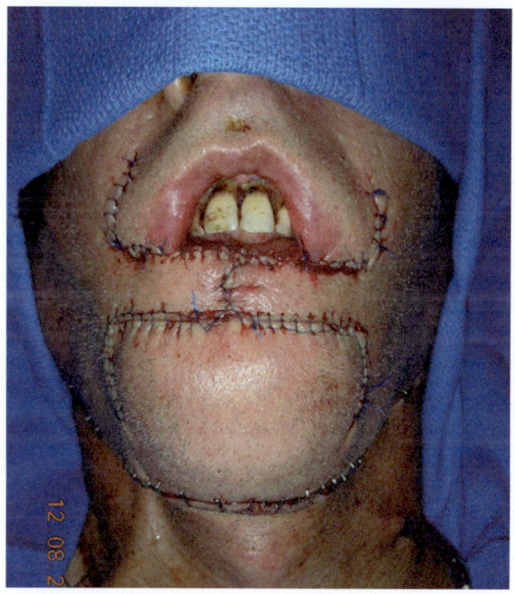

Fig. 12.2 Webster–Bernard-von burrow flap following closure

12.4.3 Subtotal Defects

12.4.3.1 Cheek Advancement Flaps

Bilateral horizontal cheek advancement flaps where described by Bernard (1852) and von Burrow (1853) for reconstruction of large lip defects [13]. Tissue is advanced from the cheek by extending incisions laterally from the commissure and excising four triangles in cases affecting the upper lip, and three triangles to close the lower lip. Webster recommended modification of this technique for lower lip defects using only partial thickness incisions and placing the triangles to be excised within the nasolabial and labiomental creases [14] (Figs. 12.1 and 12.2). This concept was further refined by Pirgousis and Fernandes for lower lip reconstruction [15] (Figs. 12.3 and 12.4).

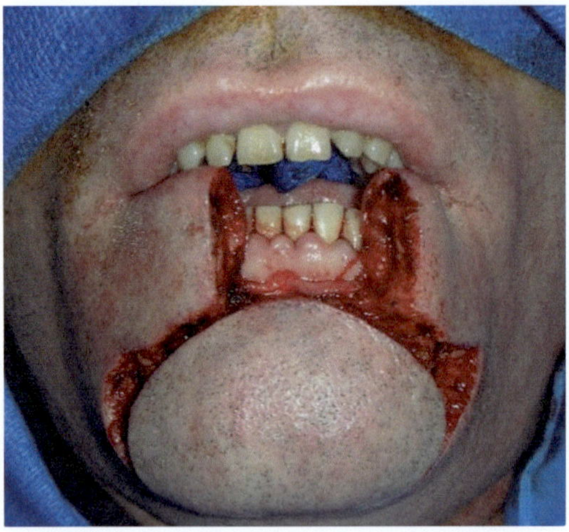

Fig. 12.3 Fernandes flap incisions following lower lip resection

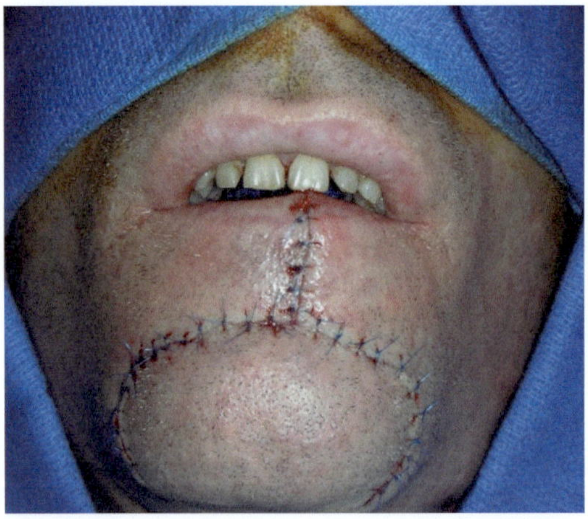

Fig. 12.4 Fernandes flap following closure

12.4.3.2 Gate Flap

Bilateral Fujimori "Gate" flaps are effectively nasolabial flaps that can be combined with advancement of the lower labial mucosa to reconstruct the entire lower lip [16]. A similar approach has been employed to reconstruct the upper lip too [17].

12.4.4 Upper Lip

12.4.4.1 Primary Closure

The upper lip is less forgiving when considering primary closure of defects. It exhibits less tissue laxity, and asymmetry is more noticeable because of deviation or distortion of the philtrum and nasal base. Defects up to around one quarter to one third of upper lip width may be satisfactorily closed, particularly if laterally situated. The philtral region is less forgiving again, and while up to around 50% can be closed primarily, there is a tendency for flattening and upwards retraction of the vermillion here.

12.4.4.2 Abbe Flap

Sabattini first reported the use of a 2-stage pedicled "lip switch" flap in 1838 [18], although the labial artery-based flap was popularized by Abbe in 1898 for reconstruction of bilateral cleft lip [19]. The lower lip flap is designed with width half that of the defect (thus the transverse discrepancy is equalized between upper and lower lips), height equal to the defect, and the pedicle lateral. The central lower lip is the preferred donor site, as it is hair-bearing in males and leaves the least visible scar. The white roll should be marked prior to incision and potential obscuration due to bleeding, edema, and pallor. The flap is raised including skin, muscle, and mucosa, but with preservation of the lateral vermilion incorporating the labial vessels. The flap is rotated and inset, taking care to reapproximate the orbicularis oris muscle and align the white roll. After 2–3 weeks, the pedicle is divided and the flap inset. For defects of the commissure, Estlander described a similar flap where the commissure is the rotation point, and therefore no secondary insetting is required.

12.4.4.3 Perialar Crescenteric Advancement

Initially described by Webster [20], a perialar incision can be made unilaterally or bilaterally to recruit lateral tissue for closure of the upper lip defects (Figs. 12.5, 12.6, and 12.7). This technique can also be combined with an Abbe flap to reconstruct the philtrum.

12.4.4.4 Reverse Karapandzic

Incisions following the melolabial groove upward to join an upper lip defect can be used to advance lateral tissue in a similar fashion as the Karapandzic flap for closure of lower lip defects.

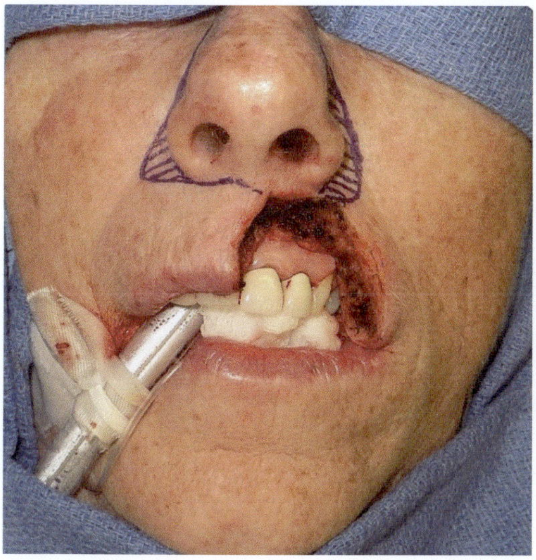

Fig. 12.5 Perialar cresenteric flap markings for and upper lip defect

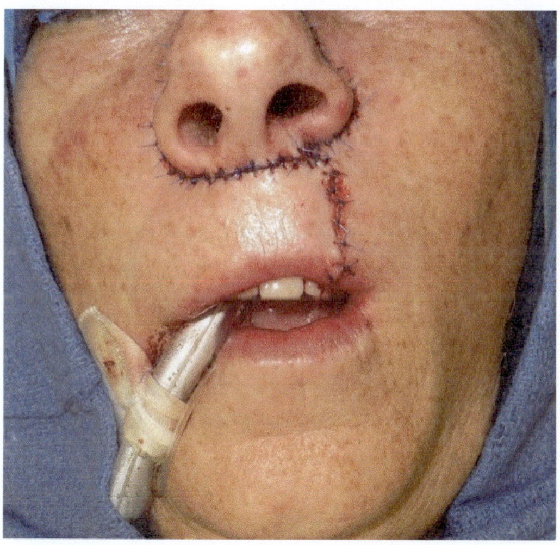

Fig. 12.6 Perialar cresenteric advancement after closure

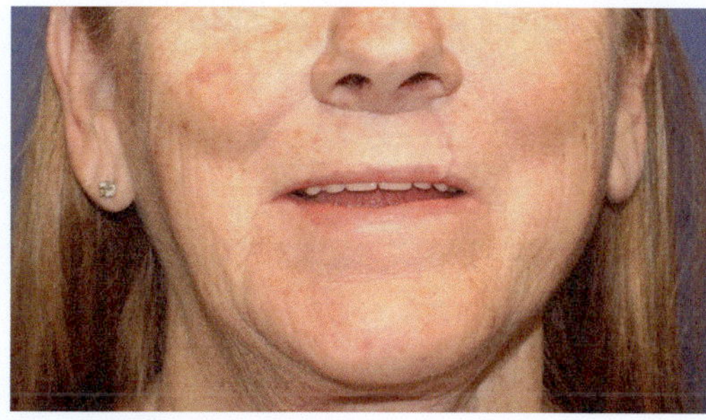

Fig. 12.7 Late postoperative appearance of perialar cresenteric advancement

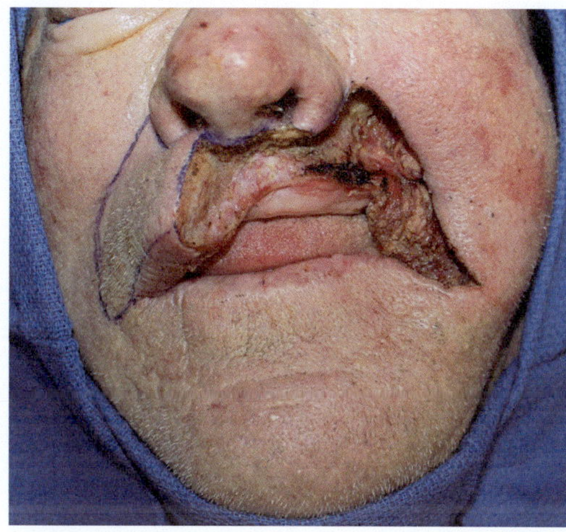

Fig. 12.8 Upper lip defect

12.4.5 Commissuroplasty

Many of the local flaps described lead to blunting of the commissure. The simplest correction is to make a horizontal full thickness incision through the blunted commissure, extending laterally to correspond with the position of the contralateral normal commissure. Epithelium superior and inferior to the incision is excised and labial mucosa advanced from intraorally to recreate the vermilion. The Gillies commissuroplasty involves excision of a triangular segment of skin lateral to the rounded commissure, to a point comparable with the normal side. A vermilion flap from the opposing lip is then lifted and rotated into this, and a mucosal flap advanced to form the vermilion of the donor site.

12.4.6 Total Lip Defects

A combination of the techniques already described can be employed to reconstruct total defects, although more commonly free tissue transfer is used. By far the most frequently used option is the radial-free flap (Figs. 12.8,

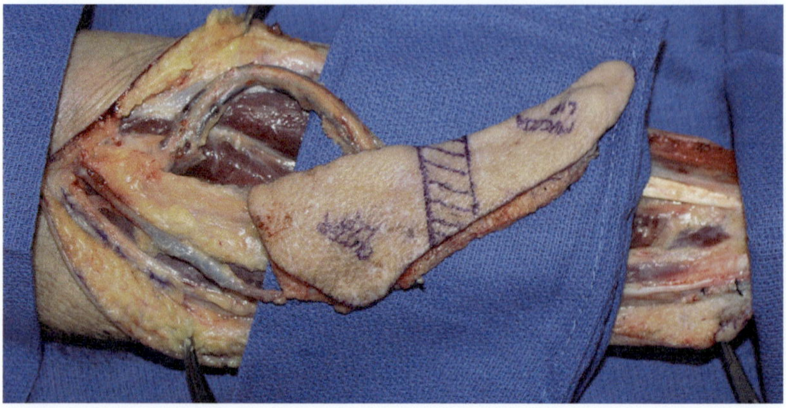

Fig. 12.9 Radial flap prior to disconnection

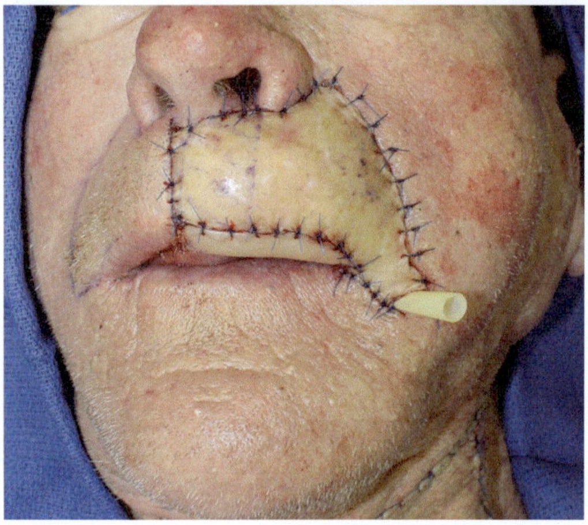

Fig. 12.10 Radial flap inset into upper lip defect

12.9, and 12.10), giving soft, pliable tissue and the option to include palmaris longus tendon [21]. The palmaris longus tendon can be utilized as a sling between the commissures, or to the malar periosteum to improve form and oral competence. The flexor carpi radialis tendon or a nonvascularized fascia lata graft can be used in a similar manner. Coaptation of the lateral antebrachial cutaneous nerve to the mental nerve has been described to restore sensation to the reconstruction [22]. Other free flaps that have been described for lip reconstruction include the gracilis for lower lip reconstruction [23–25] and temporal scalp for upper lip defects [26, 27].

12.5 Buccal Mucosa and Cheek

The function of the cheek chiefly is to bound the oral cavity and retain food between the occlusal surfaces of the teeth during mastication. However, morbidity secondary to resection of the cheek is not limited to this function. For example, a large resection closed primarily or left to heal by secondary intention can lead to trismus, particularly if postoperative radiation therapy is indicated. Small defects can be closed primarily, but larger defects limited to the inner aspect will likely benefit from resurfacing. This can be accomplished with split thickness skin grafts or buccal fad pad [28], as well as regional flaps as described in the section on reconstruction of the floor of the mouth (Fig. 12.11). Free tissue transfer for a mucosa-only defect will generally be in the form of a radial forearm flap due to its pliability and lack of bulk. Full thickness defects require consideration of reconstruction of both the intraoral and extraoral aspects of the cheek. While hybrid solutions can be considered, for example, a regional or free flap for the lateral aspect and a split thickness skin graft for the mucosal aspect, these defects are most commonly reconstructed with a folded or dual paddled flap. The intervening surface can be de-epithelialized to lie behind the oral sphincter, whether this is preserved or re-established. However, if a significant lip resection is required,

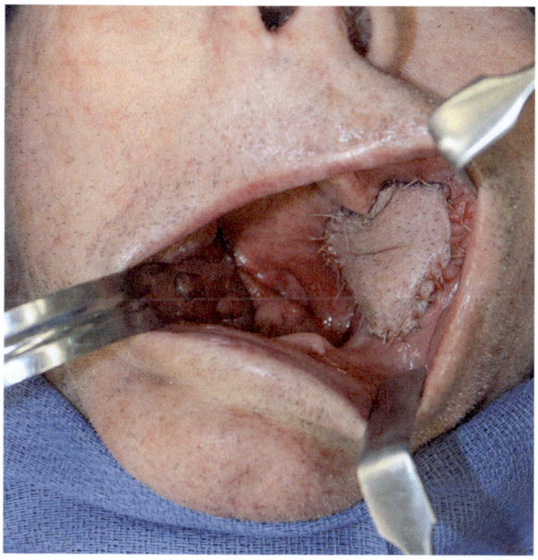

Fig. 12.11 Buccal mucosa reconstruction with submental island pedicled flap

the intervening tissue can instead be incorporated in the lip repair, keeping in mind that the greater the hiatus in the oral sphincter, the greater will be the detriment to oral competence. Both radial forearm [29] and anterolateral thigh [30] donor sites can be used for bipaddled flaps. The first is more pliable and thinner; the second can be made larger and confers less donor site morbidity, as it can generally be closed primarily.

Full thickness resections of the cheek often require sacrifice of the buccal or marginal mandibular branches of the facial nerve, with consequent paralysis of the oral aspects of facial expression. Although facial reanimation is a topic of its own, the broad strokes bear mentioning here. The simplest procedures, and often the most appropriate in the oncological setting, are the static procedures, in which the oral commissure is suspended from the deep temporal fascia by a strip of autogenous tissue, usually fascia lata, or of a prosthetic material, whether biologic (acellular dermal graft) or synthetic (PTFE, polypropylene) [31]. Dynamic procedures, which permit modulation of facial expression, involve either the restoration of nerve continuity or the interposition of innervated muscle, commonly temporalis transposition or a gracilis neuromuscular free flap [32].

12.6 Floor of Mouth

The floor of the mouth can be defined as the mucosal and muscular sling extending from the ventral surface of the tongue, bounded anteriorly and laterally by the lingual aspect of the mandibular gingiva, and posteriorly by the retromolar trigone. The mucosal layer acts as the inferior limit of the oral cavity and provides a reservoir for food during mastication. The muscles of the floor of the mouth are instrumental in deglutition. The mylohyoid, the geniohyoid, and the anterior belly of the digastric muscle draw the aerodigestive tract anteriorly and superiorly during swallowing, anchoring the tongue and increasing the diameter of the fauces. The musculature of the floor of the mouth, particularly the genioglossus, also acts as a passive sling at rest, to prevent posterior displacement of the tongue and consequent airway compromise. Finally, the range of motion of the tongue depends on adequate separation from the mandible, both laterally and medially, which is essential for speech and swallowing.

Reconstruction of the floor of the mouth should aim to restore both these functions. The tongue must be resuspended anteriorly, and sufficient tissue must be preserved or transferred to ensure adequate tongue mobility and prevent ankyloglossia. One commonly employed option for reconstruction of pure floor of mouth defects is the submental artery island flap. This flap was first described by Martin et al. in 1993 [33]. It is large, reliable, and easily raised with minimal donor site morbidity (and even improvement in cosmetic soft tissue profile). The pedicle is up to 8 cm in length, and cutaneous dimensions up to 7 × 18 cm can be harvested, sufficient to reconstruct most pure floor of mouth defects. It confers less donor morbidity than a radial forearm-free flap, which is the main alternative among the free flaps. The main proviso regarding the use of this flap is the question of oncological safety due to compromised nodal dissection of level 1. In one small series, four of nine patients undergoing SIF suffered local or regional recurrence thought to be attributable to incomplete nodal harvest [34]. On the other hand, Howard et al. found that in 50 patients undergoing SIF, all with clinically negative level I nodes, none experienced recurrence attributable to the flap [35]. It is generally accepted that the flap is contraindicated in necks with clinically positive nodes, particularly in level I. A history of radiation is a relative contraindication, though good outcomes have been described in this setting [36, 37]. Finally, since the submental vessels arise from the facial vessels, the flap cannot be performed in patients who have undergone a neck dissection with sacrifice of the facial vessels.

In patients in whom SIF is contraindicated, and those with an unfavorable defect, alternate regional flaps may be appropriate, particularly if this permits the use of nonirradiated tissue. The infrahyoid island flap [38] is of a similar size and character to the SIF and would often lie in the same radiation field. Its chief advantage over the SIF is that it obviates the question of oncological safety in level I. The supraclavicular and pectoralis major flaps are robust options and would generally lie outside any previously operated or radiated field. However, these flaps depend on a broad pedicle, which often introduces excess tissue into the defect or the tunnel from donor site to defect. Many such patients will therefore be best served with a radial forearm-free flap, which provides a thin, supple reconstruction and negligible pedicle bulk.

12.7 Tongue Reconstruction

Tongue function depends on complex interplay between sensory and motor components of both voluntary and involuntary nervous systems. Restoration of tongue function is important for mastication, deglutition and articulation, and as a result, quality of life. Evidence suggests that tongue resection has a significant effect on quality of life compared with other oropharyngeal structures, proportional to the size of resection. A reconstruction that recreates the biomechanics of the healthy tongue leads to better function and even cortical adaptation to the neotongue [39]. In terms of speech, the ability for the anterior tongue to contact the palate is particularly important. Speech therapy following tongue reconstruction should always be considered to improve proprioception of the reconstructed tongue and facilitate cortical plasticity.

12.7.1 Primary Closure

Small defects of the free oral tongue can often be closed primarily. As defect size increases, the option of healing by secondary intention should be considered as this can result in a more natural tongue morphology, while dehiscence is often the natural course for primary closure anyway.

12.7.2 Pedicled Flap Reconstruction

Where free tissue transfer is precluded, tongue defects can be reconstructed with a variety of pedicled flaps. Prior to development of free tissue transfer, the pectoralis major and deltopectoral flap were commonly used, with the facial artery myomucosal flap an option for smaller volume defects. There has recently been a renaissance in the use of other regional flaps such as submental island, supraclavicular island, trapezius island, and infrahyoid flaps.

12.7.3 Free Flap Reconstruction

Free flap reconstruction is advocated to restore form, prevent contracture, and reduce tethering in glossectomy defects one quarter of the tongue size or greater [40]. The flap should be designed to recreate premorbid morphology in all three dimensions as far as possible.

The radial forearm-free flap is the workhorse of tongue reconstruction for good reason (Fig. 12.12). It provides thin, pliable, soft tissue, and large-caliber vessels of consistent anatomy for microvascular anastomosis. Harvest can be simultaneous with resection and presents limited morbidity. Neural coaptation of the lateral antebrachial cutaneous nerve to the lingual nerve affords a sensate flap with some evidence that this helps with function and resists flap atrophy [41].

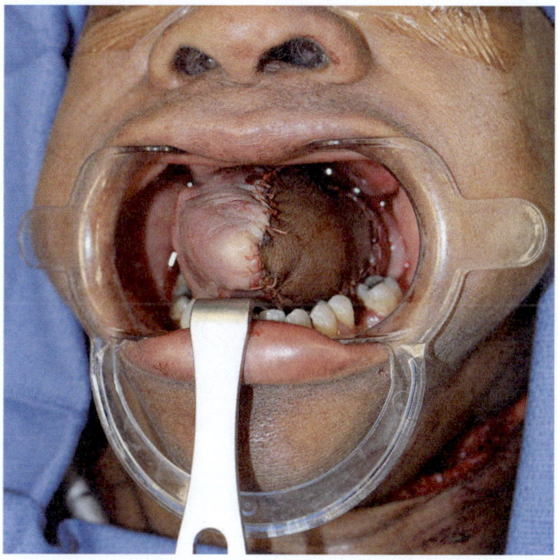

Fig. 12.12 Radial free flap to reconstruct hemiglossectomy defect

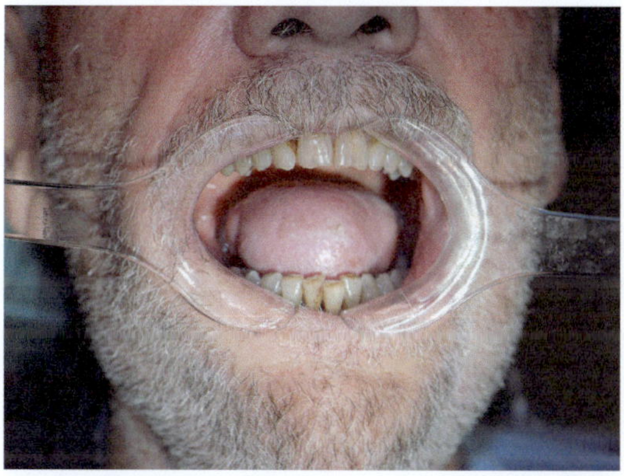

Fig. 12.13 ALT flap reconstruction following total glossectomy

Defects greater than three quarters of the tongue may benefit from reconstruction with tissue of greater substance such as anterolateral thigh (ALT) or rectus abdominis-free flaps. ALT harvest results in a more easily hidden scar, and potential sensory loss is less troublesome. Total glossectomy reconstruction is particularly challenging. Recreation of three-dimensional morphology is critical, with emphasis on height and a protuberant tip, to restore speech and swallowing function [42] (Fig. 12.13). Bulky flaps, around one third oversized to the defect are recommended to achieve this aim. When the larynx is preserved, hyolaryngeal suspension should also be considered to reduce the risk of persistent aspiration [43].

12.8 Mandibular Reconstruction

The mandible provides support for the lower third of the face and attachment for the musculature of the tongue, floor of mouth, and hyoid. Reconstruction is often necessary to restore both form and function following ablation. Additional consideration should be made for facilitation of dental rehabilitation when considering mandibular reconstruction, in the form of fixed or removable prostheses.

12.8.1 Classification of Defects

Brown et al. developed a classification system for oncological mandibular defects that is helpful in guiding reconstructive options [44]. Based on four mandibular 'corners' of the angles and canine regions, defects increase in size and complexity from class I to class IV and are subclassified by whether the condyles are included too.

The classification indicates the average length of bone required for reconstruction, and it can be appreciated that morbidity will increase with class if the defect is not reconstructed, particularly with respect to mandibular continuity.

Mandibular reconstruction may aim to restore only the hard tissue defect (autogenous bone or reconstruction bar alone) or only soft tissue, whether intra or extraoral, or both hard and soft tissue defects. In all cases, meticulous intraoral closure should be insured to reduce the risk of infection and fistulation.

12.8.2 Soft Tissue Reconstruction

Recruitment of intraoral soft tissue can permit primary closure, and often the loss of alveolar height associated with bone resection will facilitate this. The buccal fat pad can be mobilized to assist with closure of small posterolateral soft tissue defects, as can an inferiorly pedicled facial artery myomucosal flap.

Larger soft tissue defects associated with mandibular resection can be reconstructed with regional flaps such as the submental island, supraclavicular island, pectoralis major, or latissimus dorsi flap. Alternatively, free tissue transfer can be performed, most commonly radial or ALT flaps.

12.8.3 Hard Tissue Reconstruction

In some cases, restoration of mandibular continuity following segmental mandibulectomy may not be deemed necessary, particularly in elderly, edentulous patients with class 1 defects. Restoration of mandibular continuity can be achieved by a load-bearing reconstruction bar alone. However, even with good soft tissue closure, there is risk of hardware exposure, particularly if radiotherapy is to be administered. A nonvascularized bone graft, usually from the iliac crest, can be inserted with the plate, but again, considering radiotherapy is likely to be indicated within 6 weeks of surgery, this choice is precarious. Segmental defects are therefore preferably reconstructed with osseous free flaps to permit radiotherapy in the short term and facilitate future dental rehabilitation. This process has been aided greatly in recent years by the use of virtual surgical planning.

The fibular-free flap is commonly used to reconstruct mandibular defects for a number of reasons. The bone stock allows insertion of implants for dental rehabilitation, osteotomizing the bone permits restoration of mandibular form, and in class IV defects, it may be the only option to provide sufficient length of bone (Figs. 12.14 and 12.15). Additionally, the flap can include fasciocutaneous and/or muscle paddles to provide for soft tissue repair. A double-barreled bone arrangement can be used to increase mandibular height if needed.

The iliac crest arguably contributes the best bone stock in terms of both volume and quality. It can be harvested as a nonvascularized graft for smaller defects or as a free flap based on the DCIA system with or without muscle and or skin. The skin paddle is bulky and restricted in terms of its placement compared with the fibular flap, which also has a longer pedicle. The morphology of the ilium lends itself well to reconstruction of Brown Class I or II defects (Figs. 12.16 and 12.17).

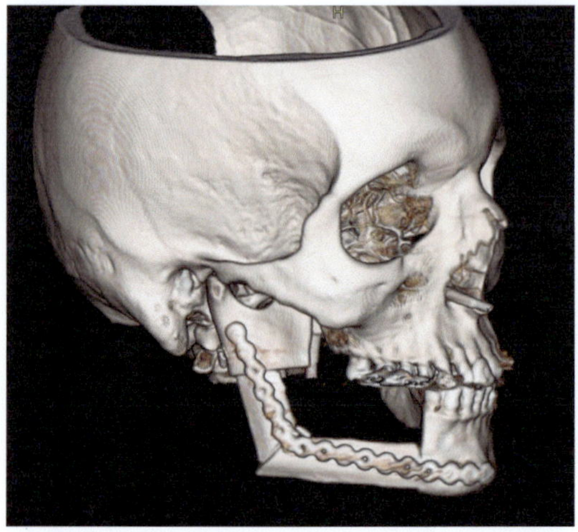

Fig. 12.14 Postoperative 3D CT of fibular flap reconstruction for Brown Class I mandibulectomy

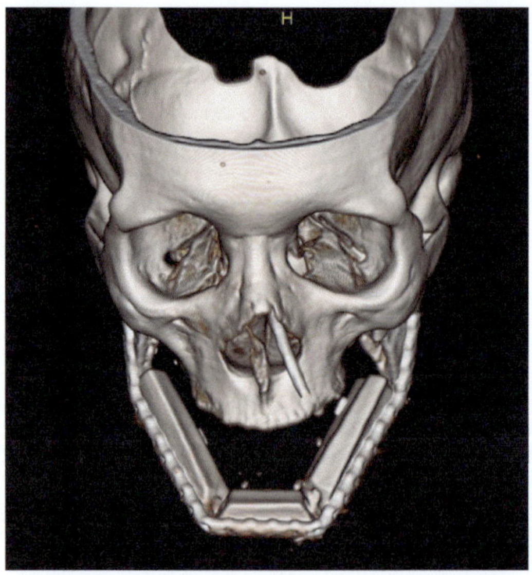

Fig. 12.15 Postoperative 3D CT of fibular free flap reconstruction for Brown class IV mandibulectomy defect

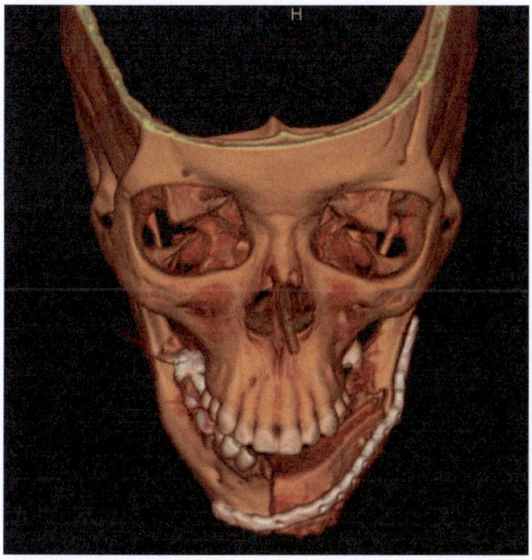

Fig. 12.16 3D CT of DCIA reconstruction of mandible

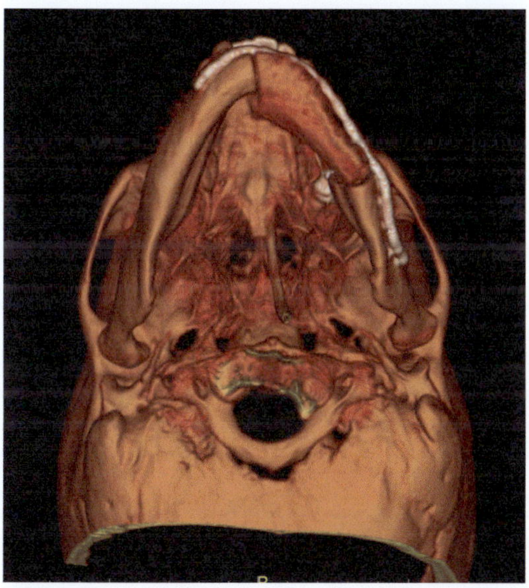

Fig. 12.17 3D CT of DCIA reconstruction of mandible. Inferior view

The lateral border of the scapula is the next most commonly used free flap in mandibular reconstruction (Fig. 12.18). It can be osteotomized, and receive implants, although not as reliably as fibula or DCIA reconstructions. Simultaneous harvest is also challenging.

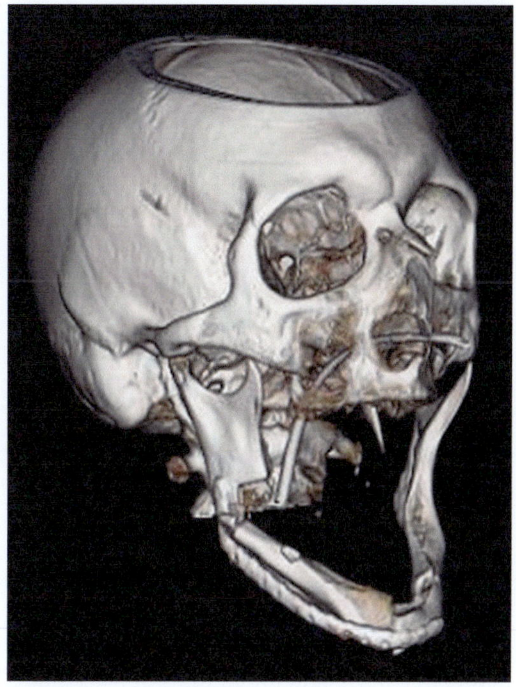

Fig. 12.18 Postoperative 3D CT of scapula flap reconstruction for Brown Class II mandibulectomy defect

12.9 Palatal and Maxillary Defects

The function of the palate is to separate the nasal passage and maxillary sinuses from the mouth and to provide a superior limit to the oral cavity. Insufficiency of this structure has predictable effects: nasal speech, difficulty propelling the food bolus posteriorly during deglutition, tendency for food to become trapped in the nasal cavity or maxillary sinus, and nasal regurgitation. Defects with greater vertical extent may also involve the orbital floor or contents. Soft palate defects result in velopharyngeal insufficiency, chiefly characterized by nasal speech, but also disposing to retrograde nasal aspiration, especially of fluids.

Maxillectomy defects have been classified by a number of authors, but arguably the most useful in terms of guiding reconstructive options is that proposed by Brown et al. [45]. The first level of classification is the vertical: Class I (low maxillectomy) defects do not cause an oronasal fistula;

class II defects do, but do not involve the orbit; class III defects involve the orbital adnexa with orbital retention; class IV defects involve orbital enucleation or exenteration; class V describes orbitomaxillary defects without oronasal fistula; and class VI describes nasomaxillary defects.

Class II–IV defects are further classified according to their horizontal extent: Horizontal class 'a' does not involve the alveolus, 'b' is a laterally located defect less than the hemipalate, 'c' is also less than half the palate, but located anteriorly, and 'd' is greater than half the palate.

Simple mucosal defects overlying the hard palate can be left to close by secondary intention. Although the process is lengthy, pain and remucosalization can be aided by an acrylic cover plate retained by bone screws or dental cribs. Most oncologic resections for lesions overlying the hard palate will require maxillectomy to obtain adequate margins. It is sometimes possible to preserve the continuity of the soft palate, thus simplifying reconstruction. Small class I defects can sometimes be closed by advancement of the buccal mucosa, since the decreased alveolar height postresection prevents excess tension. Regional pedicled flap options include buccal fat pad, facial artery myomucosal flaps, temporalis, and temporoparietal flaps. Free flaps can be subdivided into those providing hard tissue (fibula, deep circumflex iliac artery (Fig. 12.19), scapula, lateral arm, and osteocutaneous radial forearm) and those providing soft tissue alone (radial forearm (Figs. 12.20 and 12.21), rectus abdominis, free latissimus dorsi, and anterolateral thigh). Osseus flaps afford the potential for osseointegrated implant placement for dental rehabilitation (Figs. 12.22 and 12.23).

Many maxillary defects are adequately addressed with an obturator appliance, which fills the defect, re-establishes the separation between oral and nasal cavities, and can incorporate prosthetic dentition (Figs. 12.24 and 12.25). The potential advantages of an obturator are reduced operative time and morbidity due to less extensive surgery, greater ease of cavity surveillance for recurrence, and earlier restoration of dental function. On the other hand, obturators require serial revision as the cavity matures, and they can be dif-

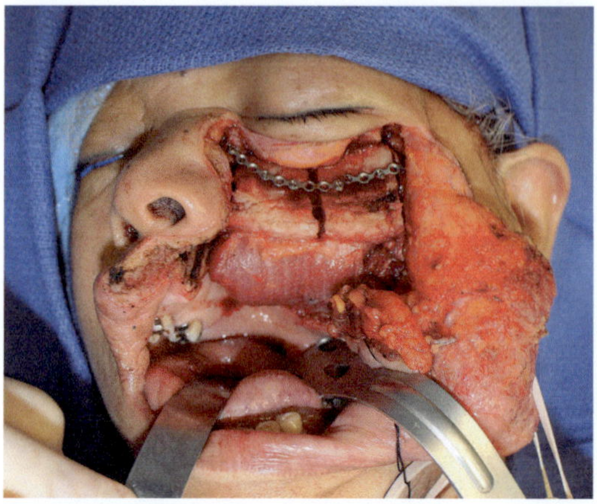

Fig. 12.19 DCIA flap inset to reconstruct Brown and Shaw class III defect

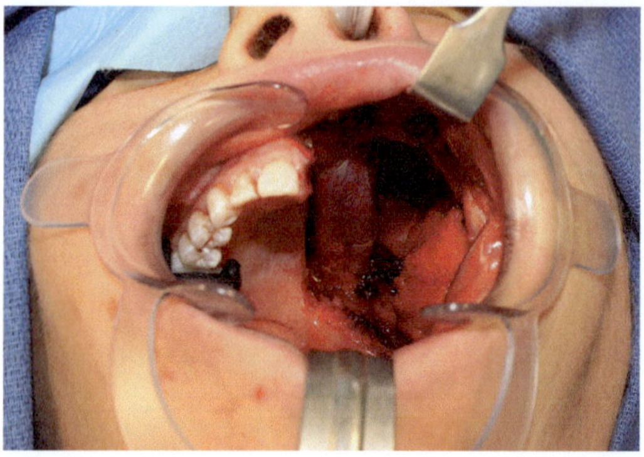

Fig. 12.20 Brown and Shaw class IIb maxillectomy defect

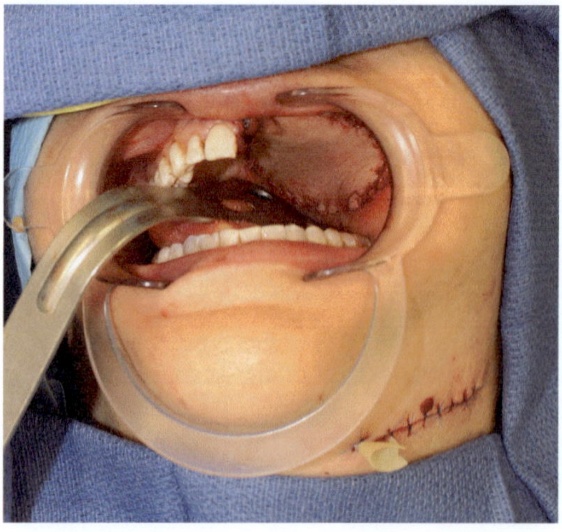

Fig. 12.21 Radial-free flap to reconstruct Brown and Shaw Class IIb defect

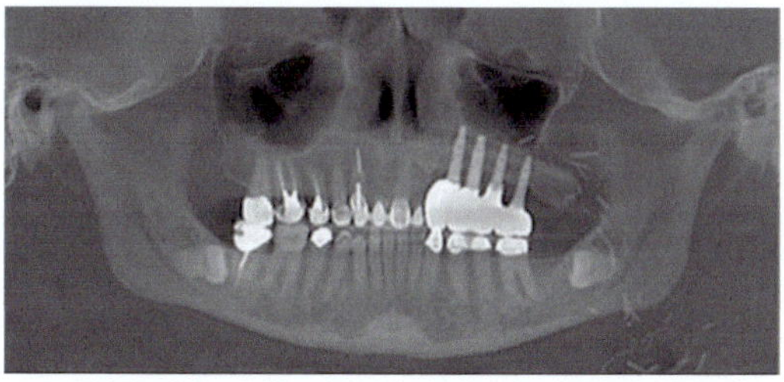

Fig. 12.22 Panoramic radiograph showing implants placed within fibula flap reconstruction of Brown and Shaw Class II maxillectomy

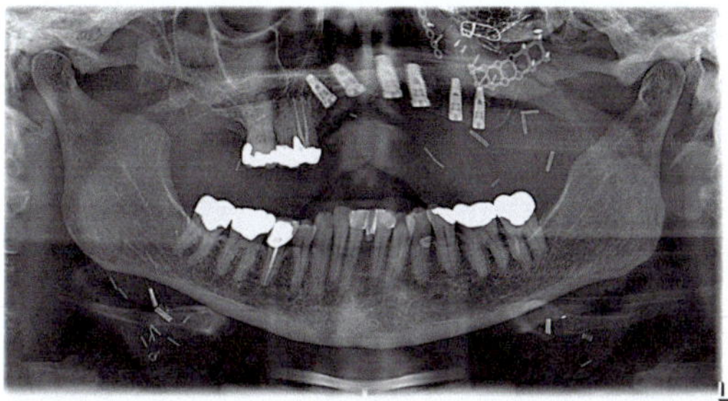

Fig. 12.23 Panoramic radiograph showing implants placed within scapula flap reconstruction of Brown and Shaw Class IV maxillectomy

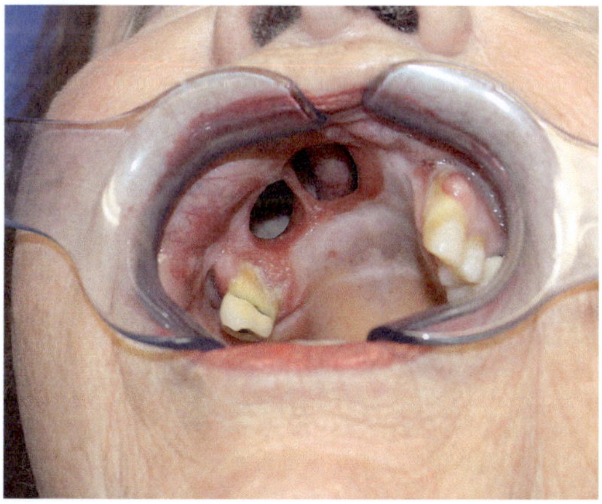

Fig. 12.24 Brown and Shaw class IIc maxillectomy defect

ficult to use in an inflamed field during radiation therapy. It is therefore not always clear whether a given defect would be better served with a free flap or an obturator. Brown et al. suggest that as a general rule, the larger the defect, the greater the potential advantages of free flap reconstruction

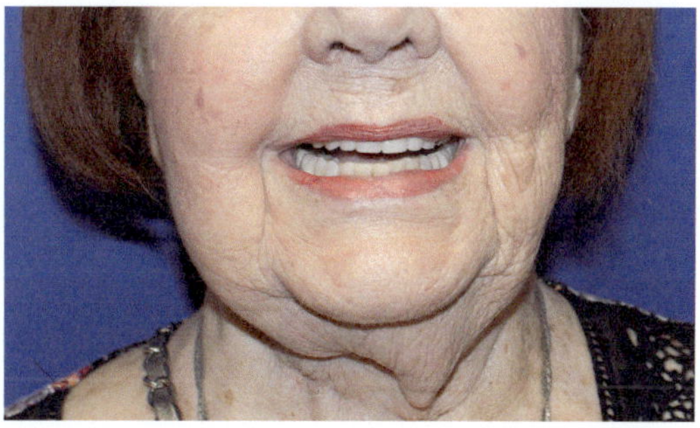

Fig. 12.25 Same patient as Fig. 12.24 with obturator in situ

[45]. Moreno et al. found that the horizontal (palatal) extent of the defect was more significant than the vertical in weighting toward flap reconstruction [46]. When an obturator is contemplated, maxillary teeth should be preserved during resection if possible, to allow for retention and stability of the obturator. When this is not feasible, obturator retention can be achieved with a two-part design or osseointegrated implants.

References

1. Ray E. Head and neck reconstructive surgery. In: Cancer treatment and research. New York, NY: Springer; 2018. p. 123–43. http://www.ncbi.nlm.nih.gov/pubmed/29435840. Accessed 3 Sep 2018.
2. Erba P, Ogawa R, Vyas R, Orgill DP. The reconstructive matrix: a new paradigm in reconstructive plastic surgery. Plast Reconstr Surg. 2010;126(2):492–8.
3. El-Marakby HH. The reliability of pectoralis major myocutaneous flap in head and neck reconstruction. J Egypt Natl Canc Inst. 2006;18(1):41–50. http://www.ncbi.nlm.nih.gov/pubmed/1723785. Accessed 31 Aug 2018.
4. Shah JP, Haribhakti V, Loree TR, Sutaria P. Complications of the pectoralis major myocutaneous flap in head and neck reconstruction. Am J Surg. 1990;160(4):352–5.
5. Zitelli JA. Wound healing by secondary intention. A cosmetic appraisal. J Am Acad Dermatol. 1983;9(3):407–15.
6. Leonard AL, Hanke CW. Second intention healing for intermediate and large postsurgical defects of the lip. J Am Acad Dermatol. 2007;57(5):832–5.
7. Jin X, Teng L, Zhang C, Xu J, Lu J, Zhang B, et al. Reconstruction of partial-thickness vermilion defects with a mucosal V–Y advancement flap based on the orbicularis oris muscle. J Plast Reconstr Aesth Surg. 2011;64(4):472–6.

8. Wagner DJD, Newman DMH. Bipedicled axial cross-lip flap for correction of major vermilion deficiency after cleft lip repair. 2017. https://doi.org/101597/1545-1569_1994_031_0148_baclff_23.co_2.
9. Ceran C, Demirseren ME, Sarici M, Durgun M, Tekin F. Tongue flap as a reconstructive option in intraoral defects. J Craniofac Surg. 2013;24(3):972–4.
10. Levi B, Ricci JA, Donelan MB. Vermillion reconstruction with anal verge transitional epithelium. J Burn Care Res. 2017;39(2):1.
11. Karapandzic M. Reconstruction of lip defects by local arterial flaps. Br J Plast Surg. 1974;27(1):93–7. http://www.ncbi.nlm.nih.gov/pubmed/4593704. Accessed 31 Aug 2018.
12. Sood A, Paik A, Lee E. Lower lip reconstruction: karapandzic flap. Eplasty 2013;13:ic17. http://www.ncbi.nlm.nih.gov/pubmed/23409208. Accessed 3 Sep 2018.
13. Bernard C. Cancer de la levre inferieure opere par un procede nouveau. Bull Mem Soc Chir. 1853;3:357–64. https://ci.nii.ac.jp/naid/10011662354/#cit.
14. Webster RC, Coffey RJ, Kelleher RE. Total and partial reconstruction of the lower lip with innervated muscle-bearing flaps. Plast Reconstr Surg. 1960;25(3):360–71.
15. Pirgousis P, Fernandes R. Reconstruction of subtotal defects of the lower lip: a review of current techniques and a proposed modification. J Oral Maxillofac Surg. 2011;69(1):295–9.
16. Fujimori R. Gate for the total reconstruction of the lower lip. Br J Plast Surg. 1980;33(3):340–5. http://www.ncbi.nlm.nih.gov/pubmed/7426811. Accessed 31 Aug 2018.
17. Aytekin A, Ay A, Aytekin O. Total upper lip reconstruction with bilateral fujimori gate flaps. Plast Reconstr Surg. 2003;111(2):797–800.
18. Agostini T. The Sabattini-Abbé flap: a historical note. Plast Reconstr Surg. 2009;123(2):767. https://insights.ovid.com/crossref?an=00006534-200902000-00051. Accessed 3 Sep 2018
19. Abbe R. A new plastic operation for the relief of deformity due to double harelip. Plast Reconstr Surg. 1968;42(5):481–3. http://www.ncbi.nlm.nih.gov/pubmed/4880838. Accessed 31 Aug 2018
20. Webster JP. Crescentic peri-alar cheek excision for upper lip flap advancement with a short history of upper lip repair. Plast Reconstr Surg. 1955;16(6):434–64.
21. Fernandes R, Clemow J. Outcomes of total or near-total lip reconstruction with microvascular tissue transfer. J Oral Maxillofac Surg. 2012;70(12):2899–906. http://linkinghub.elsevier.com/retrieve/pii/S027823911200359X. Accessed 3 Sep 2018.
22. Sakai S, Soeda S, Endo T, Ishii M, Uchiumi E. A compound radial artery forearm flap for the reconstruction of lip and chin defect. Br J Plast Surg. 1989;42(3):337–8.
23. Cordova A, D'Arpa S, Moschella F. Gracilis free muscle transfer for morpho-functional reconstruction of the lower lip. Head Neck. 2008;30(5):684–9. http://www.ncbi.nlm.nih.gov/pubmed/17979111. Accessed 3 Sep 2018.
24. Sacak B, Gurunluoglu R. The innervated gracilis muscle for microsurgical functional lip reconstruction: review of the literature. Ann Plast Surg. 2015;74(2):204–9. http://content.wkhealth.com/linkback/openurl?sid=WKPTLP:landingpage&an=00000637-201502000-00015. Accessed 3 Sep 2018.
25. Gurunluoglu R, Glasgow M, Williams SA, Gurunluoglu A, Antrobus J, Eusterman V. Functional reconstruction of total lower lip defects using innervated gracilis flap in the setting of high-energy ballistic injury to the lower face: preliminary report. J Plast Reconstr Aesthet Surg. 2012;65(10):1335–42. http://linkinghub.elsevier.com/retrieve/pii/S1748681512002471. Accessed 3 Sep 2018.
26. Lyons GB, Milroy BC, Lendvay PG, Teston LM. Upper lip reconstruction: use of the free superficial temporal artery hair-bearing flap. Br J Plast Surg. 1989;42(3):333–6. http://www.ncbi.nlm.nih.gov/pubmed/2758210. Accessed 3 Sep 2018.
27. Chang K-P, Lai C-S, Tsai C-C, Lin T-M, Lin S-D. Total upper lip reconstruction with a free temporal scalp flap: long-term follow-up. Head Neck. 2003;25(7):602–5. http://www.ncbi.nlm.nih.gov/pubmed/12808664. Accessed 3 Sep 2018.
28. Dean A, Alamillos F, García-López A, Sánchez J, Peñalba M. The buccal fat pad flap in oral reconstruction. Head Neck. 2001;23(5):383–8. http://www.ncbi.nlm.nih.gov/pubmed/11295812. Accessed 3 Sep 2018.
29. Liu F, Wang L, Pang S, Kan Q. Reconstruction of full-thickness buccal defects with folded radial forearm flaps: a retrospective clinical study. Medicine (Baltimore). 2017;96(32):e7344. http://insights.ovid.com/crossref?an=00005792-201708110-00002. Accessed 3 Sep 2018.
30. Liu Z-M, Wu D, Liu X-K, Liu W-W, Li H, Li Q, et al. Reconstruction of through-and-through cheek defects with folded free anterolateral thigh flaps. J Oral Maxillofac Surg. 2013;71(5):960–4. http://linkinghub.elsevier.com/retrieve/pii/S027823911201573X. Accessed 3 Sep 2018.
31. Liu YM, Sherris DA. Static procedures for the management of the midface and lower face. Facial Plast Surg. 2008;24(2):211–5. http://www.thieme-connect.de/DOI/DOI?10.1055/s-2008-1075836. Accessed 3 Sep 2018.
32. Coyle M, Godden A, Brennan PA, Cascarini L, Coombes D, Kerawala C, et al. Dynamic reanimation for facial palsy: an overview. Br J Oral Maxillofac Surg. 2013;51(8):679–83. https://www.sciencedirect.com/science/article/pii/S0266435613000107?via%3Dihub. Accessed 3 Sep 2018.
33. Martin D, Pascal JF, Baudet J, Mondie JM, Farhat JB, Athoum A, et al. The submental island flap: a new donor site. Anatomy and clinical applications as a free or pedicled flap. Plast Reconstr Surg. 1993;92(5):867–73.

34. Cariati P, Cabello Serrano A, Marin Fernandez AB, Perez de Perceval Tara M, Juliá MA, Ildefonso Martinez Lara M. Is submental flap safe for the oncological reconstruction of the oral cavity? J Stomatol oral Maxillofac Surg. 2018. https://linkinghub.elsevier.com/retrieve/pii/S2468785518301307. Accessed 29 Aug 2018.
35. Howard BE, Nagel TH, Donald CB, Hinni ML, Hayden RE. Oncologic safety of the submental flap for reconstruction in oral cavity malignancies. Otolaryngol Head Neck Surg. 2014;150(4):558–62. http://journals.sagepub.com/doi/10.1177/0194599814520687. Accessed 29 Aug 2018.
36. Wu Y, Tang P, Qi Y, Xu Z, He Y. Evaluation for submental island flap. Zhonghua Kou Qiang Yi Xue Za Zhi. 2002;37(6):418–20. http://www.ncbi.nlm.nih.gov/pubmed/12641952. Accessed 31 Aug 2018.
37. Taghinia AH, Movassaghi K, Wang AX, Pribaz JJ. Reconstruction of the upper aerodigestive tract with the submental artery flap. Plast Reconstr Surg. 2009;123(2):562–70. https://insights.ovid.com/crossref?an=00006534-200902000-00016. Accessed 31 Aug 2018.
38. Deganello A, Manciocco V, Dolivet G, Leemans CR, Spriano G. Infrahyoid fascio-myocutaneous flap as an alternative to free radial forearm flap in head and neck reconstruction. Head Neck. 2007;29(3):285–91. http://www.ncbi.nlm.nih.gov/pubmed/17230563. Accessed 3 Sep 2018.
39. Mosier K, Liu W-C, Behin B, Lee C, Baredes S. Cortical adaptation following partial glossectomy with primary closure: implications for reconstruction of the oral tongue. Ann Otol Rhinol Laryngol. 2005;114(9):681–7.
40. Brown L, Rieger JM, Harris J, Seikaly H. A longitudinal study of functional outcomes after surgical resection and microvascular reconstruction for oral cancer: tongue mobility and swallowing function. J Oral Maxillofac Surg. 2010;68(11):2690–700.
41. Biglioli F, Liviero F, Frigerio A, Rezzonico A, Brusati R. Function of the sensate free forearm flap after partial glossectomy. J Cranio-Maxillofac Surg. 2006;34(6):332–9.
42. Kimata Y, Sakuraba M, Hishinuma S, Ebihara S, Hayashi R, Asakage T, et al. Analysis of the relations between the shape of the reconstructed tongue and postoperative functions after subtotal or total glossectomy. Laryngoscope. 2003;113(5):905–9.
43. Weber RS, Ohlms L, Bowman J, Jacob R, Goepfert H. Functional results after total or near total glossectomy with laryngeal preservation. Arch Otolaryngol Neck Surg. 1991;117(5):512–5.
44. Brown JS, Barry C, Ho M, Shaw R. A new classification for mandibular defects after oncological resection. Lancet Oncol. 2016;17(1):e23–30. http://linkinghub.elsevier.com/retrieve/pii/S1470204515003101. Accessed 31 Aug 2018.
45. Brown JS, Rogers SN, McNally DN, Boyle M. A modified classification for the maxillectomy defect. Head Neck. 2000;22(1):17–26.
46. Moreno MA, Skoracki RJ, Hanna EY, Hanasono MM. Microvascular free flap reconstruction versus palatal obturation for maxillectomy defects. Head Neck. 2009;32(7):860–8.

Predicting Quality of Life (QoL) of Oral Cancer

13

Roderick Y. Kim, Jason N. Burkes, and Fayette C. Williams

13.1 Introduction

Surgical and adjuvant therapy for treatment of oral cancer is ultimately designed to treat, preserve, and restore patients back to a functional life. Unfortunately, quality of life (QoL) has not been a primary focus in the advancement of care for the oral cancer patient, although it often has a significant impact on the patient. QoL studies have attempted to address, in a standardized manner, the dilemma of improving the patient's subjective effect, and in objective manner, the unintended consequences of clinical treatment decisions.

The best way to deal with a problem is to prevent it from ever happening in the first place. As surgeons, this involves carefully considering all aspects of perioperative care as well as the long-term implications of the recommended treatment. Predicting the QoL life in oral cancer patients allows multiple comportments to occur:

1. Allows the surgeon to discuss candidly the limitation of ablative and reconstructive options while aligning patient expectations with the surgeon.
2. Determines the main goal of therapy since QoL is subjective and should be individualized.
3. Ultimately permits the patient to make the best-informed treatment decisions.

Therefore, before even any treatment is rendered, the patient's expectations are established. This in turn improves the overall treatment outcome by cultivating the patient expectations and motivation. Through these evidence-based practices, surgeons are better prepared to predict quality of life issues in oral cancer patients to advance the overall care of the patient.

13.2 Quality of Life (QoL)

In the treatment of oral cancer, much focus in the past has been in regards to understanding the pathophysiology, surgical, and medical management. However, it is no surprise treating cancers that arise in the oral cavity has consequences beyond the locoregional control and survival of the patient. These treatment implications include esthetics, social cues, speech, breathing, eating, and affection. Rogers in 2007 noted that, although we have improved care with multimodality methods through tumor board consensus, little

R. Y. Kim (✉) · F. C. Williams
Division of Maxillofacial Oncology and Reconstructive Surgery, John Peter Smith Health Network, Fort Worth, TX, USA
e-mail: Rkim01@jpshealth.org

J. N. Burkes
Department of Oral and Maxillofacial Surgery, Walter Reed Nation Military Medical Center, Bethesda, MD, USA

D. Kademani (ed.), *Improving Outcomes in Oral Cancer*,
https://doi.org/10.1007/978-3-030-30094-4_13

debate occurs in terms of what effect the clinicians have in health-related quality of life outcomes [1]. As we perform surgical interventions, along with adjuvant therapies, it is easy to witness the significant impact the treatments have on the physical, mental, emotional, and psychosocial well-being of the patient. Therefore, it is important for clinicians to be familiar in evidence-based QoL measurements to allow objective assessments beyond the treatment efficacy and disease outcome.

Most common QoL parameters for head and neck cancer include the University of Washington QoL (UW-QoL) and the European Organization for Research and Treatment of Cancer QoL (EORTC-QoL) [2–4]. These are considered health-related quality of life parameters (HRQOL). UW-QoL, currently in version 4, is originally described by Hassan SJ and Weymuller EA published in 1993 in the journal of Head and neck [3]. Its benefits include a short self-administered questionnaire that requires no input from the provider, guided toward head and neck cancer, and multifactorial questions that allow identification of subtle changes. A short 12-item questionnaire domains, which takes about 10 minutes to complete, the score is scaled from 0 being the worst to 100 being the best, and a composite score can be calculated by averaging each domain score. Patients can also rank the importance of the domain in their quality of life. Currently the domains include pain, appearance, activity, recreation, swallowing, chewing, speech, shoulder, taste, saliva, mood, and anxiety. In some recent studies, UW-QoL was noted to be the most frequently used HRQOL parameter [2]. Thus, it is considered an important tool for assessing the progression of disease and effectiveness of treatment, perhaps most suited for patients undergoing surgery [5].

The EORTC-QoL, specific to the cancer type, consists of 35 questions. A composite score is calculated by sum of individual scores, with 1 being the best and 4 being the worst. The domains include pain, swallowing, sense, speech, social eating, social contact, and sexuality [2, 4]. This questionnaire focuses on the symptoms and side effects of treatment. These QoL parameters allow bridging of the gap between expectations and reality, as Morton et al. noted, "a larger gap between perceived reality and one's expectation, [leads to] a poor QoL [6]."A striking example of reality versus expectation is of McNeil in the "Fireman" study [7], where patients expressed that they would rather die than have a total laryngectomy [5] due to preconceived perception of the postoperative self. The issue may in part be due to the fact during the consultation in clinic, commonly the surgery and treatment were discussed and seldomly the expectations.

In the literature, QoL scores are frequently obtained at pre-, during, and post-therapy. Having objective data to properly counsel, the patient allows for a candid conversation, alleviates patient fears regarding treatment, and establishes patient expectations. Through open communications based on evidence-based practices, the expectations of the patients and the surgeon are better aligned. This allows identification of gaps in patient's needs, which can be augmented by a multidisciplinary team consisting of a social work, nutrition, support group, psychosocial counseling, physical therapy, occupational therapy, and speech/language pathology. These personnel are all essential to address the functional and QoL changes that occur after oral cancer surgery. The ultimate goal in treating patients with oral cancer is to improve their outcome in all aspects of care, in which QoL is clearly a large factor.

13.3 Glossectomy and Reconstruction

Tongue is the most common subsite in the oral cavity for squamous cell carcinoma. Tongue cancer has implications in multiple parameters of QoL and function since speech, swallowing, oral hygiene, taste, affection, and airway are all at risk for dysfunction. Ganziano alerted in 2002 that dysphagia after surgical resection of tongue cancer can lead to malnutrition, dehydration, weight loss, functional loss, fear of eating, and drinking and thus lead to depression with decreased QoL [8]. Although traditional teaching is that 50% of the tongue can be resected without affecting speech and swallowing, there are multiple studies that describe resection of large tongue cancers with negative effects on QoL [9–11]. This was highlighted by Brown et al. in 2006, who showed speech and swallowing were worse when the tongue resection was greater than 50% [11]. These tumors are more likely to require adjuvant radiotherapy, which is known to decrease QoL [10, 12]. Interestingly, Zhang et al. have noted that as long as the tongue is replaced, it seems to decrease functional outcomes compared to preoperative function [10]. Not surprisingly, there are multiple data that show without replacement the functional outcome is worse [13, 14]. Perhaps the correct question we should ponder is, what is the QoL difference that is reasonable for the patient? Not only is it important to make sure the patient has realistic expectations of their operative course, whether this is better or worse than the expectations of the surgeon, but perhaps it is equally important that we shed light on QoL changes that will occur in some capacity with the surgery.

One aspect that we as surgeons have an integral effect on is the method of reconstruction. This includes healing by secondary intention, autologous/allogenic graft, locoregional tissue transfer, and free tissue transfer. Typically, the decision making is first formulated by the size and location of tumor—floor of the mouth (FOM), lateral, ventral, and base of tongue. The tumor size determines if a hemi, partial, subtotal, or total glossectomy is warranted. Before the popularity of vascularized free flaps, McConnel and colleagues in 1987 found reconstructed tongue defects with split-thickness skin graft (STSG) had the best outcomes for speech and swallowing after they noted tongue mobility to be the most significant factor in the determination of postoperative speech results [15]. Since then, there are increasing evidence for differences in QoL with differing reconstructive options [12, 14, 16]. Locoregional flaps have good postoperative QoL outcomes, minimize operating room time, morbidity, and postoperative care but are usually limited to T1–T2 lesions [13]. Vascularized free tissue transfer has been associated with better functional results [17]. Interestingly the bulk, size, and type of flap utilized is poorly understood for QoL with no specific amount or size criteria to obtain maximal results [14]. Yang et al. in 2016 measured the QoL difference between Pectoralis Major Pedicled Flap (PMPF) and the Anterolateral Thigh (ALT) free flap and brought to the attention how the current measure of success for reconstruction was based only the survival of the flap, rather than the patient's QoL [18]. They also noted that although PMPF as a locoregional flap provided ample reliable soft tissue, but it was limited by pliability, restriction in arc of rotation, and poor esthetics. Recently with the popularity of free tissue transfers, investigators are attempting to answer if there is superiority between the kind of free tissue transfers. Yuan et al. compared the functional difference between the ALT-free flap and radial forearm-free flap (RFFF) for reconstruction of tongue defects [17]. They used UW-QoL and EORTC-QoL to discuss differences between RFFF and the ALT-free flap. The results showed the QoL and oral function improved from 6 to 12 months postoperatively for both RFFF and the ALT-free flap reconstructions. The authors noted the ALT-free flap required longer operative time and was better suited for larger tongue defects requiring tissue bulk while most partial tongue defects were better reconstructed with RFFF.

Overall, the literature rather seems to suggest that significant implications for QoL lies within radiotherapy, cancer stage, and socioeconomic status rather than the type of tongue reconstruction [10, 12, 18]. Unfortunately, the long-term QoL data are still lacking, and further investigations, prospective in nature, could provide better insight concerning the superiority of particular tongue reconstructive methods.

13.4 Maxillectomy

Another location of oral cancer that affects a multitude of QoL domains is the maxilla. Maxilla affects chewing, swallowing, speech, and facial esthetics. There are classifications from Brown and Shaw, as well as Okay for prosthetically derived classification of maxillectomy defects [19, 20]. These defect classifications, which the details are beyond the scope of this chapter, have been utilized in numerous studies on QoL. Additionally, obturators have been classified by the obturator functioning scale (OFS), which has domains of ability to eat, speak, satisfaction with lip position, cosmetic effect, and lubrication of mouth with saliva [21].

A controversial topic concerning the maxillectomy is the reconstruction of the defect with obturator reconstruction versus locoregional/ free flap reconstruction. Conventional teaching cautioned the flap reconstruction, as surveillance of tumors was difficult and only large tumors would be noted as a recurrence. Having the convenience and assurance of open, visible surgical site allowed easy surveillance and outweighed obturator issues of poor fit, expenses, and frequent visits with the prosthodontist. For those proponents of obturators, Signetmartin et al. in 2015 studied the understandability of speech after maxillectomy obturator placement. They noted the obturator is considered one of the most efficient rehab tools, immediately enhancing intraoral function and decreases cosmetic deformity by supplying missing teeth and soft tissue support [22]. Particularly they showed 2B defects or lower had better obturator function and QoL, but postoperative radiation caused overall lower QoL. In contrast, in patients who have poor manual dexterity and cannot clean the crusting obturators, the obturator may be nonfunctional [23] and could lead to a poor QoL. Although the overall QoL noted in the literature for obturators is good, if the patient had postoperative radiation, it was associated with a poorer QoL due to hyposalivation, lack of social eating, and poor understandability. A comparative study by Genden et al., evaluating the functional outcomes of hard palate defects reconstruction with RFFF and obturator, showed equivalent success in diet, mastication, articulation, appearance, speech, and taste. The RFFF, however, had improved satisfaction scores and social scores [24]. In contrast, Brandao et al. performed a study specifically addressing obturator versus free tissue transfer [25]. Their data showed although free flaps provide a definitive reconstruction with good results in small defects, it is associated with increased hospital stay and morbidity. They reiterate the point that larger defects are more difficult to fit obturators and associated with problems of leakage and hypernasal speech. Yet, their main outcome showed that obturator restores QoL almost completely, while free flaps do not. Furthermore, people with large obturators cope and ultimately assimilates to the prosthesis, but free flap patients do not always get used to their reconstruction, leading to poorer QoL. They concluded that obturator, if available, shortens therapy time, restores function, and is still one of the most promising ways of improving QoL.

Therefore, in terms of the literature, similar to reconstructive option for tongue defects, there is yet to be comprehensive data that favor one method of reconstruction for maxillectomy defects. It is important to note that oral rehabilitation following ablation plays a key role in promoting QoL and self-esteem even if chewing is not improved [1]. The surgeon and the patient, based on the patient's goals, expectations, and changes of QoL, need to establish a coordinated treatment plan.

13.5 Dental Implants

The surgical management of oral, head, and neck malignancies frequently results in deterioration of oral function, speech, and swallowing. Rehabilitation of the orofacial form aspires not only to restore oral function but also to improve speech, swallowing, and facial appearance. The use of vascularized free flaps for reconstruction significantly diminishes disfigurement of these patients and provides a foundation for restoring oral function. Unfortunately, the resulting neo-oral structures can be suboptimal [26] and often unfavorable for prosthodontic rehabilitation. To facilitate oral rehabilitation in this situation, the placement of endosseous implants for support of a fixed prosthesis has been found to optimize function, esthetics, and quality of life (QoL) [27–31].

Dholam et al. found most head and neck cancer patients reported improved QoL in function, pain, in addition to psychological and social disabilities with any prosthetic rehabilitation [32]. Nonetheless the ability of oral function is significantly worse in patients without implant-supported overdenture. Ablative techniques often further complicate satisfactory retention and stability of oral prosthesis necessitating the application of implants for retention. The McGill consensus statement concerning overdentures for the general population in 2002 concluded there was overwhelming evidence for two-implant overdentures as the first choice of treatment in edentulous mandibles [33]. In support of the McGill statement, the York census statement concluded in 2009 the QoL, and patient satisfaction was greater in mandibular implant-retained overdentures when compared to dentures without retention [34]. Intriguingly, the number of implants installed does not appear to influence the QoL or denture satisfaction in patients [27, 29, 31].

The placement of dental implants in the head and neck cancer patient can be achieved during the primary ablative/reconstructive surgery (PARS) or secondarily during post-radiotherapy (PR) surveillance. Since the majority of osseointegration occurs within 6 weeks following implant placement [35], some authors advocate implant placement at the end of the ablative/reconstruction procedure when postoperative radiotherapy is indicated [29, 36, 37]. This is mainly due to evidence showing primary placement of implants for oral rehabilitation to be optimal when placed into vascularized bone at the time of the PARS as a two-stage implant technique [26, 29, 31, 36]. To minimize complications during radiotherapy, the implants are covered by soft tissue at time of primary placement. The second stage of implant exposure with abutment placement is completed 6 months after completing radiation therapy [28]. This allows the patient to regain oral function with an implant-retained prosthesis in as little as 10 months after the initial ablative procedure. Patients who underwent immediate implant placement during PARS followed by postoperative radiotherapy were found to have an equal chance of one-year implant survival after prosthesis placement as noncancer/nonradiated patients [29, 37]. Some of the main advantages of PARS implant placement include avoidance of additional surgical procedures, risk minimization associated with implant placement in irradiated tissues, as well as restoring oral function sooner to assist in rehabilitation of speech and swallowing. There are risks involved with PARS dental-implant placement, though these have been found to be low incidence when compared to placement of dental implants in irradiated tissues. These risks, while marginal include poor anatomical positioning of the implant, possible delay in postablative chemoradiation therapy, possibility of recurrent disease, and risk of postradiation treatment complications [29, 38].

Radiation worsens treatment outcomes in regard to oral function, pain, and jaw opening. However, it's no longer considered a contraindication for placement of dental implants. The placement of implants in irradiated bone secondarily during PR surveillance has an 84.3% success rate [39]. Claudy et al. found in a systematic review and meta-analysis approximately 34% higher risk in implant failure if the implants were placed within 12 months of completion of radiotherapy [40]. The time delay for PR dental-implant placement can require patients to wait 18 months or more after initial treatment to obtain an implant-retained prosthesis [26, 29, 31, 38, 41]. Site placement has been found to influence PR implant placement with higher implant failure rates associated with irradiated maxilla [42]. Interestingly, Curi et al. found higher PR implant failure rates among older females as well as conventional conformal radiotherapy modality when compared to intensity-modulated radiotherapy (IMRT) [38]. An additional risk factor for increased P-RS implant failure is total radiation therapy dosages greater than 50 Gy.

13.6 The Patient

Management of the patient after treatment has traditionally concentrated on survival, locoregional disease control, and function [14], but social well-being, psychological [43], and vocational restoration [44] are emerging as critical factors in treatment success. QoL is a crucial factor in treatment outcomes and is subjectively determined by the patient. Valdez and Brennan explained QoL as "an abstract, subjective, and multidimensional conceptualization of a patient's perception of self" [2]. It subjectively improves with time following acute oncological treatment as the patient learns to manage both physical and somatic dysfunctions, notwithstanding continuing dysfunction [45]. Nevertheless, establishing a QoL closest to the predisease state is vital to the overall well-being of the patient.

Psychological morbidity is a significant contributor to the overall health and QoL of the patient [46]. Head and neck cancer (HNC) patients are more disposed to psychological distresses (PD) when compared to other types of cancer patients [43, 47]. PD is an undifferentiated amalgamation of symptoms varying from anxiety, depression, functional disabilities, and cognitive challenges to behavioral deficits [48, 49]. The situation can lead to significant impairment of daily living and social functions. Predictive factors are influenced by the combined psychosocial aspects when patients are not married and live alone [50–52]. Additional contributor to the PD is financial hardship obtained from treatment cost, medical debt, and reduced income [53, 54]. The definitive course of PD is largely undetermined when left untreated, but suggestive of a natural continuum to major depression disorder [49].

The prevalence of major depression disorder (MDD) among HNC patients vary from 3.7% to 20% [55]. Following cancer diagnosis and acute treatment, the incidence of MDD in HNC patients within the first year is 15–50% [43, 56] with peak symptoms occurring within 2–3 months following diagnosis [43] and a suicide rate more than four times the rate of the general population [57]. Depression is a well-documented contributor to reduced treatment compliance and poor prognosis. It is an independent determinant of QoL in HNC patients associated with poorer quality of life, weaken immune system, increased hospital length of stay, and impaired abilities to perform activities of daily living (ADLs) [43, 49]. Unfortunately, physicians have a marked tendency to underestimate the severity of depression in cancer patients resulting in inadequate treatment [46, 50, 58].

In addition to the psychological morbidities and psychosocial challenges of HNC patients, there are many physical and financial consequences that impact the patient's quality of life. As previously mentioned, the most notable of these physical effects involve the esthetics of the face, speech, voice, and swallowing. These physical toxicities, notably radiation as mentioned throughout this chapter, frequently contribute to development of malnutrition and loss of muscle mass. Protein calorie malnutrition, low body mass index, and weight loss leads to poor QoL, reduced survival, and impedes all cancer therapies (surgery, chemotherapy, radiotherapy) [51, 59]. All cancer patients should be screened routinely for malnutrition to optimize nutritional status, treatment modalities, and improve their QoL.

13.7 Conclusion

There is no doubt oral cancer and surgical intervention has significant impact on the QoL of patients. The QoL of the patient will evolve from initial diagnosis, during treatment, and post-treatment surveillance. Patient-reported QoL outcomes have the potential to provide more individualized treatment and care, as the decisions are determined by the QoL issues most important to the patient. QoL is an important tool for evaluation of patient as well as influencing the treatment outcome. It should be a critical part of surgeon's care for the patient, as much as the scalpel.

References

1. Rogers SN, Ahad SA, Murphy AP. A structured review and theme analysis of papers published on 'quality of life' in head and neck cancer: 2000–2005. Oral Oncol. 2007;43(9):843–68.
2. Valdez JA, Brennan MT. Impact of oral cancer on quality of life. Dent Clin N Am. 2018;62(1):143–54.
3. Hassan SJ, Weymuller EA. Assessment of quality of life in head and neck cancer patients. Head Neck. 1993;15(6):485–96.

4. Aaronson NK, Ahmedzai S, Bergman B, Bullinger M, Cull A, Duez NJ, Filiberti A, Flechtner H, Fleishman SB, de Haes JC, Kaasa S. The European Organization for Research and Treatment of Cancer QLQ-C30: a quality-of-life instrument for use in international clinical trials in oncology. J Natl Cancer Inst. 1993;85(5):365–76.
5. Parikh SL, Chen AY. Quality of life in head and neck cancer. In: Eisele DW, Smith RV, editors. Complications in head and neck surgery. 2nd ed. Philadephia, PA: Mosby; 2009. p. 215–8.
6. Morton RP, Davies DM, BAKER J, Baker GA, Stell PM. Quality of life in treated head and neck cancer patients: a preliminary report. Clin Otolaryngol Allied Sci. 1984;9(3):181–5.
7. McNeil BJ, Weichselbaum R, Pauker SG. Speech and survival: tradeoffs between quality and quantity of life in laryngeal cancer. N Engl J Med. 1981;305(17):982–7.
8. Gaziano JE. Evaluation and management of oropharyngeal dysphagia in head and neck cancer. Cancer Control. 2002;9(5):400–9.
9. Lazarus CL, Husaini H, Anand SM, Jacobson AS, Mojica JK, Buchbinder D, Urken ML. Tongue strength as a predictor of functional outcomes and quality of life after tongue cancer surgery. Ann Otol Rhinol Laryngol. 2013;122(6):386–97.
10. Zhang L, Huang Z, Wu H, Chen W, Huang Z. Effect of swallowing training on dysphagia and depression in postoperative tongue cancer patients. Eur J Oncol Nurs. 2014;18(6):626–9.
11. Brown JS, Rogers SN, Lowe D. A comparison of tongue and soft palate squamous cell carcinoma treated by primary surgery in terms of survival and quality of life outcomes. Int J Oral Maxillofac Surg. 2006;35(3):208–14.
12. Yang ZH, Chen WL, Huang HZ, Pan CB, Li JS. Quality of life of patients with tongue cancer 1 year after surgery. J Oral Maxillofac Surg. 2010;68(9):2164–8.
13. Boyapati RP, Shah KC, Flood V, Stassen LF. Quality of life outcome measures using UW-QOL questionnaire v4 in early oral cancer/squamous cell cancer resections of the tongue and floor of mouth with reconstruction solely using local methods. Br J Oral Maxillofac Surg. 2013;51(6):502–7.
14. Breeze J, Rennie A, Dawson D, Tipper J, Rehman KU, Grew N, Pigadas N. Patient-reported quality of life outcomes following treatment for oral cancer. Int J Oral Maxillofac Surg. 2018;47(3):296–301.
15. McConnel FM, Pauloski BR, Logemann JA, Rademaker AW, Colangelo L, Shedd D, Carroll W, Lewin J, Johnson J. Functional results of primary closure vs flaps in oropharyngeal reconstruction: a prospective study of speech and swallowing. Arch Otolaryngol Head Neck Surg. 1998;124(6):625–30.
16. Villaret AB, Cappiello J, Piazza C, Pedruzzi B, Nicolai P. Quality of life in patients treated for cancer of the oral cavity requiring reconstruction: a prospective study. Acta Otorhinolaryngol. 2008;28(3):120.
17. Yuan Y, Zhang P, He W, Li W. Comparison of oral function: free anterolateral thigh perforator flaps versus vascularized free forearm flap for reconstruction in patients undergoing glossectomy. J Oral Maxillofac Surg. 2016;74(7):1500–e1.
18. Yang Y, Li F, Li W. Factors that affect the quality of life of patients with oral cancer who have had their defects reconstructed immediately after excision of the tumour. Br J Oral Maxillofac Surg. 2016;54(4):410–4.
19. Brown JS, Shaw RJ. Reconstruction of the maxilla and midface: introducing a new classification. Lancet Oncol. 2010;11(10):1001–8.
20. Okay DJ, Genden E, Buchbinder D, Urken M. Prosthodontic guidelines for surgical reconstruction of the maxilla: a classification system of defects. J Prosthet Dent. 2001;86(4):352–63.
21. Kornblith AB, Zlotolow IM, Gooen J, Huryn JM, Lerner T, Strong EW, Shah JP, Spiro RH, Holland JC. Quality of life of maxillectomy patients using an obturator prosthesis. Head Neck. 1996;18(4):323–34.
22. Seignemartin CP, Miranda ME, Luz JGC, Teixeira RG. Understandability of speech predicts quality of life among maxillectomy patients restored with obturator prosthesis. J Oral Maxillofac Surg. 2015;73(10):2040–8.
23. Rosenthal E, Couch M, Farwell GD, Wax MK. Current concepts in microvascular reconstruction. Otolaryngol Head Neck Surg. 2007;136(4):519–24.
24. Genden EM, Wallace DI, Okay D, Urken ML. Reconstruction of the hard palate using the radial forearm free flap: indications and outcomes. Head Neck. 2004;26(9):808–14.
25. Brandão TB, Vechiato Filho AJ, de Souza Batista VE, de Oliveira MCQ, Santos-Silva AR. Obturator prostheses versus free tissue transfers: a systematic review of the optimal approach to improving the quality of life for patients with maxillary defects. J Prosthet Dent. 2016;115(2):247–53.
26. Urken ML, Buchbinder D, Weinberg H, Vickery C, Sheiner A, Parker R, Schaefer J, Som P, Shapiro A, Lawson W, Biller HF. Functional evaluation following microvascular oromandibular reconstruction of the oral cancer patient: a comparative study of reconstructed and nonreconstructed patients. Laryngoscope. 1991;101(9):935-950.
27. Kumar VV, Jacob PC, Ebenezer S, Kuriakose MA, Kekatpure V, Baliarsing AS, Al-Nawas B, Wagner W. Implant supported dental rehabilitation following segmental mandibular reconstruction-quality of life outcomes of a prospective randomized trial. J Cranio-Maxillofac Surg. 2016;44(7):800–10.
28. Hayter JP, Cawood JI. Oral rehabilitation with endosteal implants and free flaps. Int J Oral Maxillofac Surg. 1996;25(1):3–12.
29. Schoen PJ, Raghoebar GM, Bouma J, Reintsema H, Burlage FR, Roodenburg JLN, Vissink A. Prosthodontic rehabilitation of oral function in head–neck cancer patients with dental implants placed

simultaneously during ablative tumour surgery: an assessment of treatment outcomes and quality of life. Int J Oral Maxillofac Surg. 2008;37(1):8–16.
30. Karayazgan-Saracoglu B, Atay A, Korkmaz C, Gunay Y. Quality of life assessment of implant-retained overdentures and fixed metal-acrylic resin prostheses in patients with marginal mandibulectomy. J Prosthet Dent. 2017;118(4):551–60.
31. Korfage A, Raghoebar GM, Slater JJH, Roodenburg JL, Witjes MJ, Vissink A, Reintsema H. Overdentures on primary mandibular implants in patients with oral cancer: a follow-up study over 14 years. Br J Oral Maxillofac Surg. 2014;52(9):798–805.
32. Dholam KP, Dugad JA, Sadashiva KM. Impact of oral rehabilitation on patients with head and neck cancer: a study using the Liverpool Oral Rehabilitation Questionnaire and the Oral Health Impact Profile-14. J Prosthet Dent. 2017;117(4):559–62.
33. Feine JS, Carlsson GE, Awad MA, Chehade A, Duncan WJ, Gizani S, Head T, Lund JP, MacEntee M, Mericske-Stern R, Mojon P. The McGill consensus statement on overdentures. Mandibular two-implant overdentures as first choice standard of care for edentulous patients. Int J Oral Maxillofac Implants. 2002;17(4):601.
34. Thomason JM, Feine J, Exley C, Moynihan P, Müller F, Naert I, Ellis JS, Barclay C, Butterworth C, Scott B, Lynch C. Mandibular two implant-supported overdentures as the first choice standard of care for edentulous patients—the York Consensus Statement. Br Dent J. 2009;207(4):185.
35. Schoen PJ, Reintsema H, Raghoebar GM, Vissink A, Roodenburg JLN. The use of implant retained mandibular prostheses in the oral rehabilitation of head and neck cancer patients. A review and rationale for treatment planning. Oral Oncol. 2004;40(9):862–71.
36. Sclaroff A, Haughey B, Gay WD, Paniello R. Immediate mandibular reconstruction and placement of dental implants: at the time of ablative surgery. Oral Surg Oral Med Oral Pathol. 1994;78(6):711–7.
37. Schepers RH, Slagter AP, Kaanders JHAM, Van den Hoogen FJA, Merkx MAW. Effect of postoperative radiotherapy on the functional result of implants placed during ablative surgery for oral cancer. Int J Oral Maxillofac Surg. 2006;35(9):803–8.
38. Curi MM, Condezo AFB, Ribeiro K, Cardoso CL. Long-term success of dental implants in patients with head and neck cancer after radiation therapy. Int J Oral Maxillofac Surg. 2018;47(6):783–8.
39. Nobrega AS, Santiago JF Jr, de Faria Almeida DA, dos Santos DM, Pellizzer EP, Goiato MC. Irradiated patients and survival rate of dental implants: a systematic review and meta-analysis. J Prosthet Dent. 2016;116(6):858–66.
40. Claudy MP, Miguens SAQ Jr, Celeste RK, Camara Parente R, Hernandez PAG, da Silva AN Jr. Time interval after radiotherapy and dental implant failure: systematic review of observational studies and meta-analysis. Clin Implant Dent Relat Res. 2015;17(2):402–11.
41. Marker P, Siemssen SJ, Bastholt L. Osseointegrated implants for prosthetic rehabilitation after treatment of cancer of the oral cavity. Acta Oncol. 1997;36(1):37–40.
42. Colella G, Cannavale R, Pentenero M, Gandolfo S. Oral implants in radiated patients: a systematic review. Int J Oral Maxillofac Implants. 2007;22(4):616.
43. Lydiatt WM, Moran J, Burke WJ. A review of depression in the head and neck cancer patient. Clin Adv Hematol Oncol. 2009;7(6):397–403.
44. Shah JP, Patel SG, Singh B. Head and neck surgery and oncology. Amsterdam: Elsevier Health Sciences; 2012.
45. Morton RP. Studies in the quality of life of head and neck cancer patients: results of a two-year longitudinal study and a comparative cross-sectional cross-cultural survey. Laryngoscope. 2003;113(7):1091–103.
46. Singer S. Quality of life issues. In: Vermorken JB, Budach V, Leemans CR, Machiels JP, Nicolai P, O'Sullivan B, editors. Critical issues in head and neck oncology: key concepts from the fifth THNO meeting. New York, NY: Springer; 2016. p. 275–80.
47. Singer S, Krauß O, Keszte J, Siegl G, Papsdorf K, Severi E, Hauss J, Briest S, Dietz A, Brähler E, Kortmann RD. Predictors of emotional distress in patients with head and neck cancer. Head Neck. 2012;34(2):180–7.
48. Neilson K, Pollard A, Boonzaier A, Corry J, Castle D, Smith D, Trauer T, Couper J. A longitudinal study of distress (depression and anxiety) up to 18 months after radiotherapy for head and neck cancer. Psycho-Oncology. 2013;22(8):1843–8.
49. Drapeau A, Marchand A, Beaulieu-Prévost D. Epidemiology of psychological distress. In: Mental illnesses-understanding, prediction and control. London: InTech; 2012.
50. Kugaya A, Akechi T, Okuyama T, Nakano T, Mikami I, Okamura H, Uchitomi Y. Prevalence, predictive factors, and screening for psychologic distress in patients with newly diagnosed head and neck cancer. Cancer. 2000;88(12):2817–23.
51. Carrera PM, Kantarjian HM, Blinder VS. The financial burden and distress of patients with cancer: understanding and stepping-up action on the financial toxicity of cancer treatment. CA Cancer J Clin. 2018;68(2):153–65.
52. de Oliveira RL, dos Santos RF, de Carvalho SHG, Agripino GG, Canto MMN, de Vasconcelos Carvalho M, Marinho SA, Gallottini M, de Santana Sarmento DJ. Prospective evaluation of quality of life in patients with head and neck cancer. Oral Surg Oral Med Oral Pathol Oral Radiol. 2017;123(3):350–7.
53. Tarsitano A, Pizzigallo A, Ballone E, Marchetti C. Health-related quality of life as a survival predictor for patients with oral cancer: is quality of life associated with long-term overall survival? Oral Surg Oral Med Oral Pathol Oral Radiol. 2012;114(6):756–63.
54. Yabroff KR, Dowling EC, Guy GP Jr, Banegas MP, Davidoff A, Han X, Virgo KS, McNeel TS, Chawla

N, Blanch-Hartigan D, Kent EE. Financial hardship associated with cancer in the United States: findings from a population-based sample of adult cancer survivors. J Clin Oncol. 2016;34(3):259.

55. Ringash J, Bernstein LJ, Devins G, Dunphy C, Giuliani M, Martino R, McEwen S. Head and neck cancer survivorship: learning the needs, meeting the needs. Semin Radiat Oncol. 2018;28(1):64–74.
56. Sehlen S, Lenk M, Herschbach P, Aydemir U, Dellian M, Schymura B, Hollenhorst H, Dühmke E. Depressive symptoms during and after radiotherapy for head and neck cancer. Head Neck. 2003;25(12):1004–18.
57. Zeller JL. High suicide risk found for patients with head and neck cancer. JAMA. 2006;296(14): 1716–7.
58. Passik SD, Dugan W, McDonald MV, Rosenfeld B, Theobald DE, Edgerton S. Oncologists' recognition of depression in their patients with cancer. J Clin Oncol. 1998;16(4):1594–600.
59. Cereda E, Cappello S, Colombo S, Klersy C, Imarisio I, Turri A, Caraccia M, Borioli V, Monaco T, Benazzo M, Pedrazzoli P. Nutritional counseling with or without systematic use of oral nutritional supplements in head and neck cancer patients undergoing radiotherapy. Radiother Oncol. 2018;126(1):81–8.

MIX
Papier aus verantwortungsvollen Quellen
Paper from responsible sources
FSC® C105338

If you have any concerns about our products,
you can contact us on
ProductSafety@springernature.com

In case Publisher is established outside the EU,
the EU authorized representative is:
Springer Nature Customer Service Center GmbH
Europaplatz 3, 69115 Heidelberg, Germany

Printed by Libri Plureos GmbH
in Hamburg, Germany